The American Medical Association

HOME MEDICAL LIBRARY

YOUR CHILD'S HEALTH

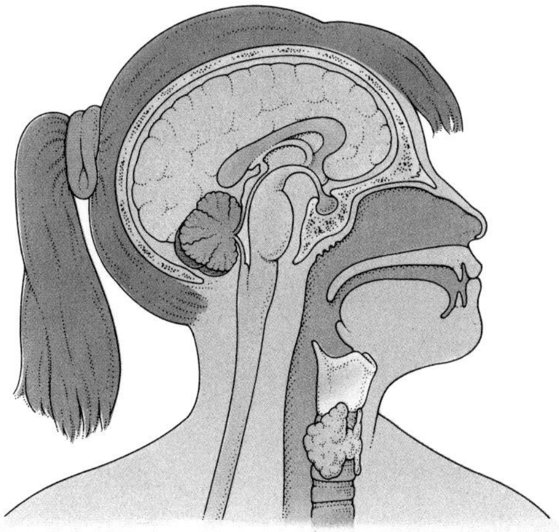

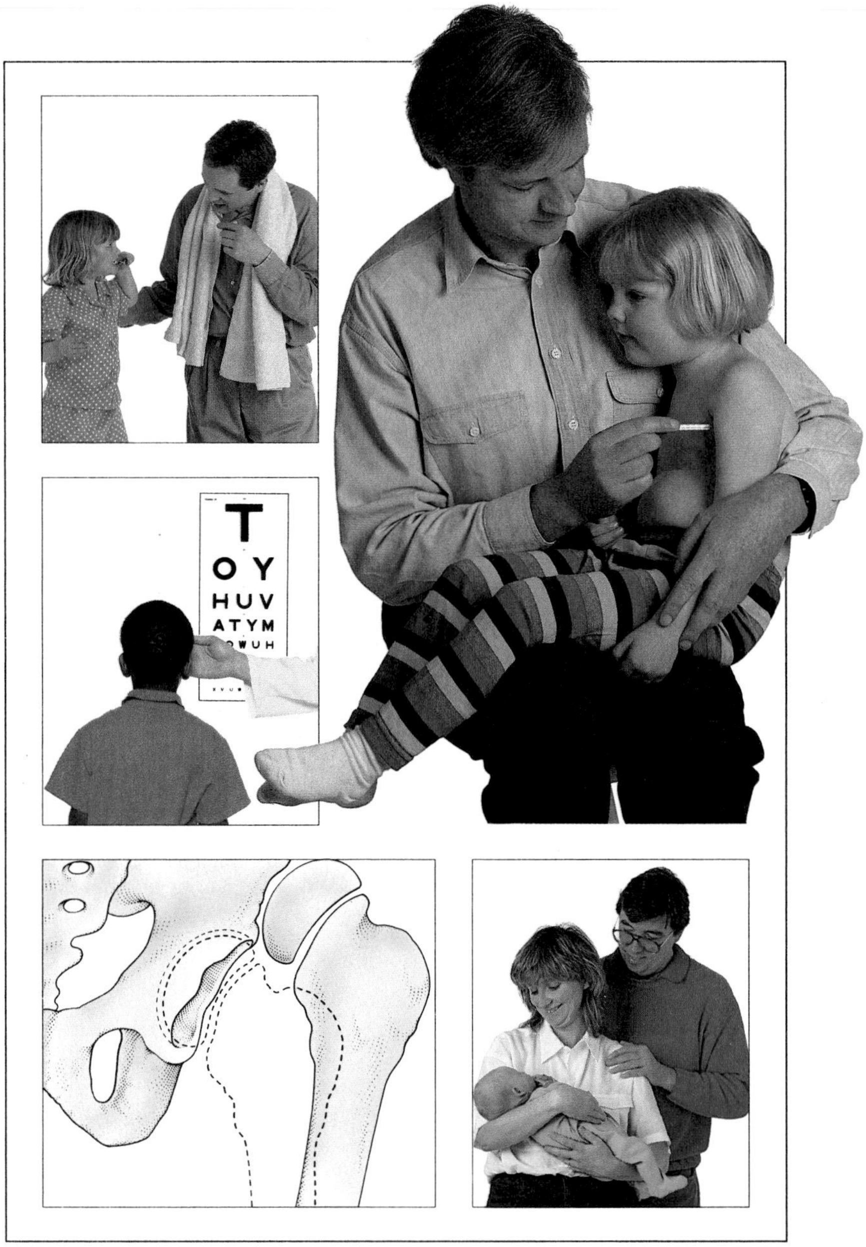
T
O Y
HUV
ATYM

THE AMERICAN MEDICAL ASSOCIATION

YOUR CHILD'S HEALTH

Medical Editor
CHARLES B. CLAYMAN, MD

THE READER'S DIGEST ASSOCIATION, INC.
Pleasantville, New York/Montreal

The AMA Home Medical Library was created and produced
by Dorling Kindersley, Ltd., in association with the
American Medical Association.

 Published in the
United States by The Reader's Digest Association, Inc.,
Pleasantville, New York/Montreal

Manufactured in the United States of America

The information in this book reflects current medical knowledge. The recommendations and information are appropriate in most cases; however, they are not a substitute for medical diagnosis. For specific information concerning your personal medical condition, the AMA suggests that you consult a physician.

The names of organizations, products, or alternative therapies appearing in this book are given for informational purposes only. Their inclusion does not imply AMA endorsement, nor does the omission of any organization, product, or alternative therapy indicate AMA disapproval.

The AMA Home Medical Library is distinct from and unrelated to the series of health books published by Random House, Inc., in conjunction with the American Medical Association under the names "The AMA Home Reference Library" and "The AMA Home Health Library."

Library of Congress Cataloging in Publication Data

Your child's health / medical editor, Charles B. Clayman.
p. cm. — (The American Medical Association home medical library)
At head of title: The American Medical Association.
Includes index.
ISBN 0-89577-492-5
1. Pediatrics—Popular works. 2. Children—Health and hygiene—Popular works. 3. Prenatal care—Popular works. I. Clayman, Charles B. II. Series.
RJ61.Y7 1993
618.92—dc20 92-38562

FOREWORD

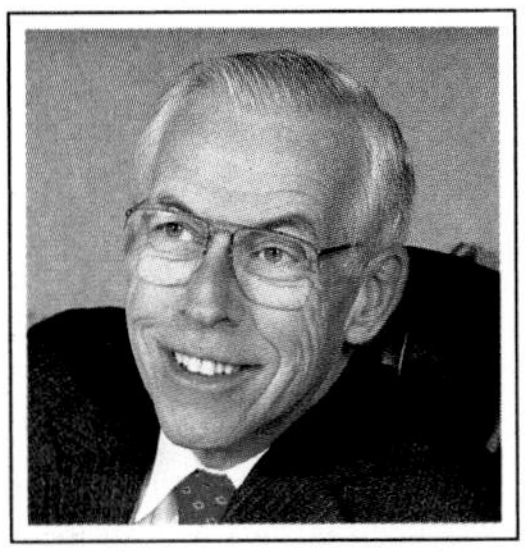

Few experiences in life bring as much delight as having a baby. Holding your baby for the first time, watching him or her grow, and marveling at each new skill learned bring immense satisfaction. Although most parents want to provide the best care for their children, many parents lack practical information about specific aspects of child health, such as feeding patterns and sleep requirements. They are not certain about when their baby should begin to walk and talk. When their child gets sick, they may not know the best way to handle the situation.

This volume of the AMA Home Medical Library provides you with current, reliable information about how to care for your healthy child and what to do when your child gets sick. We describe the routine checkups your child should have to monitor his or her growth and development. We also present the most up-to-date schedule of immunizations recommended by pediatricians to protect your child from once-common childhood infectious diseases, such as measles, whooping cough, and diphtheria. We describe the illnesses now common in childhood, explain their treatments, and tell you how to care for a sick child. A safe and nurturing upbringing is essential for a child's physical and emotional development. This volume explains how you can provide a safe and caring environment, whether or not you work outside the home.

As new research findings emerge about the importance of preventive health care, we understand better than ever before that childhood lays the foundation for a person's physical, mental, and emotional health in adulthood. We hope this volume of the AMA Home Medical Library will help you learn how to start your child on a lifetime of good health.

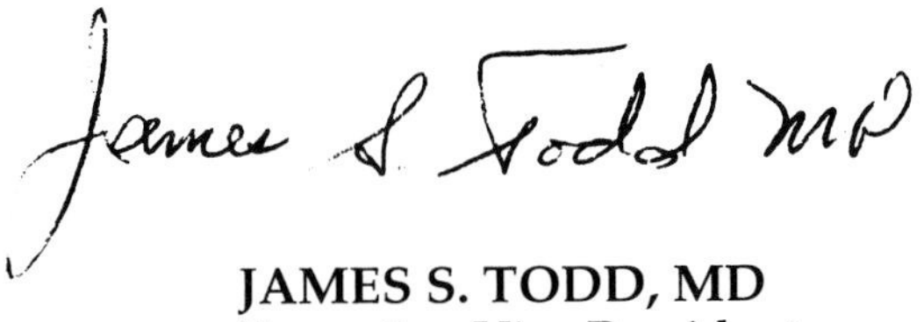

JAMES S. TODD, MD
Executive Vice President
American Medical Association

DORLING KINDERSLEY

Editorial Director Jonathan Reed; **Series Editor** Robert Dinwiddie; **Senior Editor** Francis Ritter
Editors Karen Bessant, Edda Bohnsack, Maxine Lewis, Caroline Macy, Dr. Fiona Payne, Joanna Thomas
Production Manager Ian Paton; **Editorial Assistant** Margaret Little
Design Director Ed Day; **Series Art Editor** Simon Webb; **Art Editors** Tony Foo, Karin Murray
Designers Wayne Blades, Joanna Cameron, Sean Edwards, Sara Hill, Jenny Hobson, Virginia Walter
Picture Research Julia Tacey

CONTENTS

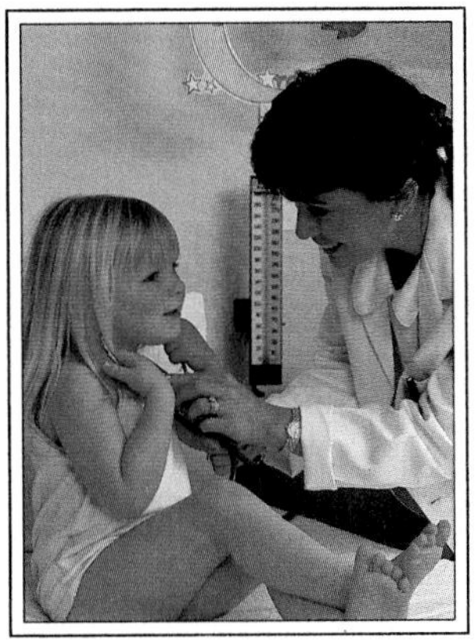

CHAPTER ONE

CHILDREN AND HEALTH

kill 400 children under the age of 4 years. These fatalities account for 40 percent of all deaths of children in this age group. This figure represents 50 percent of all deaths in children aged 5 to 14.

Chronic childhood diseases

Chronic diseases not caused by infection are still common in children. About one child in 100 is born with a serious physical disorder, such as congenital (present at birth) heart disease or spina bifida (a defect of the spinal column). A similar number of babies are born with a genetic defect that causes chronic (long-term) ill health, such as the lung and digestive disorder cystic fibrosis or the blood-clotting disorder hemophilia.

Many more children develop chronic diseases, such as asthma (affecting one child in 10) or diabetes, at some time during childhood. Cancer is the second most frequent cause of death in children aged 1 to 14, accounting for about 10 percent of all deaths in this age group. Both genetic and environmental influences play a role in childhood illnesses.

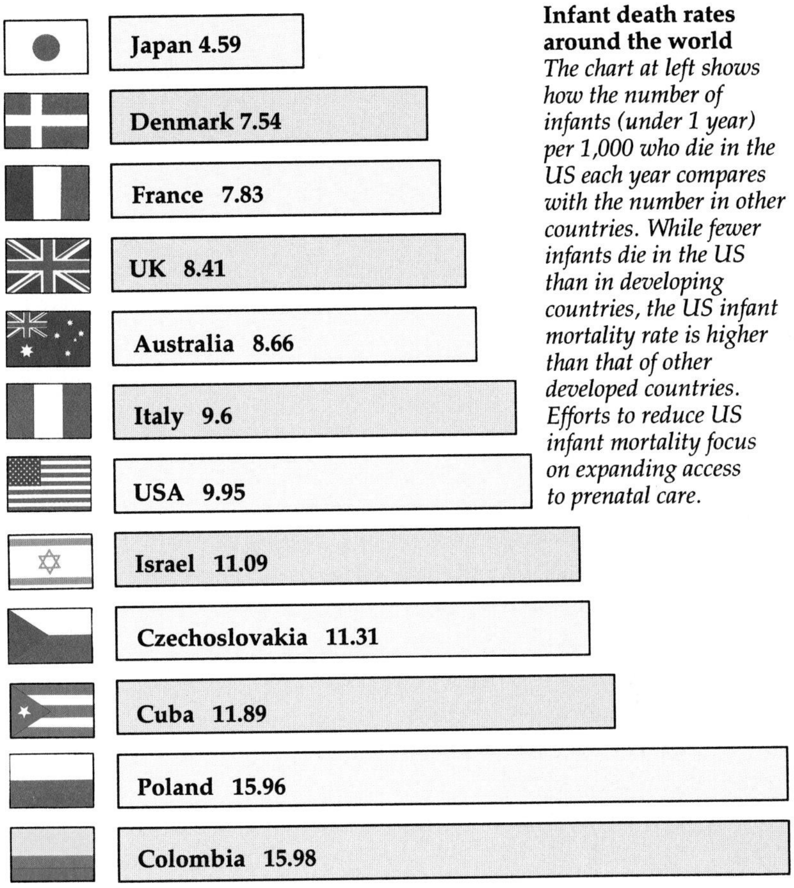

Infant death rates around the world
The chart at left shows how the number of infants (under 1 year) per 1,000 who die in the US each year compares with the number in other countries. While fewer infants die in the US than in developing countries, the US infant mortality rate is higher than that of other developed countries. Efforts to reduce US infant mortality focus on expanding access to prenatal care.

MAJOR CAUSES OF DEATH IN CHILDREN AGED 1 TO 14 IN THE US

Accidental death is number one
The pie chart at right clearly shows that accidents far outnumber all other single causes of death in the 1 to 14 year age group.

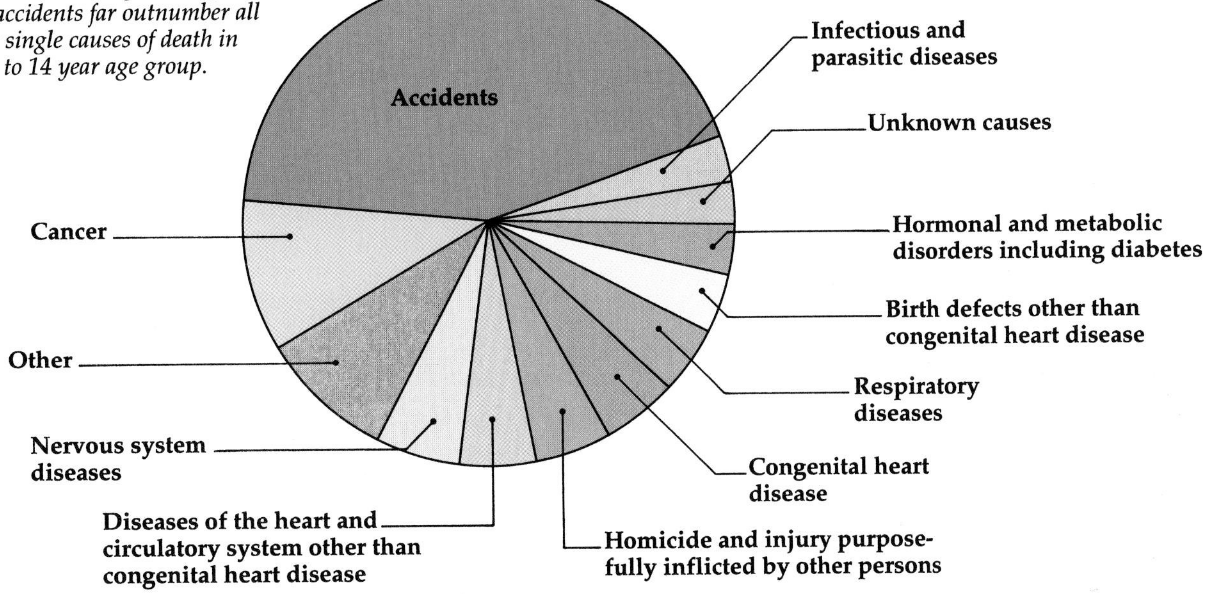

FOUNDATIONS OF GOOD HEALTH

A couple can favorably influence their child's health before birth in many important ways. In fact, parents-to-be can take steps to ensure their child's healthy fetal development even before conception. Once a healthy baby has been born, the most hazardous part of his or her life is over.

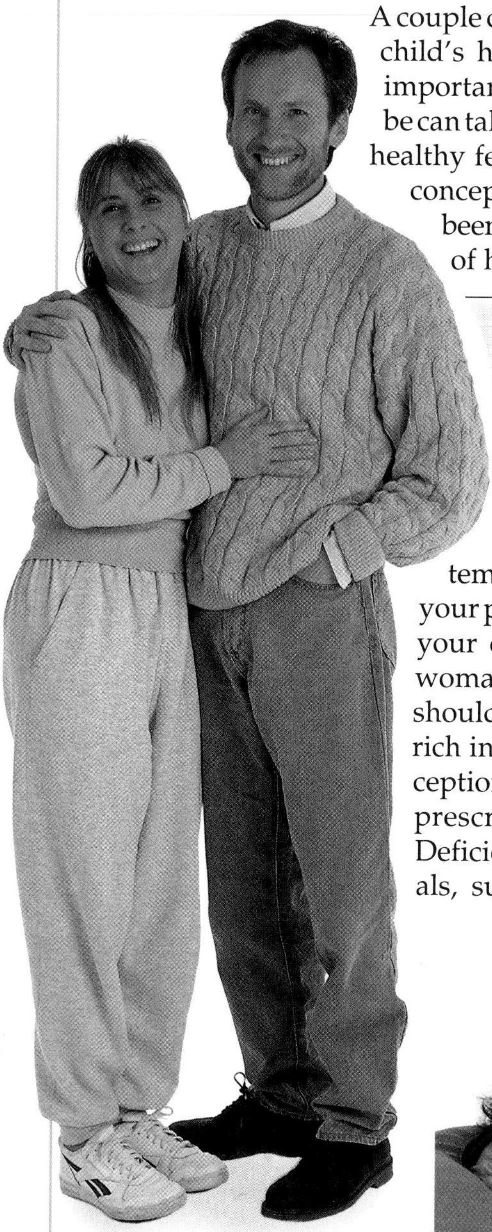

Planning a family
If you plan to have children, talk to your doctor about the steps you can take to ensure that your pregnancy develops normally and your baby is born in good health.

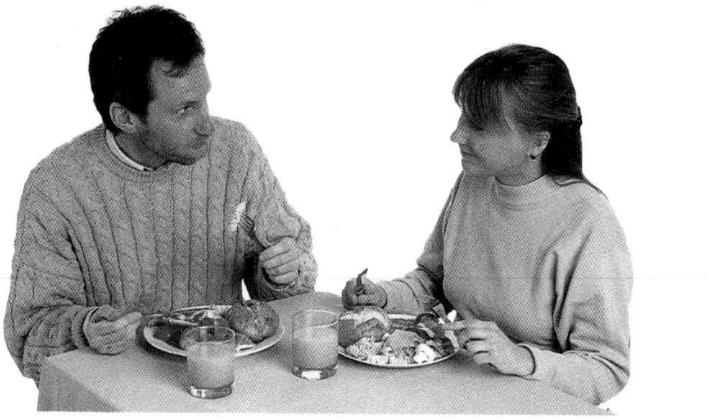

A nutritious diet
During pregnancy, both the mother and her developing fetus benefit from a nutritious, balanced diet. The prospective father, too, should be in good physical condition so he can participate in the demanding first weeks of the baby's life.

PREPARING FOR PARENTHOOD

Most couples cannot anticipate the demands that the arrival of a new baby will place on them. Before attempting to get pregnant, you and your partner should each make sure your own health is at its peak. A woman contemplating pregnancy should eat nutritious foods that are rich in calcium and iron. After conception, your doctor will probably prescribe a vitamin supplement. Deficiencies of vitamins and minerals, such as folic acid, have been linked to developmental defects, such as spina bifida, in which one or more of the spinal vertebrae develop incompletely.

During the critical first months of pregnancy, the mother's health can affect the development of the fetus. If the woman has a chronic illness, such as diabetes, she should work with her doctor to make sure that it is under control months before conception. She should also ask her doctor about the effects that any prescribed or over-the-counter medications may have on the fetus. Any woman planning to become pregnant should be immunized against infections, especially rubella (German measles),

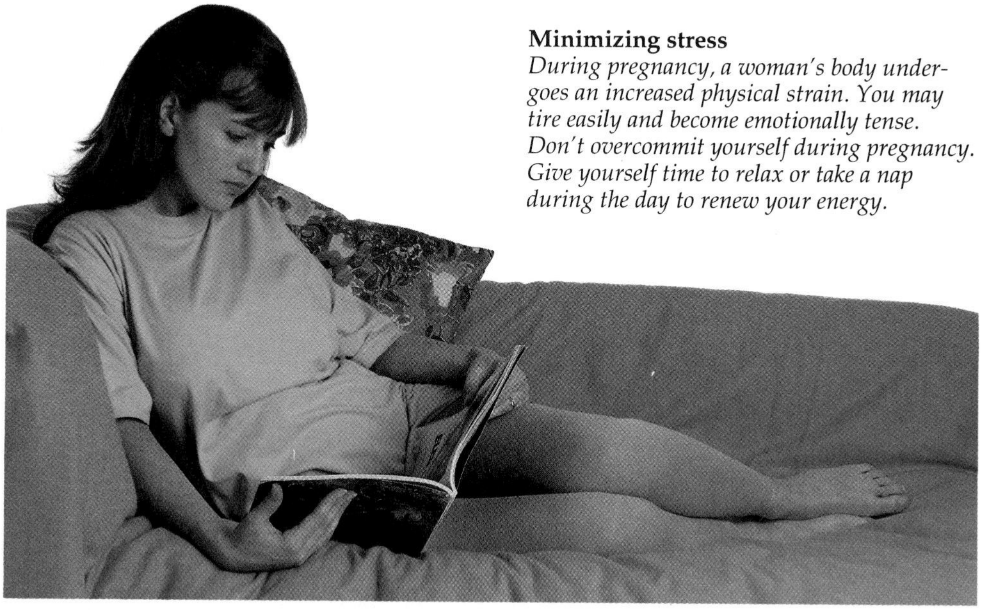

Minimizing stress
During pregnancy, a woman's body undergoes an increased physical strain. You may tire easily and become emotionally tense. Don't overcommit yourself during pregnancy. Give yourself time to relax or take a nap during the day to renew your energy.

which can cause severe birth defects, before she conceives, unless she is already immune. After pregnancy occurs, she should also avoid contact with people who have illnesses such as measles, so she does not transmit the virus to the fetus and risk a developmental defect.

Months before she conceives, a woman should quit smoking and avoid drinking alcoholic beverages. Cigarette smoking can cause low birth weight, premature birth, miscarriage, and stillbirth. Even small amounts of alcohol, especially if consumed daily, can affect the development of the fetus, or cause birth defects or miscarriage. Drinking alcohol during pregnancy can cause a disorder known as fetal alcohol syndrome, which causes physical and mental retardation.

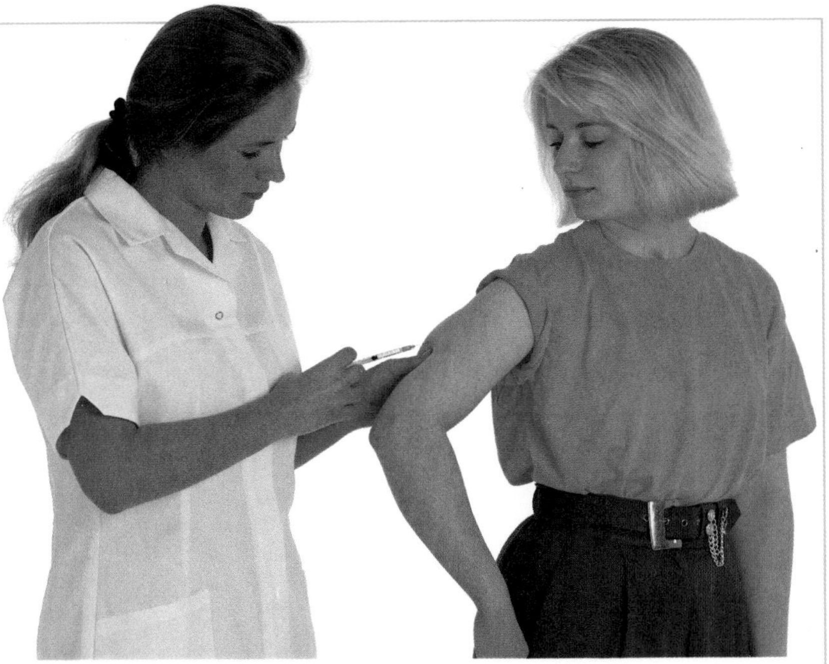

Immunization
A woman who has been immunized against a disease, such as rubella, ensures that the fetus will not be at risk from infection during pregnancy. Any inoculations should be given well before conception occurs.

Age of the parents

Parental age is an important factor to consider when contemplating pregnancy, because several chromosomal abnormalities occur more frequently in children born to parents who are over the age of 35. For example, achondroplasia, a rare form of dwarfism, occurs more often when the father is over 35. Down's syndrome, a chromosomal defect that causes mental and physical handicaps, is more common when the mother is over 35. Prospective parents who are over 35 should discuss prenatal chromosomal evaluation of the fetus with their obstetrician (a doctor who specializes in childbirth). The doctor will perform the evaluation using either amniocentesis, a procedure that can detect abnormalities using fetal cells found in the fluid that surrounds the fetus, or chorionic villus sampling, which tests for abnormalities using a small sample of tissue taken from the placenta.

Risk of a genetic disorder

The risk of a genetic disorder is higher than average in people whose close relatives have had stillborn infants, who have relatives with a genetic disease, or whose ethnic or racial background places them at high risk for a genetic disorder. Doctors recommend that these people consult a genetic counselor before starting a family.

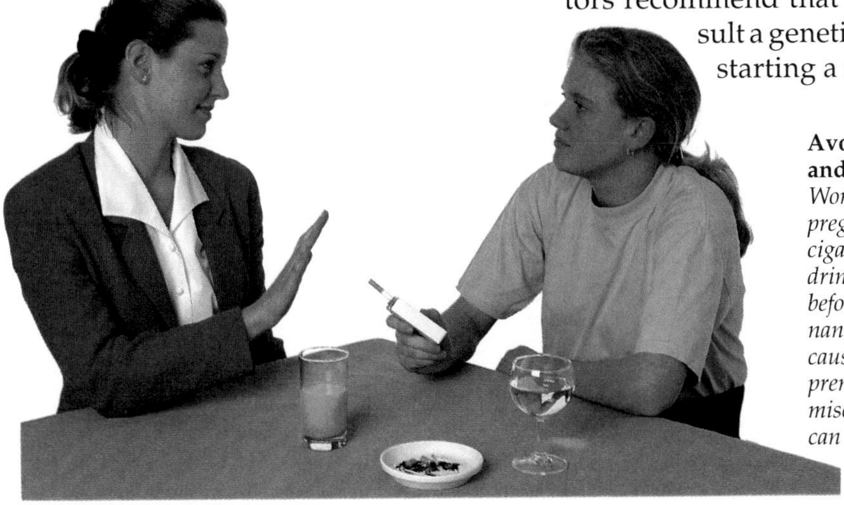

Avoiding tobacco and alcohol
Women who plan to become pregnant should avoid cigarette smoking and drinking alcoholic beverages before and during pregnancy. Use of tobacco can cause low birth weight, premature birth, and miscarriage. Use of alcohol can cause birth defects.

BREAST-FEEDING

Breast milk provides the best nutrition for your baby. It also boosts your baby's immunity to disease. Babies are not allergic to breast milk, but many babies become allergic to formula. Breast-fed babies almost never get constipated and they rarely become overweight. Breast-feeding can also help the mother's uterus contract and regain its shape. Breast-feeding also fosters a strong bond between you and your baby.

GIVING YOUR CHILD A HEALTHY HEAD START

At 1 month of age, a healthy baby has a life expectancy of about 78 years if she is a girl and 72 years if he is a boy. To some extent, the ability to remain healthy is a matter of the child's constitution: some babies are born with great natural resistance to disease; others are frail. But parents can influence the health of their children in many ways. Parents can instill positive, health-conscious behavior patterns in a child that he or she can continue to follow into adulthood.

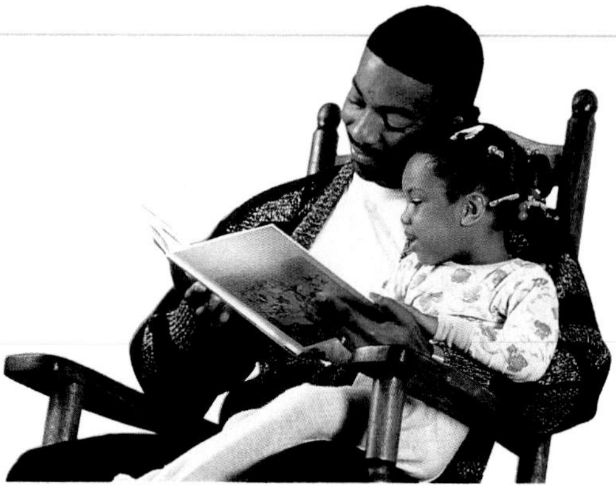

Emotional security
The most valuable things you can give your child are your time and your full attention. But full-time parenting has become a luxury in the US. Two thirds of mothers work outside the home. One fifth of all children do not have a father living at home. To help give your child a stable emotional base, make sure that the people who care for your child when you are not at home are attentive and nurturing.

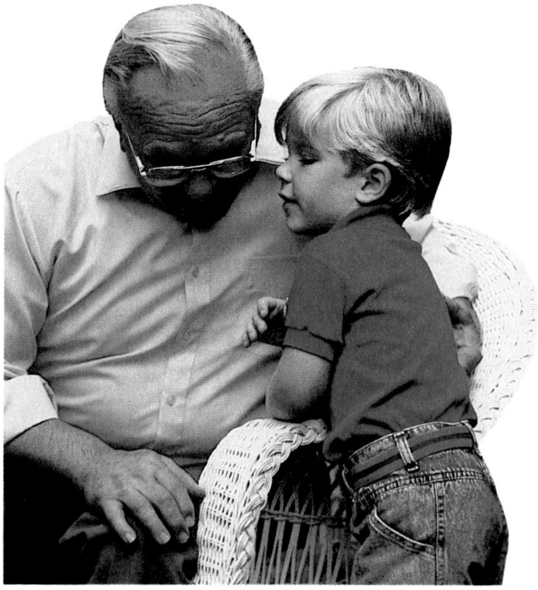

Communication
Parents and other care givers need to have frequent, extended conversations with their preschool children every day. Young children ask many questions and need simple, sensible, but brief answers. The essence of adult-child communication is for the child to talk and the adult to listen. This interaction helps prepare a child for the challenges of school.

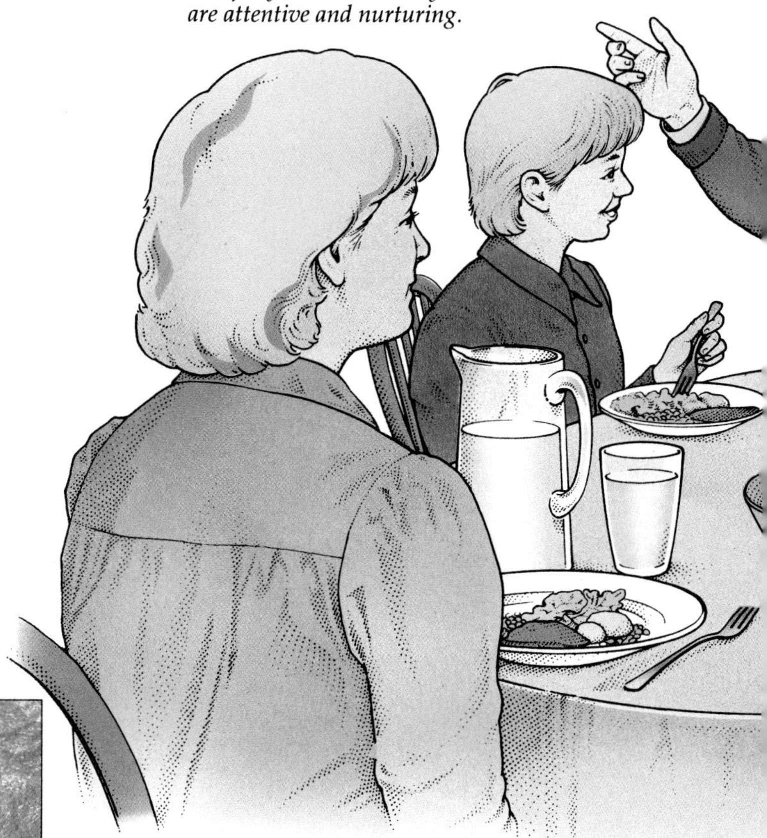

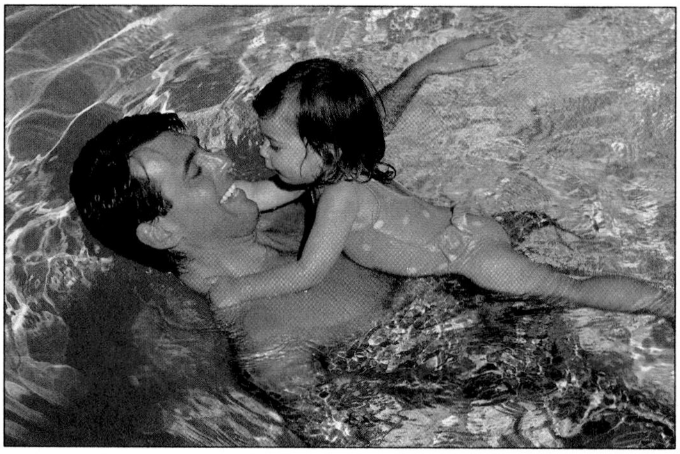

Frequent exercise
Regular, vigorous exercise is vital for growing children. Exercise strengthens a child's heart and lungs and encourages the development of his or her physical coordination. Lack of exercise is an important cause of childhood obesity. A child who is overweight at 7 years of age is much more likely to be overweight as an adult than is a child of normal weight.

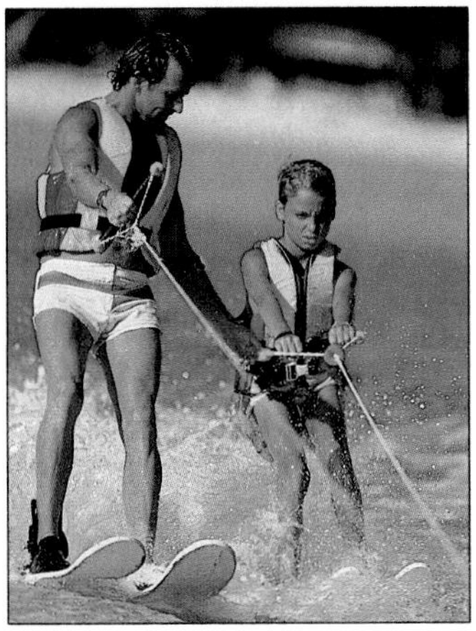

A safe environment

Help your child understand safety-conscious behavior. The risk of an accident diminishes greatly when children use safety helmets for bicycling, seat belts in cars, and life jackets for all water sports. Children participating in sports and other outdoor activities should always be supervised by an adult. Check your home regularly for potential hazards.

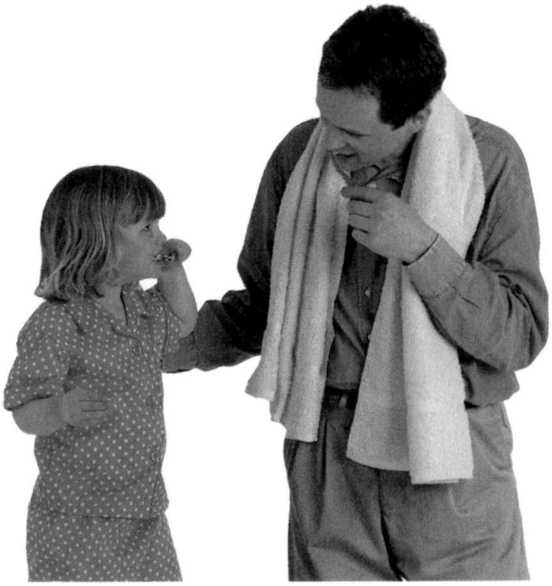

Regular meals

Children who become accustomed to eating regular meals are less likely to snack as adults. Most snack foods contain too much fat, refined sugar, and salt and lack fiber and unrefined carbohydrates. If your children ask for food between meals, offer them a variety of fruits, vegetables, or other nutritional foods.

Hygiene

Parents can help their children avoid some disorders, such as rashes, by encouraging daily bathing from the first year of life. Teach your child how to use a toothbrush properly and show him or her how to use dental floss to prevent cavities and gum disease. Babies tend to put objects into their mouths, so playthings should be cleaned thoroughly to prevent illness through contamination from these objects.

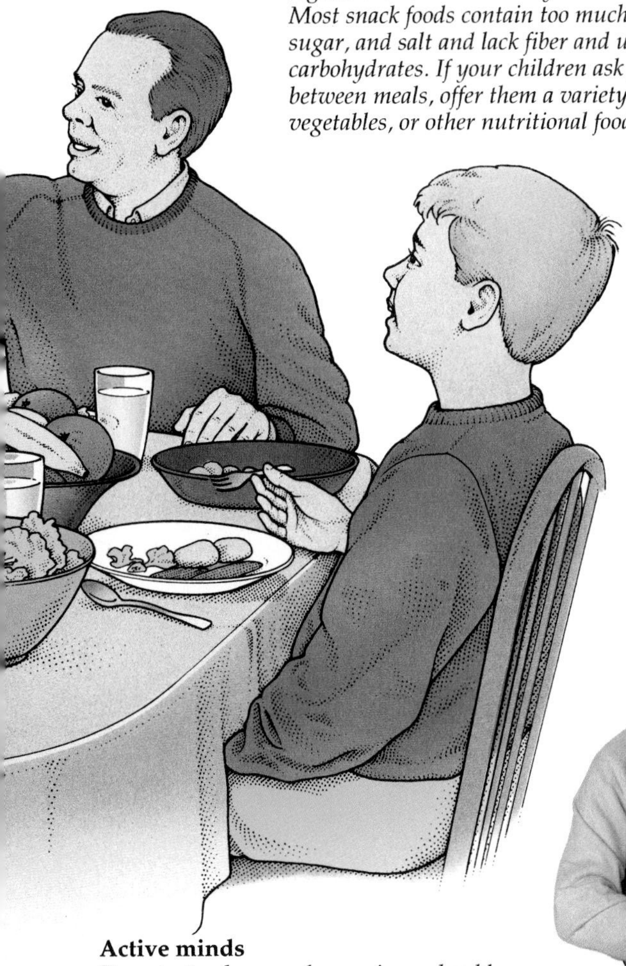

A healthy diet

Children who grow up eating a balanced diet that contains no more than 30 percent fat, with a high proportion of whole grains and fresh fruits and vegetables, tend to practice healthy eating habits as adults. They also reduce their risk of coronary heart disease and cancer.

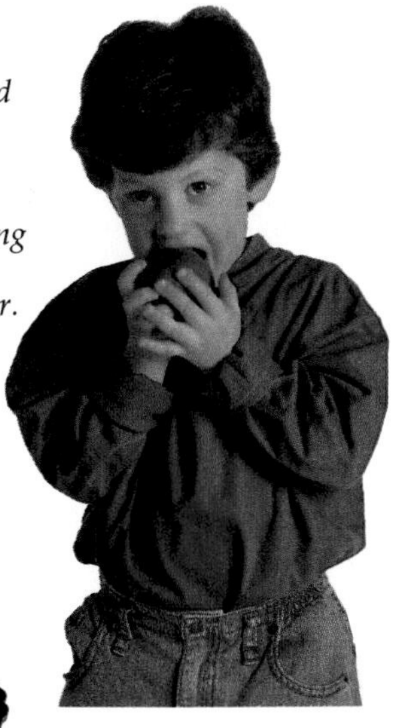

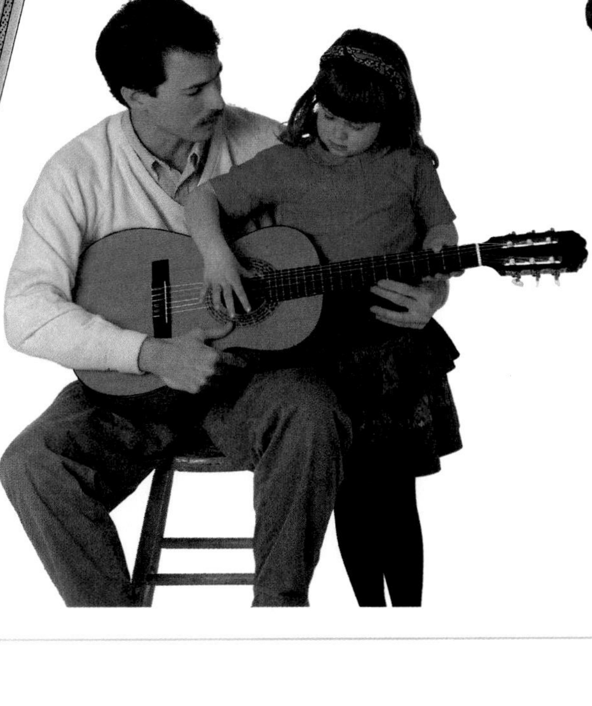

Active minds

Parents, teachers, and care givers should involve children in activities that are mentally stimulating. Minimize your child's time in front of the television. Children of all ages need a variety of activities so that they can develop all aspects of their intellect, including language skills, mathematical ability, creativity, visual/spatial abilities, and musical aptitude.

CHAPTER TWO

INFANCY

THE TRANSITION from inside the uterus to the outside world is the most critical event in a person's life. The first day of life holds a greater risk of death than does any other day, despite continuing medical advances. A baby must undergo phenomenal physiological changes on his or her day of birth. First, he or she must make the journey through the birth canal or survive cesarean section. Then the baby's body must change quickly to adapt to its new environment. For example, the ability to breathe air requires a complete change in the way blood circulates through the newborn baby's body. In addition, the newborn baby must avoid several new threats, such as infectious organisms and hypothermia (a below-normal body temperature), to which newborns are especially susceptible. Today, most babies in the US are born healthy. After the doctor examines your baby in the delivery room, he or she will give your baby to you so that you can see and hold your child for the first time. This time provides an intimate opportunity for you and your partner to bond with your newborn. At first, your baby may look different from the way you expected. The features of a newborn baby can vary considerably; many new parents seek reassurance from their doctor that their baby is normal.

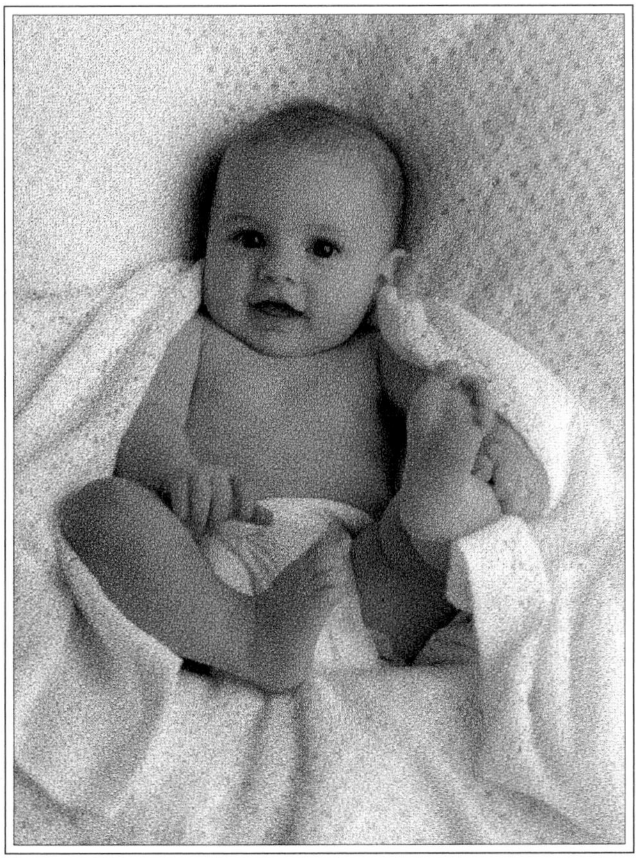

This chapter tells you what to expect when your baby arrives. It explains the demands of parenthood and describes the changes – both physical and mental – that occur in your baby as he or she develops during the first year of life. The chapter discusses high-risk infants, including those who are premature, of low birth weight, born to mothers with illnesses such as diabetes, or exposed to drugs or alcohol. It also discusses life-threatening conditions, such as respiratory distress syndrome and a type of brain hemorrhage, that develop in some babies after birth and the recent advances in the medical treatment of such conditions. To help you learn how to care for your baby, the next section describes the clothing and equipment you will need for your child and explains how to care for him or her during the first year of life. This section also gives practical advice on feeding and bathing your baby and tells you how to establish your baby's sleeping pattern and daily routine. Finally, we describe the minor conditions that doctors typically see in young babies and list the warning signs that could alert you to the presence of a more serious disorder. When a newborn baby joins your family, your entire life changes. The information provided in this chapter will help guide you through this important period safely.

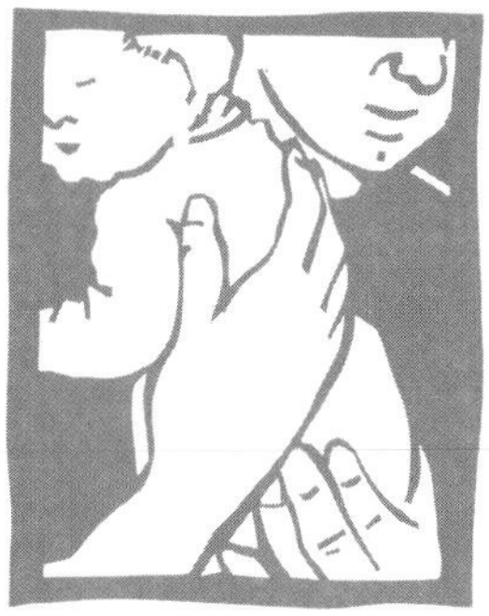

GETTING TO KNOW YOUR BABY

AT FIRST, your new baby may look and behave differently from the way you expected. Because all the systems of the baby's body may not yet be working effectively, you might notice blemishes and variations in skin color, which are usually normal. Comfort and play with your baby as much as possible in the first few weeks. You will soon become familiar with your baby's behavior and will be able to interpret his or her signals.

Babies are born with the ability to make certain automatic movements, called reflexes. For example, your baby will close his or her eyes when the eyelids are touched. This reflex protects the baby's eyes. Other reflexes include the walking reflex, in which a baby moves his or her legs in a stepping motion if held under the arms on a firm surface, and the Moro or startle reflex, in which the baby flings out his or her arms and legs in response to a sudden movement or a loud noise. These reflexes vary in intensity during the early months and usually disappear by the age of 4 months when the nervous system has developed.

APGAR SCORE

Immediately after birth, the delivery team will assess your baby's condition with the Apgar scoring method, devised by American anesthesiologist Virginia Apgar. The baby's breathing, heart rate, skin color, movements, and response to stimulation are individually evaluated and given a score from 0 to 2. The sum of these scores gives the overall Apgar score (maximum of 10). Babies are scored 1 and 5 minutes after delivery, and most healthy babies score between 7 and 10 at each interval. A score lower than 7 suggests the need for further medical intervention. If the score does not improve after clearing the baby's airway and giving oxygen, the baby may need emergency lifesaving measures.

The rooting reflex
If you stroke your newborn's cheek, he or she will turn his or her head in the direction of your finger and open his or her mouth. Your baby makes this movement when searching for a breast on which to start feeding. Your baby instinctively knows how to suck.

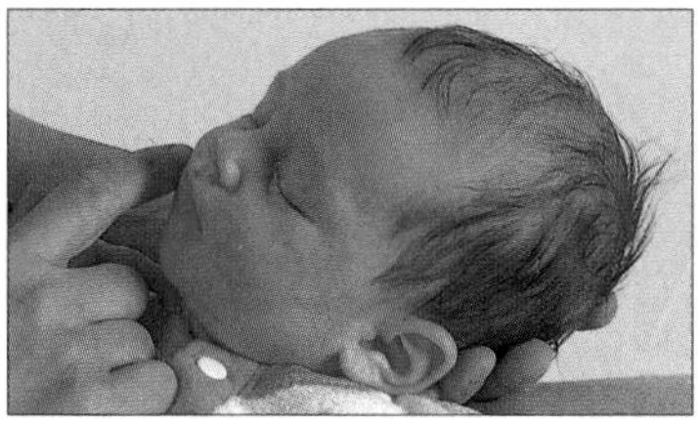

The grasping reflex
Your baby's fingers will automatically tighten around anything that is pressed into the palm. This reflex is so strong that your baby's entire weight can be supported if he or she grasps your fingers. The baby usually loses this reflex by 3 months of age.

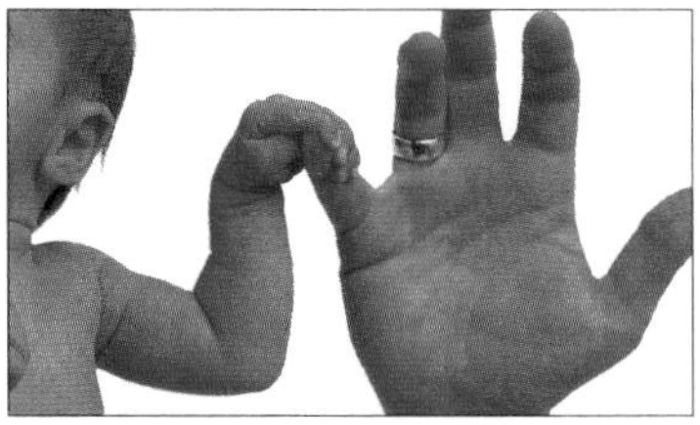

Meconium
At birth, your baby's bowel movements consist of a dark, sticky substance called meconium. Bowel movements change color once your baby starts to eat.

Hands and feet
Your baby's hands and feet may be bluish because the nervous system and circulation are not yet fully functional. If you change your baby's position, his or her hands and feet should turn pink. The baby's hands will be clenched into fists.

Genitals
Genitals look disproportionately large in babies. A girl may have a discharge from the vagina, from the withdrawal of her mother's hormones following birth. In most boys, testicles lie in the scrotum at birth but may be located in the groin and usually descend within several months.

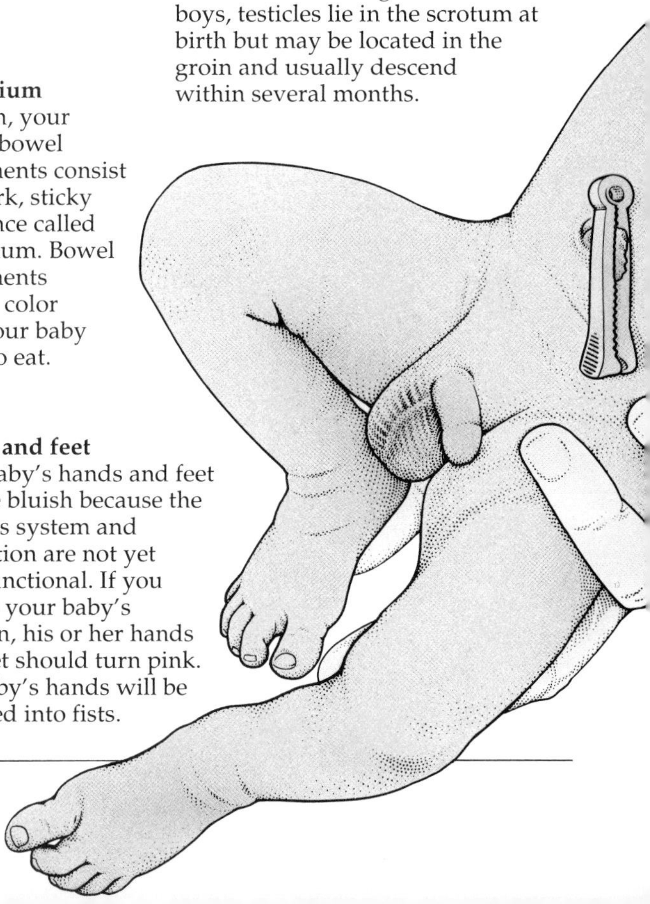

PHYSICAL FEATURES OF THE NEWBORN

At birth, most babies are covered with a white, cheesy substance called vernix that protects the skin while the baby is inside the uterus and acts as a lubricant during delivery. You may think your newborn baby's body looks out of proportion. The baby's abdomen may seem distended, and the head may be large in relation to the rest of the body. In contrast, the baby's arms and legs may look too thin. Don't worry – all of these body proportions are normal. Even a newborn's facial features may look wrinkled or unusual.

Mouth
Your baby's tongue may seem anchored to the floor of his or her mouth so that the tip looks slightly forked. This trait is common in newborns. As your baby gets older, the tongue will grow forward. Small gray-white areas may also appear on the baby's gums or palate – these will soon disappear.

Head
Your baby's head may be misshapen at birth. This is normal; the shape of the head is altered when the separate bones of the skull squeeze together to make delivery easier. The baby's head regains its normal shape within 2 weeks. If your doctor delivers the baby with forceps, the baby may have red marks on either side of the head, but these rapidly disappear.

Hair
At birth, some babies have a full head of hair; others are completely bald. Downy hair (lanugo) covers the bodies of some babies, especially those born prematurely. It generally rubs off within 2 weeks but may persist for a few more weeks.

Eyes
Most babies have blue eyes at birth. True eye color takes about 6 months to develop. Squinting is common in newborns because they do not have full control of the muscles that move their eyeballs. Most babies stop squinting within a few months. Your baby may also have puffy eyelids and bruising around the eyes. Your doctor will check your baby's eyes to rule out infection and any other problems present at birth.

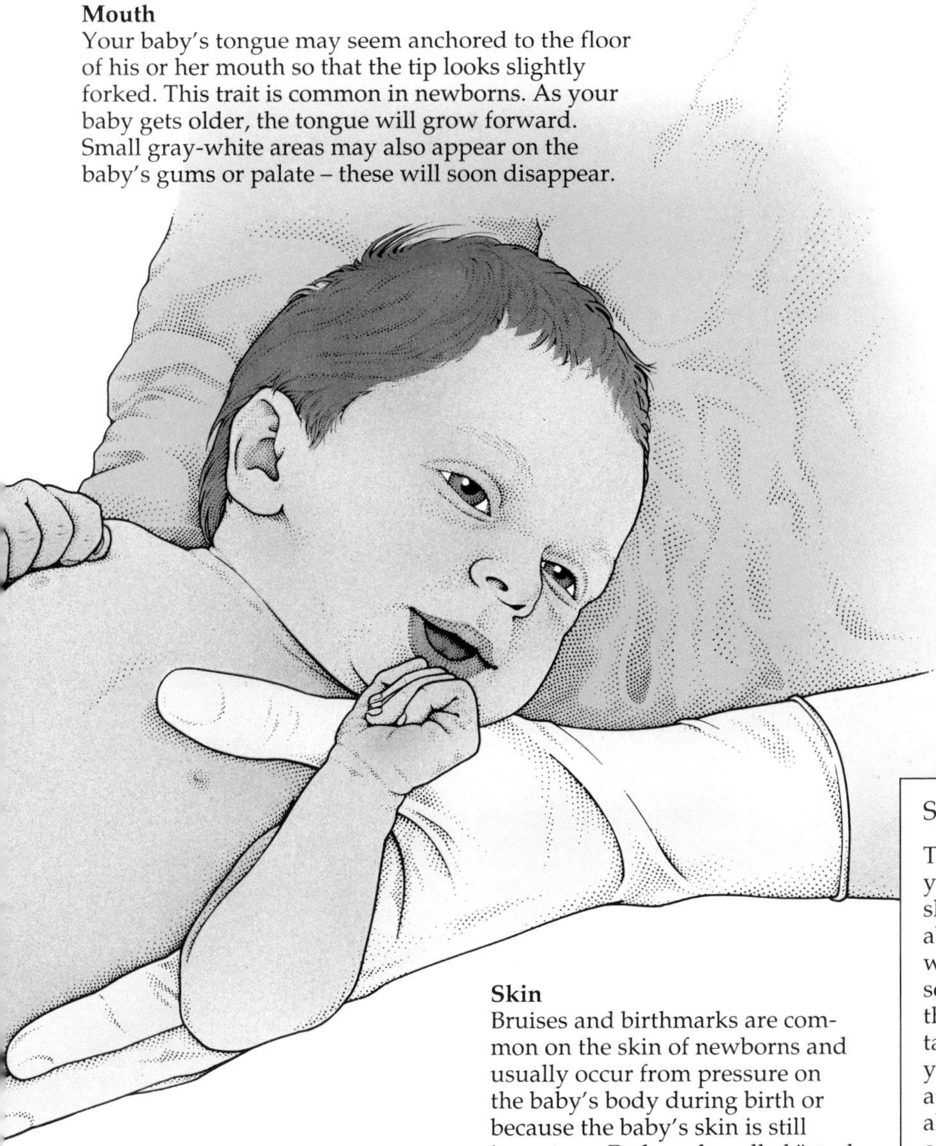

Skin
Bruises and birthmarks are common on the skin of newborns and usually occur from pressure on the baby's body during birth or because the baby's skin is still immature. Red marks called "stork bites" frequently appear on the eyelids and neck. Rashes and peeling skin may appear, especially on the hands and feet. Few of these blemishes are permanent.

Breasts
Your baby's breasts will probably be swollen and may secrete a little milk. This phenomenon is produced by hormones that the mother secretes during pregnancy. The swelling should decrease within a few weeks.

SOFT SPOTS

The soft spot (fontanelle) on the top of your baby's head is present because the skull bones do not join until your baby is about 2 years old. Normal handling and washing of the baby will not harm the soft spot. If you notice that the skin over the area is taut or if it bulges, call your doctor immediately. Your baby may also have a soft spot on the back of the head. It closes by 3 to 4 months of age.

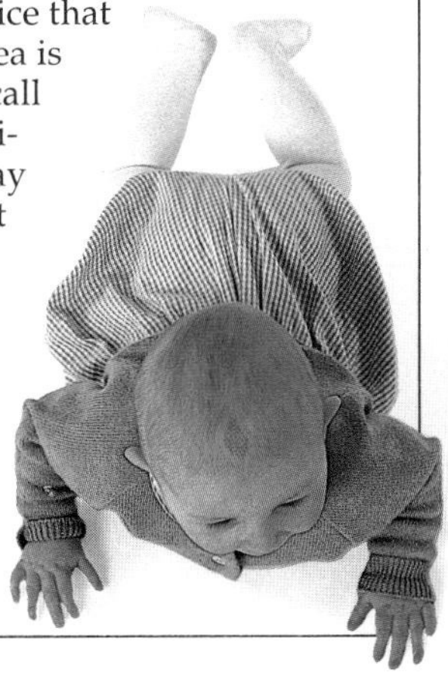

INITIAL CHECKUPS

Your doctor or a pediatrician (a doctor who specializes in the care of children) examines your baby in the delivery room. He or she will perform a more detailed examination before you leave the hospital. The doctor usually allows you and your partner to be present so that you can ask questions. The doctor performs a similar follow-up examination about 2 to 4 weeks later. If your baby has any abnormality, it almost certainly will be detected at this stage. In addition to performing the external examinations described at right, your doctor or pediatrician will routinely screen your baby for some internal disorders during the first week of life. For example, doctors test all babies for disorders of metabolism such as phenylketonuria, an inherited disorder that causes a buildup of an amino acid in the body, leading to mental retardation; congenital hypothyroidism, characterized by mental retardation and stunted growth; and galactosemia, an enzyme deficiency that causes the sugar galactose to accumulate in the blood.

The Guthrie and thyroid tests
These tests are usually performed 2 days after birth. A blood sample is taken from the baby's heel. The blood is tested for phenylketonuria, a rare cause of mental retardation, and congenital hypothyroidism, a form of thyroid deficiency. A child with either disorder can develop normally if diagnosed and treated promptly. The blood is also screened for disorders such as sickle cell anemia.

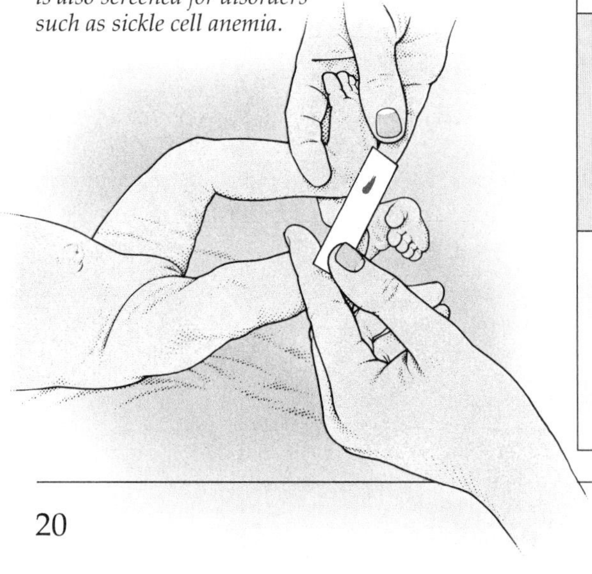

PHYSICAL EXAMINATIONS

In the examinations done just after birth and at 2 to 4 weeks, the doctor checks your baby from head to toe to make sure that he or she has no abnormalities.

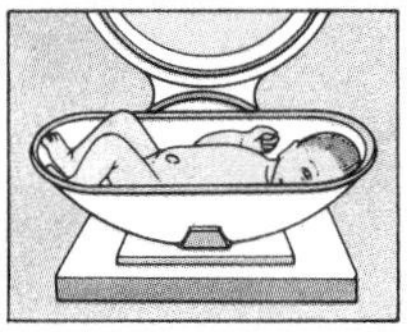

Immediately after birth, the doctor weighs your baby and measures his or her length. After this initial examination, your baby will be weighed and measured at regular intervals to make sure he or she is gaining weight and growing adequately.

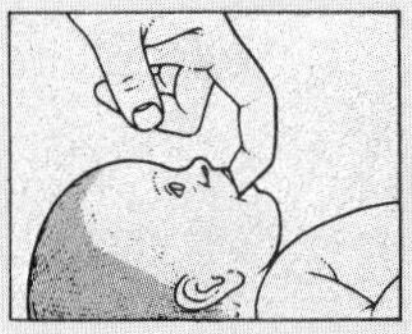

The doctor inspects the baby's mouth and feels the palate to detect clefts and to make sure that it is intact. After measuring the circumference of your baby's head, he or she checks the fontanelles (soft spots). The doctor also examines the eyes and ears for abnormalities.

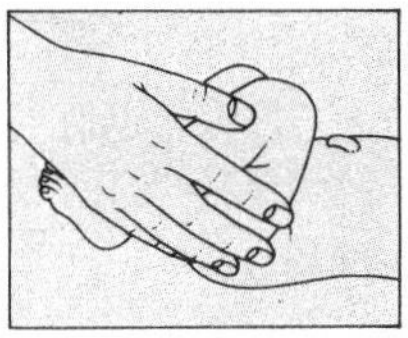

The doctor checks your baby's posture and the length of the limbs and moves the limbs to make sure they are aligned. He or she also checks the hips for dislocation. The doctor tests the baby's reflexes and strength to evaluate the muscular and nervous systems.

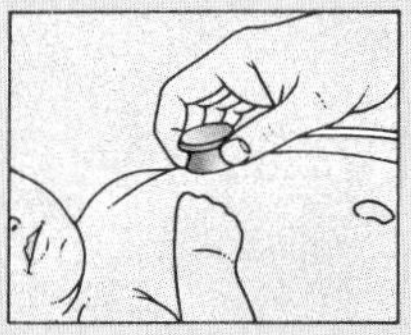

The doctor listens to the heart and lungs. Heart murmurs are common among newborn babies in the first 24 to 48 hours of life and do not usually indicate a defect. Persistent murmurs or abnormal heart sounds require follow-up examination.

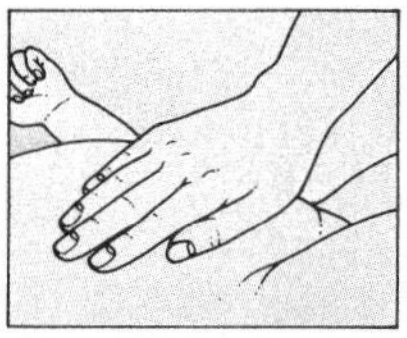

By putting his or her hands on your baby's abdomen, the doctor can check for organ enlargement or the presence of any masses. He or she checks the baby's groin for the presence of a normal pulse in the main artery leading to the legs and to detect any hernias.

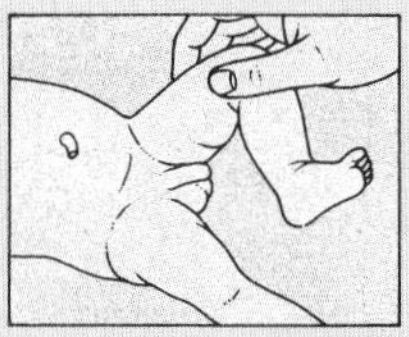

The doctor checks the baby's genitals for any abnormality. If the baby is a boy, the doctor examines his testicles to make sure they have descended into the scrotum. If the baby is a girl, the doctor carefully inspects the folds of the labia and checks the clitoris.

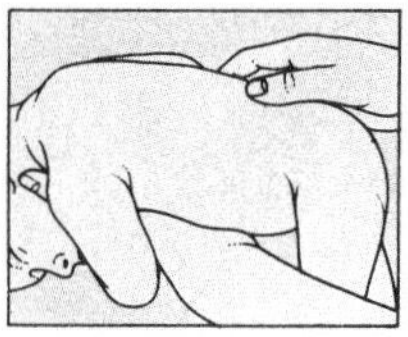

The doctor checks the curvature of the spine and makes sure that all the vertebrae are in place by running his or her thumb down the baby's back. Any lumps, hairy patches, colored areas of skin, or cavities may indicate a spinal abnormality that needs further investigation.

Birth defects

Congenital abnormalities (birth defects) refer to abnormalities present at birth, although their effects may not be manifested until later in life. Birth defects affect about 2 to 4 percent of all pregnancies in the US. Doctors check all newborns for birth defects immediately after birth. About two thirds of these conditions are minor and either disappear or can be treated with simple surgery. Minor problems include protruding flaps of skin, birthmarks, and clubfoot (a condition in which the ankle is bent in an abnormal position). Other birth defects are more serious and may require major surgery to correct them. Serious abnormalities that are present from birth include cleft lip and palate, spina bifida (a split in the spinal column), genital and digestive tract abnormalities, limb deformities, and heart defects.

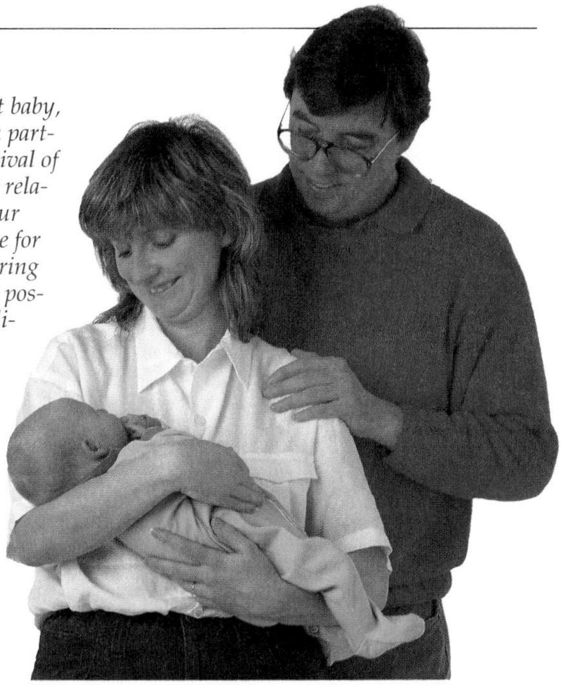

Becoming a family
When you have your first baby, everything changes. Both partners may feel that the arrival of the baby has altered their relationship. But you and your partner need to make time for each other. Take turns caring for your baby as much as possible. Sharing responsibilities is more fair and also fosters a close and happy family relationship.

LIVING WITH YOUR BABY

Nothing can prepare you for the exhausting demands of having your first baby. Suddenly, you are no longer just a partner in a relationship. You are responsible for a new human being. Caring for your new baby requires love, attention, and responsiveness. But you will be exhausted from childbirth, and your baby's cries will deprive you of much-needed sleep. You may feel that you have been thrown into a situation about which you know very little, even if you have read a great deal about the subject. Don't worry if you feel inadequate as a parent at first; you will soon learn the best way to respond to your own baby's needs. Gradually, your days will become more ordered as your baby settles in and you are able to establish a routine.

Changes in your baby

Your baby will change from a totally dependent newborn during the first few weeks of life into a mobile, playful, and sociable little person with a distinct personality by the time he or she is 1 year old. After just a few months, some of your baby's permanent characteristics, such as eye and hair color, will appear.

Babies grow rapidly in the first year of life. Overall increases in size and weight are enormous. The change in proportions will be striking. Compared with the rest of the baby's body, the head does not look as large at 1 year as it did at birth. Each time you visit your pediatrician, he or she will measure your baby's height and weight and plot the measurements on growth charts. These charts enable your doctor to ensure that your baby is growing at a normal rate. The doctor also assesses your baby's mental and emotional development.

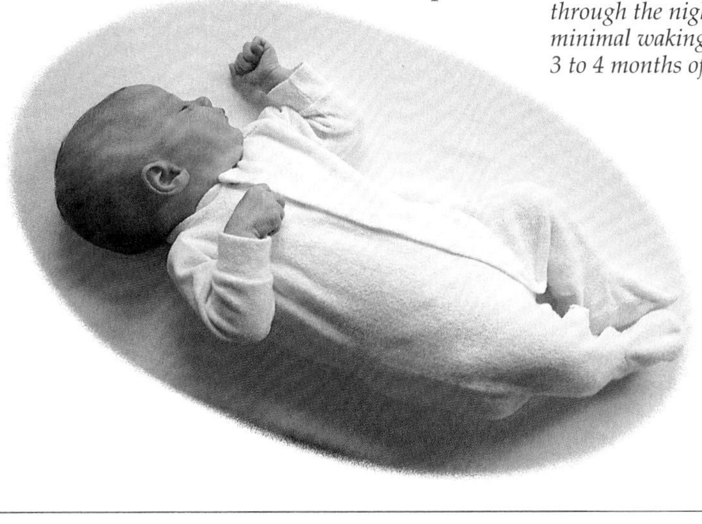

Sleeping patterns
At first, your newborn will sleep for up to 16 hours a day, often in short intervals. By about 3 months, your baby will stay awake longer during the day. Between 3 and 5 months, you should establish a bedtime routine to associate nighttime with sleeping. Many children become accustomed to a bedtime and sleep through the night with minimal waking by 3 to 4 months of age.

YOUR BABY'S DEVELOPMENT

Watching your baby grow and learn is a fascinating and joyful experience. During the first year of life, your baby develops rapidly and reaches a series of distinct milestones. It is possible to forecast when most babies will arrive at these developmental milestones. But don't worry if your baby does not reach each milestone by the average age shown here – some babies learn certain skills more quickly than others. Babies progress at their own pace and in their own time; those who develop late catch up quickly with their peers. If you have any serious concerns about your baby's development, talk to your doctor.

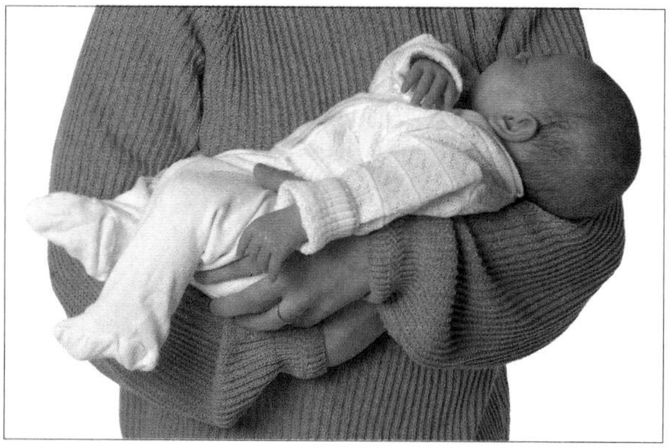

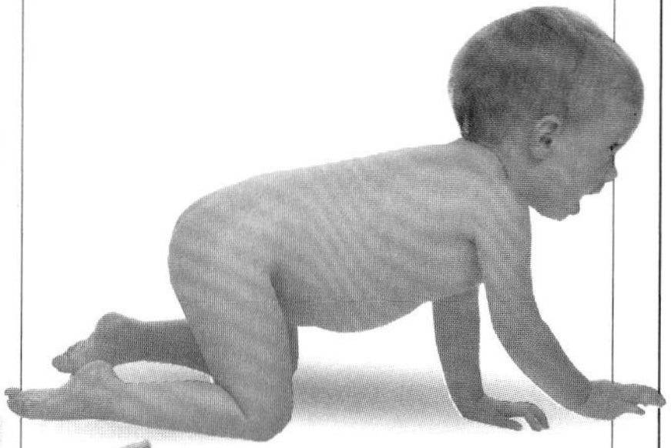

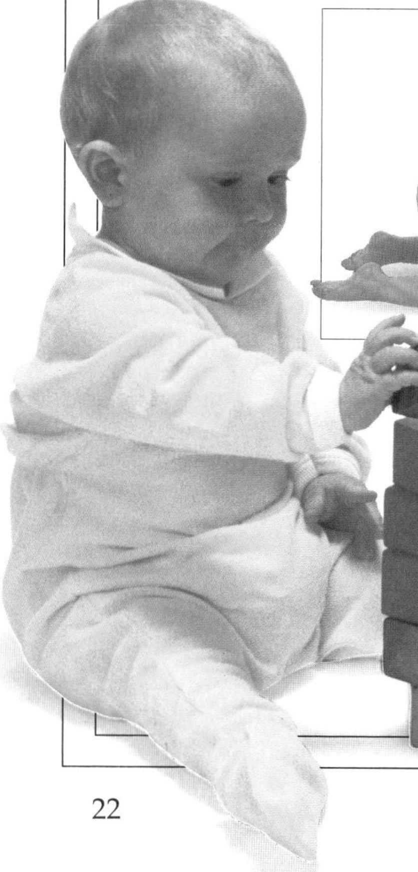

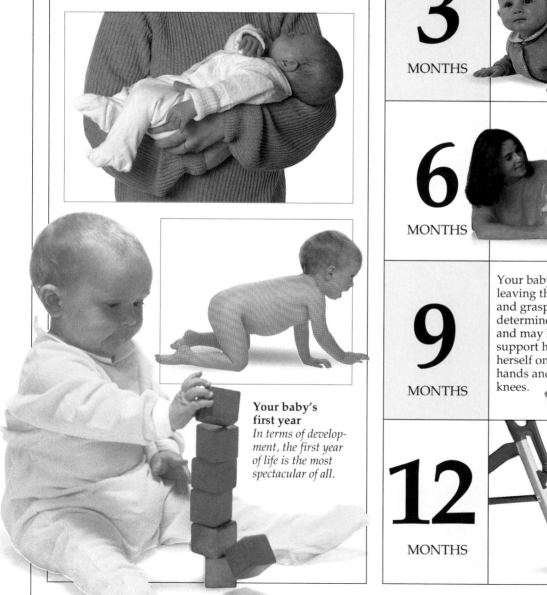

Your baby's first year
In terms of development, the first year of life is the most spectacular of all.

	MOVEMENT AND COORDINATION
1 MONTH	By 1 month, your baby no longer looks like a newborn, although his or her legs are still bent. The baby may be able to lift his or her head. 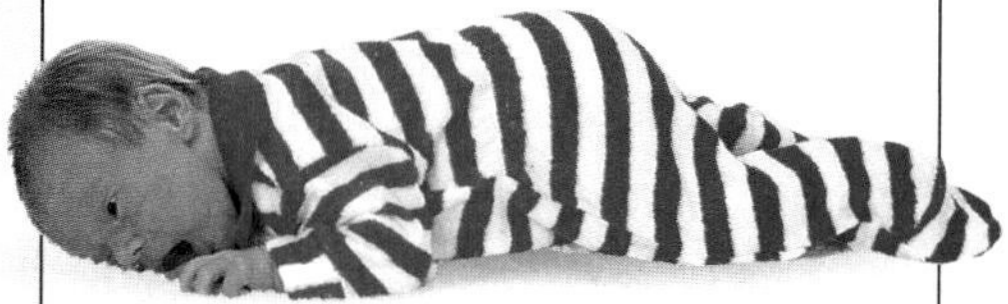
3 MONTHS	Your baby's body is straighter, and the legs are extended. The baby can hold up his or her head. 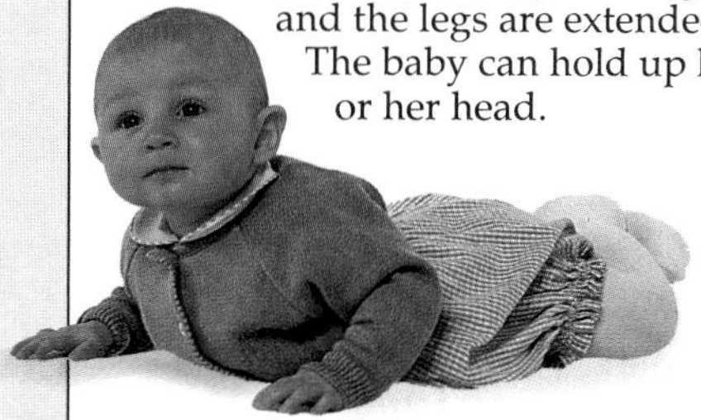
6 MONTHS	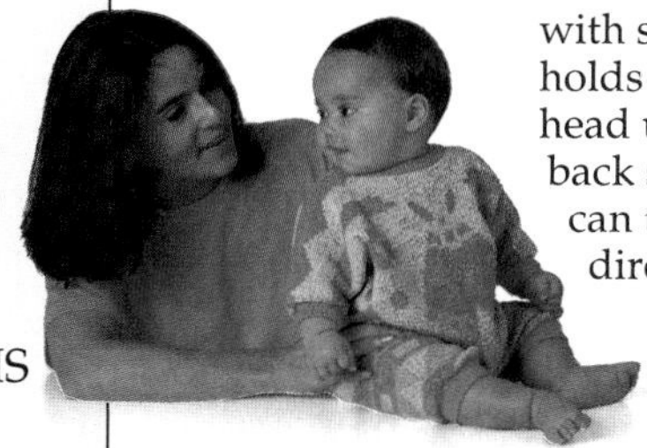 Your baby sits with support, holds his or her head up with the back straight, and can twist in all directions.
9 MONTHS	Your baby sits without support, leaving the arms free to reach and grasp. He or she also makes determined efforts to crawl and may be able to support himself or herself on the hands and knees. 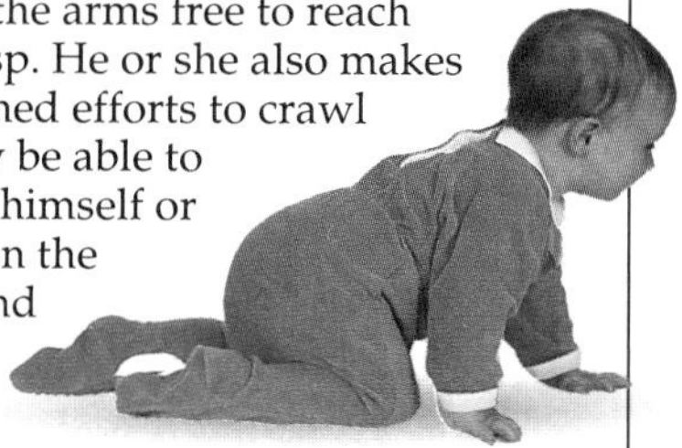
12 MONTHS	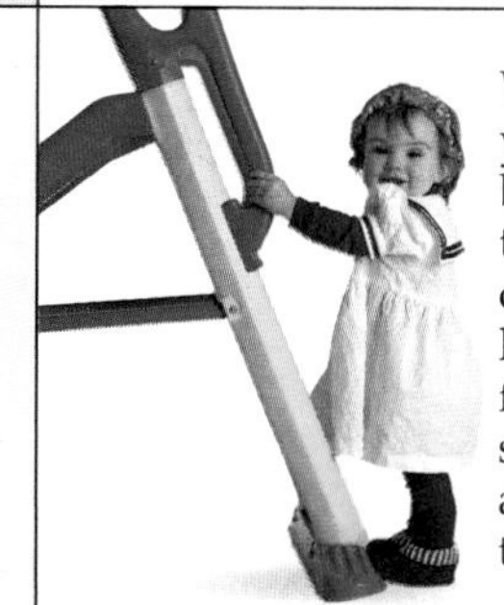 While holding your hands, your baby can probably take a few steps or can move around holding onto furniture. He or she can pull up to a standing position with support.

VISION AND MANIPULATION	HEARING AND SPEECH	PLAY AND SOCIAL SKILLS
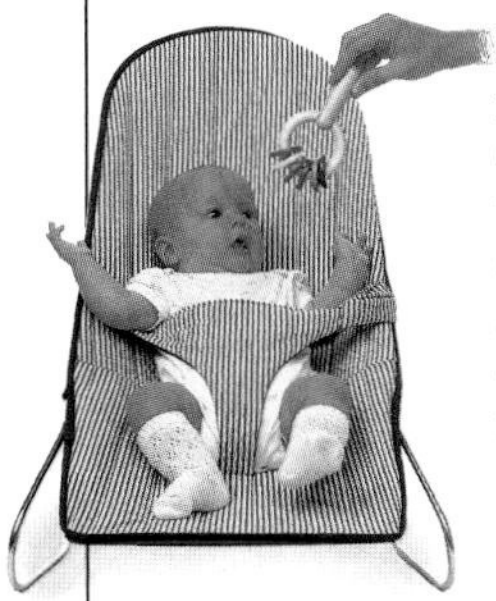 Your baby's pupils react to light, and he or she turns the head toward light. He or she watches your face when you talk and follows a moving object placed in the immediate field of vision.	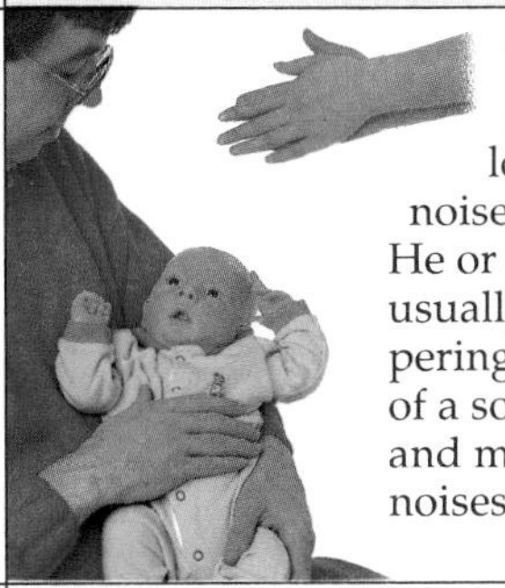 Your baby is startled by loud, sudden noises and may cry. He or she will usually stop whimpering at the sound of a soothing voice and makes throaty noises when content.	Your baby generally sleeps when not being fed or held. He or she stops crying when picked up and spoken to. His or her hands are normally closed but grasp onto a finger if you touch the palm. 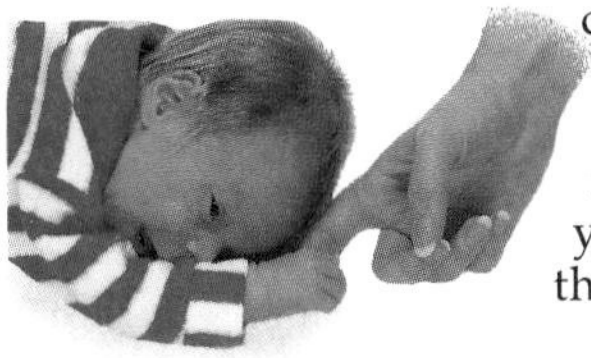
Your baby can move the head to gaze around and follows most of your movements. The baby can clasp and unclasp the hands and can press the palms together. 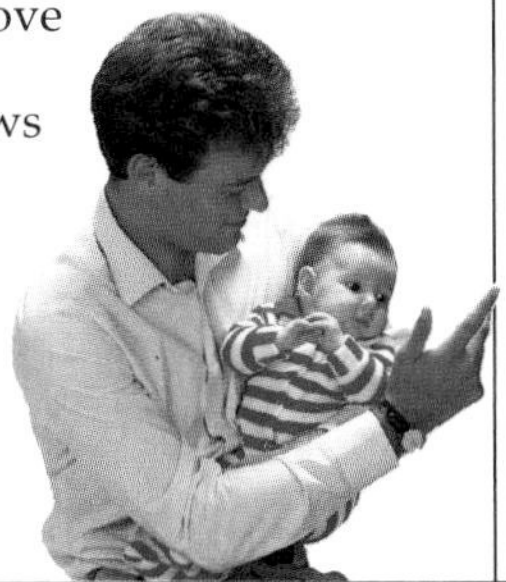	The baby cries when uncomfortable and chuckles or coos when content. While listening to an interesting sound, he or she remains quiet. 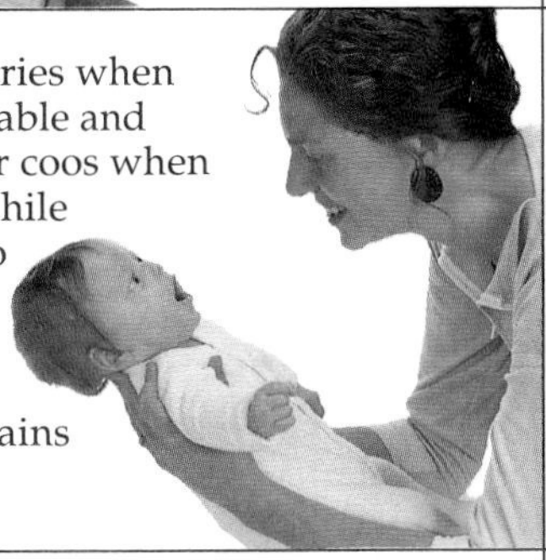	Your baby begins to react to familiar surroundings and now responds with obvious pleasure to friendly handling. 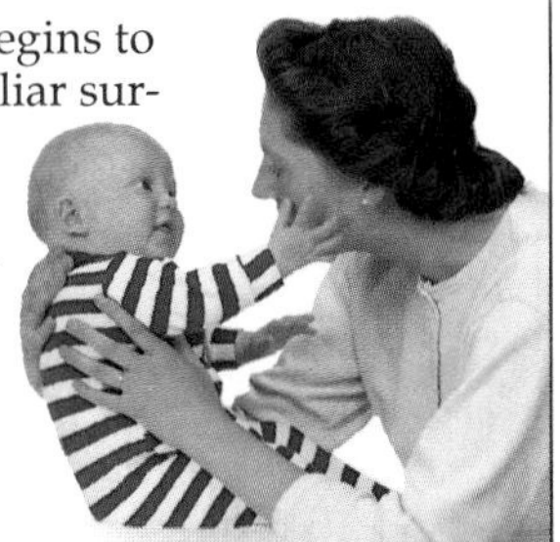
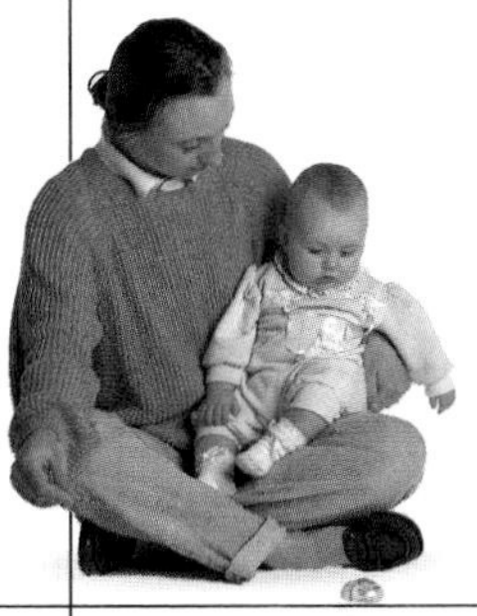 When something attracts his or her attention, your baby now moves the head eagerly. He or she can watch a ball roll up to 6 feet away and can hold an object between the finger and thumb.	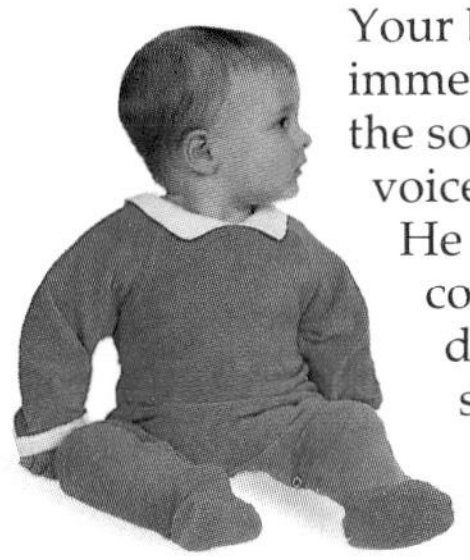 Your baby now turns immediately toward the sound of a familiar voice across a room. He or she can make cooing noises and double-syllable sounds.	Your baby now reaches for and grasps small toys, bringing everything up to the mouth. If offered a rattle, the baby shakes it to make a sound. He or she is occasionally shy, especially if the mother is out of sight. 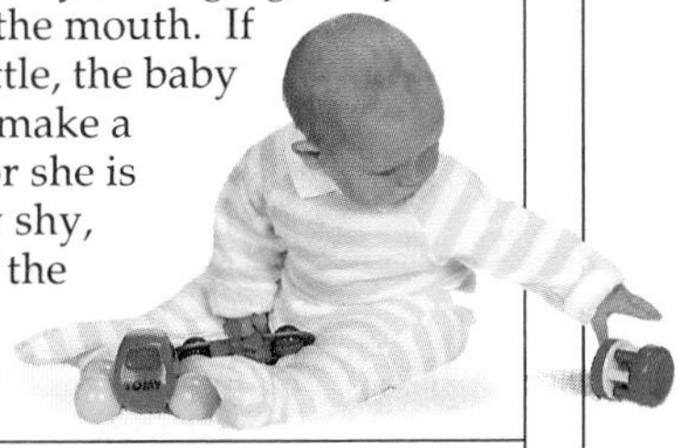
Your baby can look for dropped toys and can point to distant objects. He or she can also transfer objects from one hand to the other. 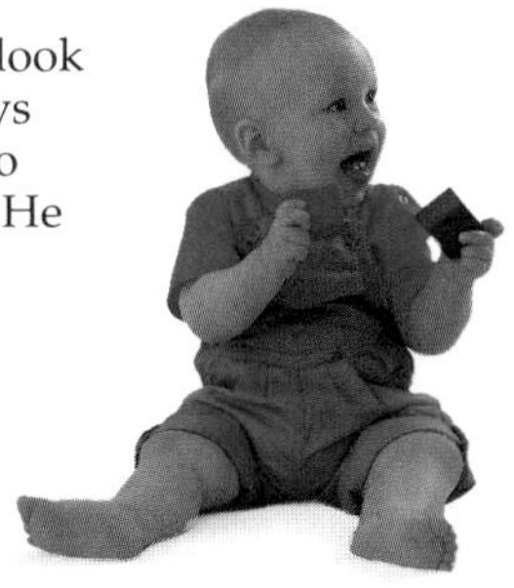	Your baby turns toward soft sounds up to 3 feet away from either ear and babbles contentedly. He or she now knows how to shout to attract attention. 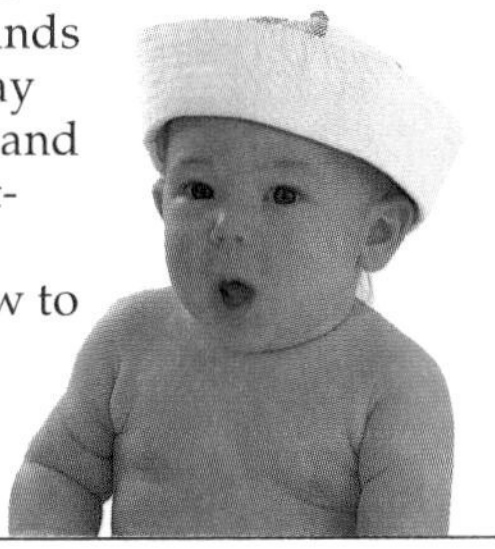	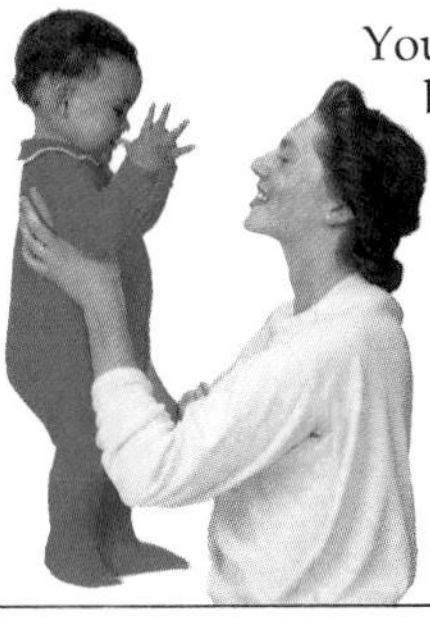 Your baby holds, bites, and chews solid food and holds a cup or bottle. He or she can discern strangers. The baby can imitate hand-clapping and peek-a-boo.
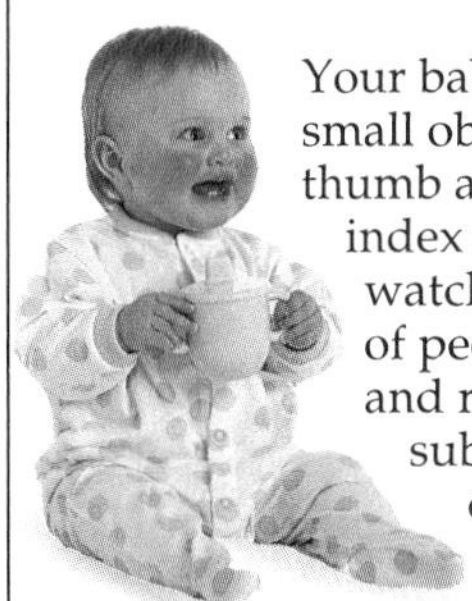 Your baby can pick up small objects between the thumb and the tip of the index finger. He or she watches the movements of people and objects and recognizes familiar subjects from a distance of 20 feet or more.	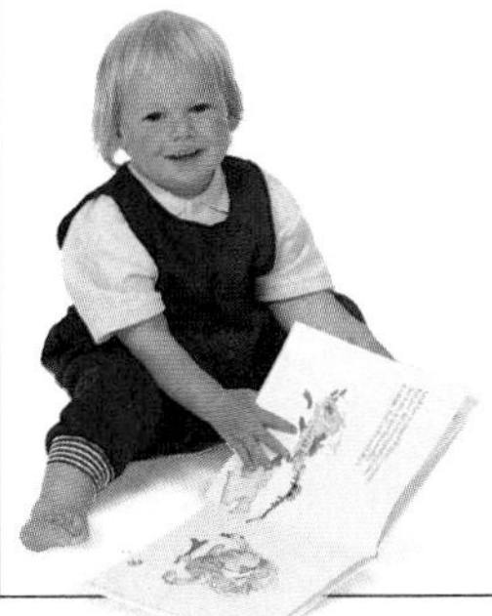 Your baby now turns immediately at the sound of his or her name, babbles incessantly, and begins to understand simple commands.	Your baby drinks from a cup with little help and holds a spoon but cannot yet use it unaided. He or she helps with dressing by holding out the arms for sleeves and the feet for shoes. 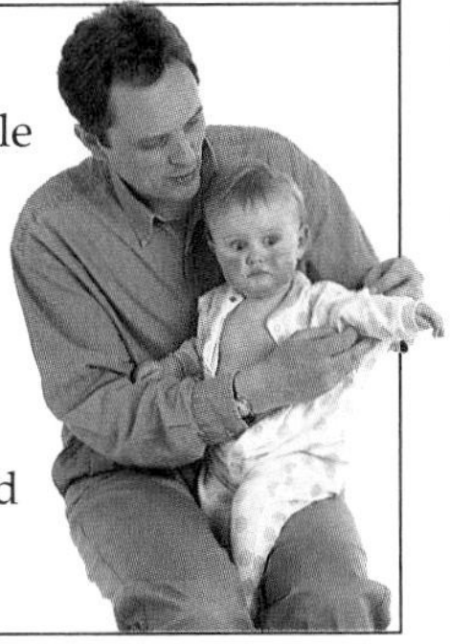

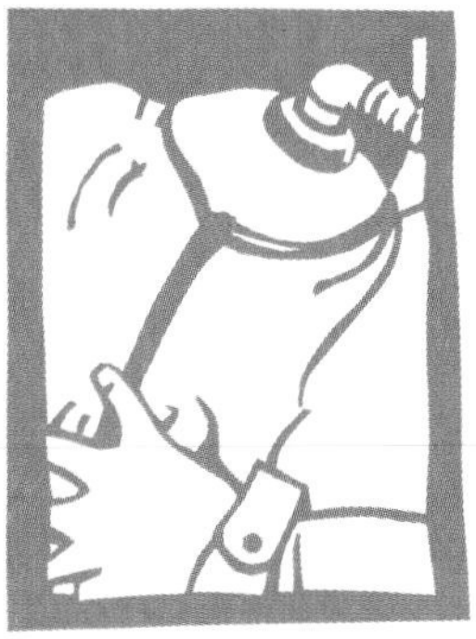

HIGH-RISK INFANTS

HIGH-RISK INFANTS enter the world with a tenuous hold on life. But advances in the medical care of newborns during the past 30 years have dramatically improved the outlook for high-risk infants. More than 90 percent of babies who are born after the seventh month of pregnancy now survive without serious long-term problems. But many need intensive medical care.

High-risk infants include those born prematurely, those of low birth weight, infants whose mothers had an infection or illness during pregnancy, and infants born in a multiple pregnancy, such as twins or triplets. Babies are said to be premature when they are born before 37 weeks of pregnancy have elapsed. Pregnancy usually lasts about 40 weeks. In the US, 7 percent of all newborns have a low birth weight (less than 5½ pounds); two thirds of them are premature.

Premature babies are at greater risk of developing problems after birth than are full-term babies. Premature babies usually cannot maintain a stable temperature. They do not suck well and need help with feeding. Their lungs are immature, predisposing them to breathing difficulties. Premature babies are also more vulnerable to infection than are full-term babies.

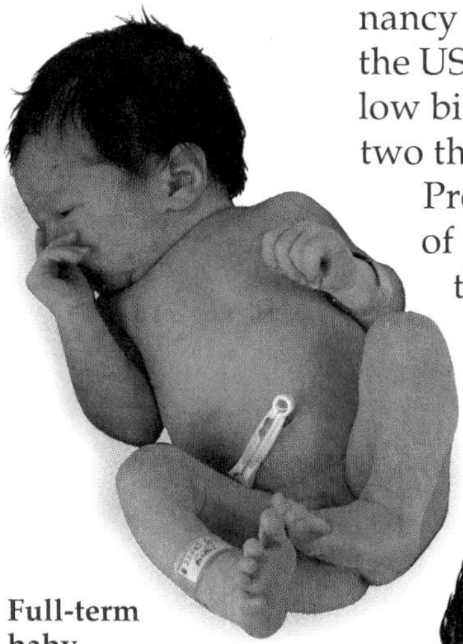

Full-term baby

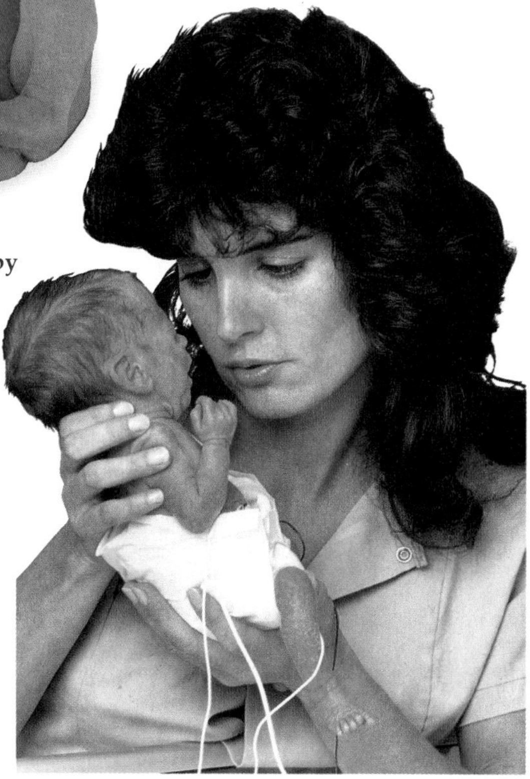

Premature baby

Premature babies
Premature babies are smaller and thinner than full-term babies. The poor muscle tone of premature babies gives them a "floppy" appearance. Fine, downy hair covers the skin of premature babies, especially on their backs. Their skin is thinner, redder, and more fragile than that of full-term babies. These differences increase with the degree of prematurity.

BREATHING DIFFICULTIES

Premature babies, infants born of diabetic mothers, and second-born twins are more likely to develop respiratory distress syndrome than are other babies. Boys develop the syndrome more often than girls. Respiratory distress syndrome occurs when the baby's immature lungs cannot produce sufficient amounts of a substance called surfactant, a lubricant that helps the tiny air sacs in the lungs to expand and remain expanded after birth. Babies with respiratory distress syndrome usually begin breathing rapidly during the first few hours after birth. Their ribs and chest appear to be sucked inward as they breathe, and they emit grunting sounds. Without treatment, a baby with respiratory distress syndrome does not get enough oxygen, begins to turn blue, and may die. Respiratory distress syndrome usually worsens during the first 48 to 72 hours of life and then improves during the next few days.

Treating respiratory distress

If your baby has respiratory distress syndrome, you should talk with the pediatrician and the intensive care nurses about the course and management of the illness. Doctors treat mild respiratory distress by putting the baby's head inside a hood in which the level of oxygen is controlled. Most babies with respiratory distress require breathing assistance from a ventilator. Connected to a tube placed in the baby's windpipe, the ventilator controls the rate of breathing and the amount of oxygen that the baby receives. When a doctor sees that respiratory distress syndrome is likely to occur, he or she may give replacement surfactant to a premature baby at birth.

The doctor takes frequent blood samples to make sure that the baby is getting enough oxygen and is eliminating carbon dioxide. The blood is usually taken from an artery in the baby's arm or from the baby's umbilical stump.

INTRAVENTRICULAR HEMORRHAGE

In very small premature babies, usually those born before 34 weeks of pregnancy have elapsed or weighing less than 4 pounds, the tiny blood vessels that line the brain can sometimes rupture and bleed. This bleeding, called intraventricular hemorrhage, is more common in babies who have undergone injury or infection at birth, who have been deprived of oxygen for long periods during birth, or who are in shock at birth.

Pediatricians can detect intraventricular hemorrhages by performing an ultrasound scan (an imaging technique that uses high-frequency sound waves) of the baby's brain. Most intraventricular hemorrhages cause no immediate or long-term problems. But a severe hemorrhage can block the circulation of fluid inside the baby's brain and cause it to accumulate – a condition called hydrocephalus. To reduce the swelling caused by this condition, doctors may have to perform surgery to drain the excess fluid. In a very few babies, a large hemorrhage can cause permanent brain damage, leading to limb weakness or stiffness, developmental delay, or death.

INTENSIVE CARE FOR BABIES

Very small or sick babies are often placed in a newborn intensive care unit. The babies lie inside an incubator or an Ohio bed (see below). They may be connected to machines that monitor their vital signs, provide food, or aid breathing. If the vital signs change, alarms warn the medical staff.

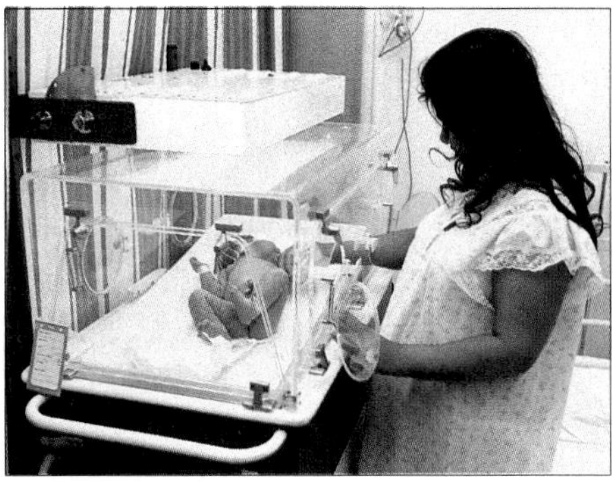

An incubator
An incubator keeps the air around the baby at a constant temperature and protects the baby against infectious organisms. Doctors usually give premature infants antibiotics for the first 48 hours of life, or until tests show that no infections are present.

Providing life support
The immature organs of a critically ill baby do not always function effectively. To ensure that a premature baby's liver and kidneys are working, intensive care nurses regularly take blood samples for analysis from the umbilical cord, or from a tube in the baby's arm called an arterial line.

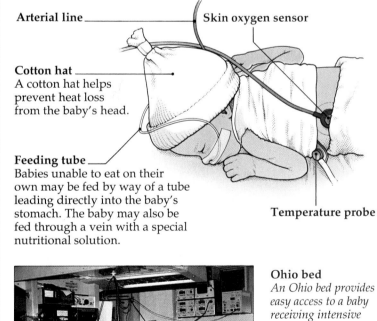

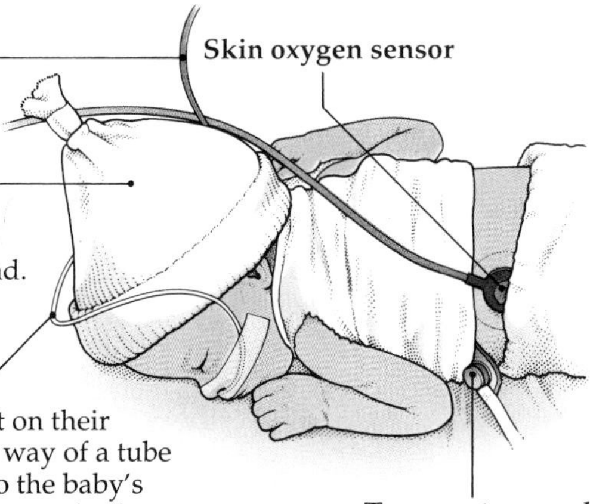
Arterial line
Skin oxygen sensor
Cotton hat
A cotton hat helps prevent heat loss from the baby's head.
Feeding tube
Babies unable to eat on their own may be fed by way of a tube leading directly into the baby's stomach. The baby may also be fed through a vein with a special nutritional solution.
Temperature probe

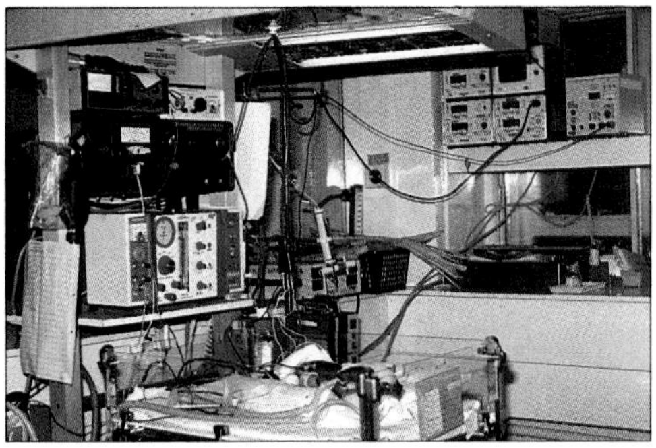

Ohio bed
An Ohio bed provides easy access to a baby receiving intensive care. The design of the bed provides plenty of space around the baby for the equipment needed to support life. It also maintains the infant's body temperature.

SMALL FULL-TERM BABIES

Some full-term babies weigh less than $5^1/_2$ pounds at birth. Such a low birth weight can reflect poor growth throughout pregnancy or, more commonly, slow growth in late pregnancy. If a baby has grown slowly throughout pregnancy, he or she will probably not exhibit "catch-up" growth quickly after birth. But babies whose growth slows only in late pregnancy usually make up for this lack of growth in the first 6 months of life.

FEEDING

Many premature babies cannot suck or swallow well enough to feed themselves. A mother can feed a premature baby through a small tube that the doctor passes through the baby's mouth or nose and into the digestive tract. Although breast milk is the ideal food for all babies, it sometimes must be supplemented with a formula specially designed to meet the increased nutritional needs of a premature baby.

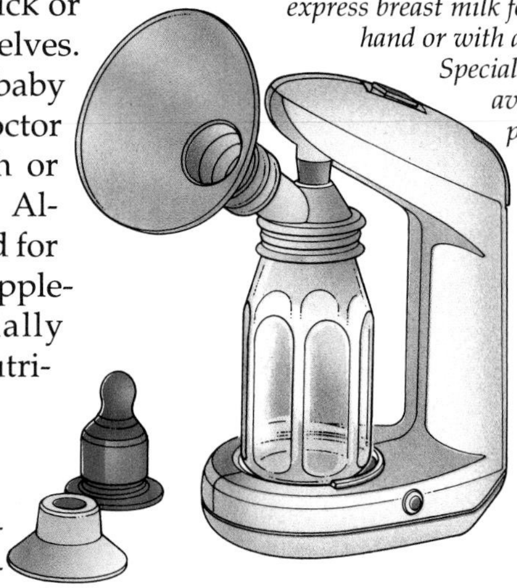

Expressing breast milk
Premature babies who cannot suck well can sometimes receive breast milk through a feeding tube (see below left). You can express breast milk for this purpose by hand or with a pumping device. Special formulas are also available for feeding premature infants.

Digestive problems

Premature babies often have a temporary paralysis of the gastrointestinal tract that can distend the stomach and intestines and cause vomiting. These babies receive food intravenously (through a tube inserted in a vein) until the doctor is sure that the gastrointestinal tract is functioning.

A baby who has blood in his or her stool along with a distended abdomen may have necrotizing enterocolitis, a serious inflammation of the intestines that causes bloody diarrhea, anemia, dehydration, and death. Babies with this condition receive food intravenously and are given antibiotics to fight off the infection. Surgical removal of the inflamed intestine may be necessary.

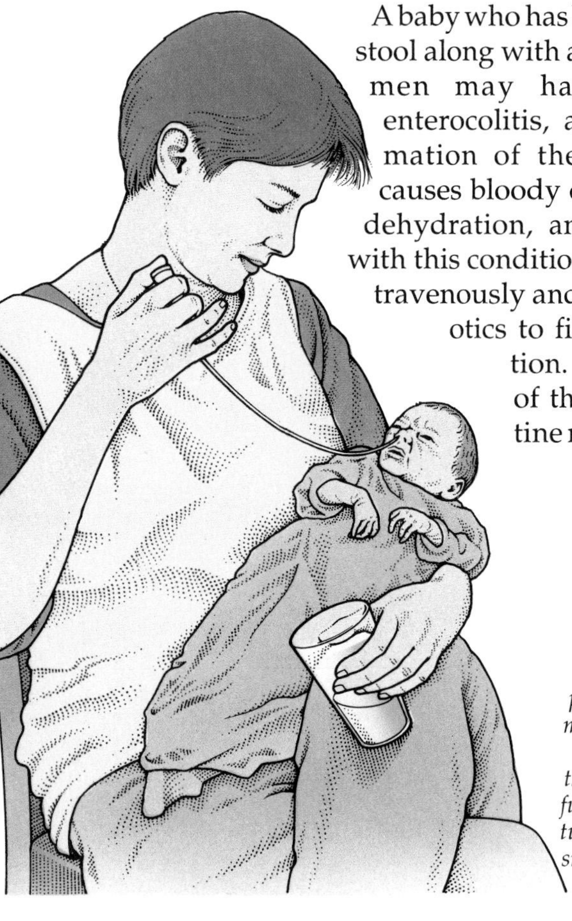

Feeding
Mothers can feed their premature babies breast milk or formula through a tube that passes into the baby's stomach. Like full-term babies, premature babies initially need small amounts of food at hourly intervals.

OUTLOOK FOR PREMATURE BABIES

Unless a premature baby experiences a serious complication, such as a severe brain hemorrhage, the outlook for the development of normal mental and motor skills is excellent. But parents should remember to gauge the development of their baby by his or her corrected age – the age calculated from birth minus the number of weeks he or she was born prematurely, until the baby reaches the chronological age of 2. For example, a 7- to 10-week-old baby who was born 8 weeks prematurely is about the same "age" in developmental terms as a full-term baby who has just been born.

Medical advances have made survival possible for extremely tiny $1\frac{1}{2}$-pound babies (born at 25 or 26 weeks of pregnancy). But many such babies have serious problems and face a high risk of developmental delay. Minor difficulties include weakness and learning problems; major complications include deafness, blindness, and muscle stiffness and rigidity (cerebral palsy). The care of such extremely small premature babies can place an enormous emotional and financial strain on parents.

JAUNDICE

Jaundice, a yellow coloring of the skin and whites of the eyes, is caused by the buildup of a pigment called bilirubin, which is released when red blood cells are broken down in the spleen. This red blood cell breakdown is a normal process that accelerates immediately after birth. About 50 percent of full-term newborn babies become jaundiced if the bilirubin level in their blood becomes higher than normal. If the level becomes very high, a risk of brain damage exists.

Treating jaundice
Doctors treat jaundice by increasing the amount of fluids given and by placing the baby under a lamp that radiates ultraviolet B light. For babies with very severe jaundice, doctors may order a blood transfusion, which replaces the baby's entire blood supply.

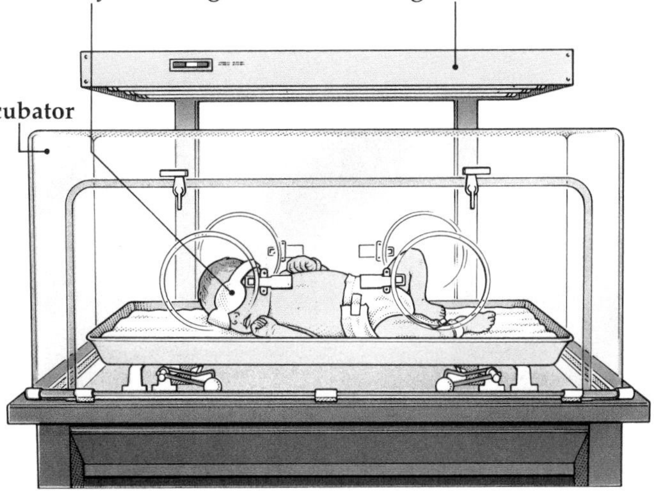

BIRTH INJURIES

Some babies are deprived of oxygen for a time during birth or fail to begin to breathe just after birth. Oxygen deprivation can cause a "floppy" appearance or feeding problems. If the oxygen deprivation is severe, it can also cause seizures, stiffness, irritability, and irregularity of the heartbeat. Infants deprived of oxygen during birth may need care in a neonatal intensive care unit. If the baby's condition returns to normal by 1 week of age, the baby is eating well, and his or her symptoms subside, then the outlook for normal development is excellent.

Other birth injuries include facial or scalp bruising and marks, which are often caused by forceps used during delivery, and temporary paralysis of the arm. All of these problems usually resolve on their own without long-term implications for the baby's future health.

INFANTS OF DIABETIC MOTHERS

Temporary diabetes is a common complication of pregnancy. Babies born to diabetic mothers are usually large; have an increased risk of respiratory distress syndrome, jaundice, and heart disease; and may have a low level of sugar in their blood. For this reason, doctors closely monitor blood sugar levels in babies born of diabetic mothers during the first few days of life. These babies also need frequent feedings to maintain normal blood sugar levels.

EFFECTS OF DRUG USE

Smoking during pregnancy is linked to low birth weight. Prolonged exposure of the fetus to alcohol can cause developmental delay and heart defects. Other drugs, such as heroin or cocaine, used during pregnancy can cause addiction and withdrawal symptoms in newborns.

Contact with parents
Most premature babies can be cuddled and held. When cuddling is not permitted, parents can touch and reassure their baby through openings in the sides of the incubator or by talking to and touching the infant in an Ohio bed.

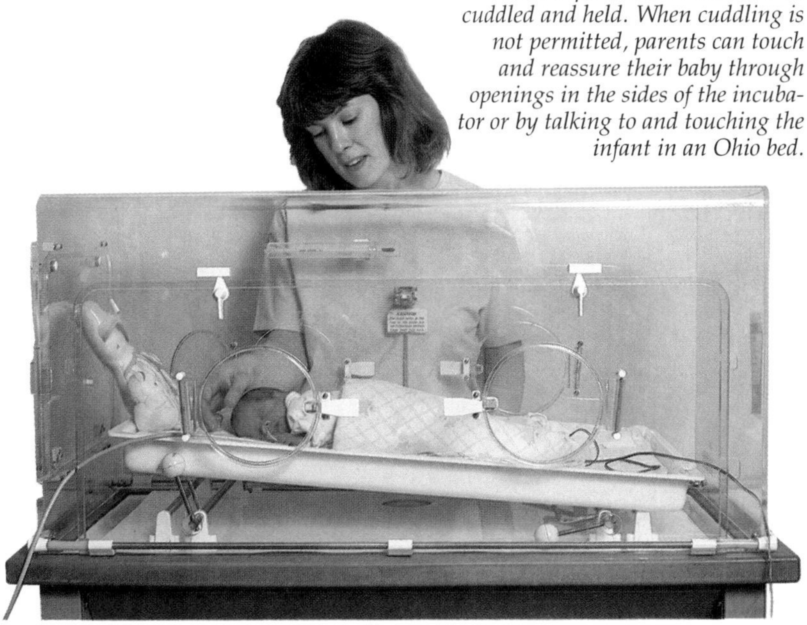

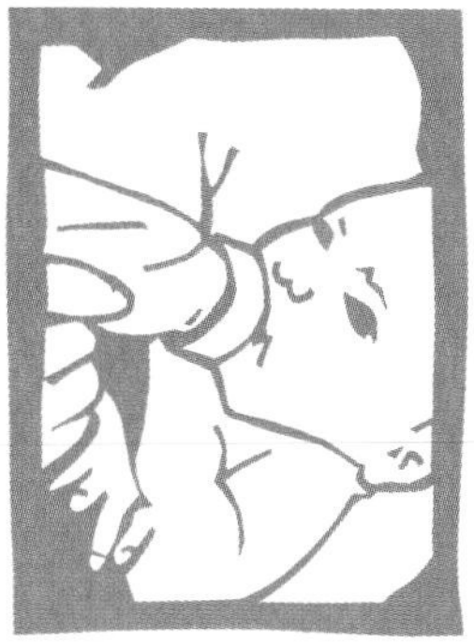

CARING FOR YOUR BABY

HAVING A BABY is a big responsibility. Caring for your new baby will probably take most of your time and energy. You may find the first few weeks following childbirth surprisingly tiring. To help this important time run smoothly, start thinking about what your baby will need well before your due date.

The first few days that you and your baby spend at home will be much easier if everything you need is at hand. In the weeks before your baby's birth, buy only essential items, such as a crib and a car seat. Then add other items, such as toys, after the birth. You do not need to buy a wide variety of clothes for your newborn. He or she will outgrow them quickly. The complete set of clothing and equipment you need for a newborn baby is often called a layette.

CHOOSING THE LAYETTE

The most important factor to consider when choosing a layette is safety. Make sure that the items you have are suitable for your child's age and conform to product safety standards.

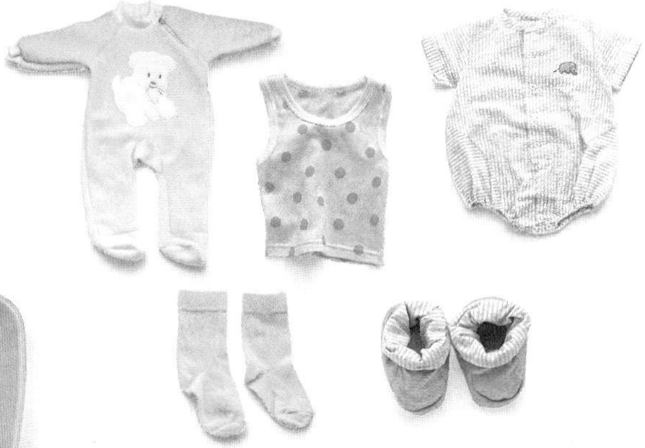

Clothing
Try not to underdress or overdress your baby. If you don't think you need a sweater, your baby probably doesn't either. Basic clothing should include several wide-necked t-shirts and one-piece sleepers, a sweater, soft socks, and a hat. You will also need cloth or disposable diapers (see page 30) and a few receiving blankets.

Car safety seat
Motor-vehicle accidents represent the biggest threat to child safety in the US. Laws in all 50 states now require the use of a car safety seat when you transport your baby in your car. For your newborn, choose a small, portable car seat that provides the best fit for younger babies. The car seat should face the back of the car so that it can support the infant's body and head in the event of a collision.

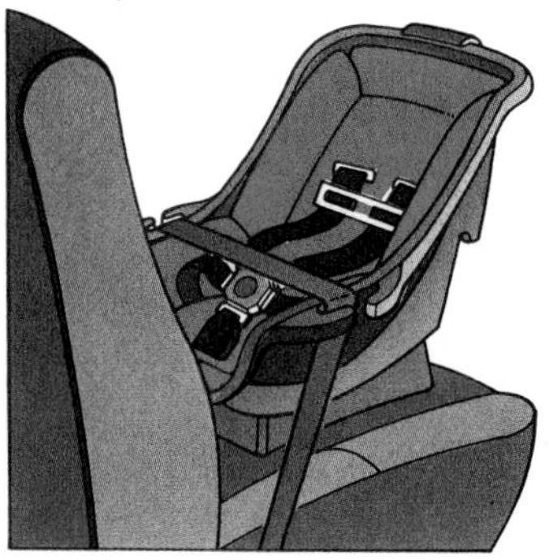

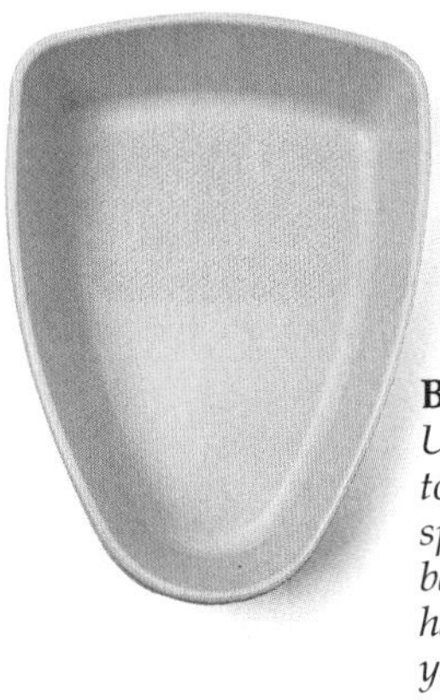

Baby bathtub
Until your baby is old enough to bathe in the family bathtub, a special plastic baby tub will make bathtime easier for you. It should have a textured bottom to prevent your baby from slipping.

Bottle-feeding equipment
If you choose to bottle-feed, you will need at least eight bottles with extra nipples and cans of formula (powder, concentrate, or ready-made). Until your baby is about 5 months old, you should use a bottle sterilizer to destroy bacteria. You can also sterilize bottles and nipples in a pan of boiling water.

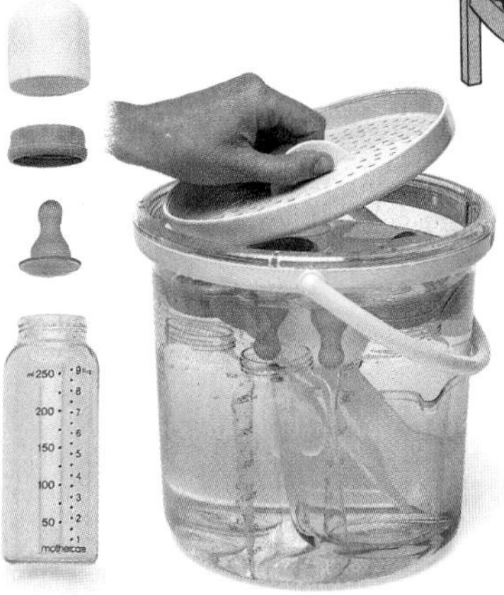

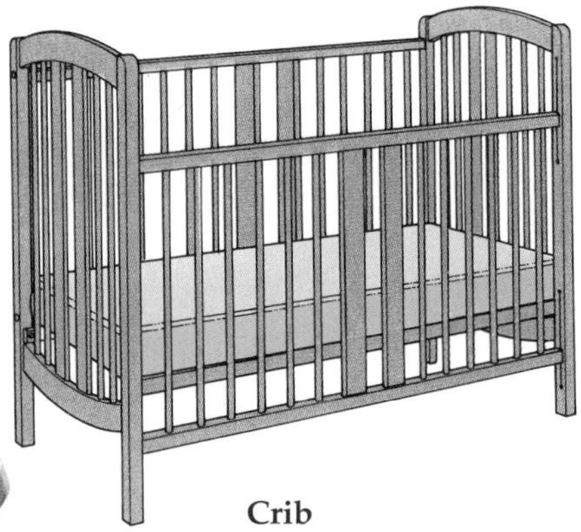

Crib
Choose a drop-sided crib with bars that are close enough together to prevent your baby from trapping his or her head between them – no more than $2^{3}/_{8}$ inches apart. In some cribs, the mattress can be lowered as your baby grows and becomes more mobile.

HANDLING YOUR BABY

If you are a first-time parent, you may be afraid to pick up your new baby, thinking you might somehow hurt him or her. Don't hesitate to hold your child – right from the start, your baby needs closeness and comfort as much as he or she needs food, warmth, and sleep. To make your baby feel secure, cradle him or her in the crook of your arm against your body or upright against your shoulder, supporting the head with your other arm. Remember that a newborn cannot hold up his or her head. You must always support the baby's head and neck when you hold him or her for the first month or two. Make sure that all of your movements are slow and gentle.

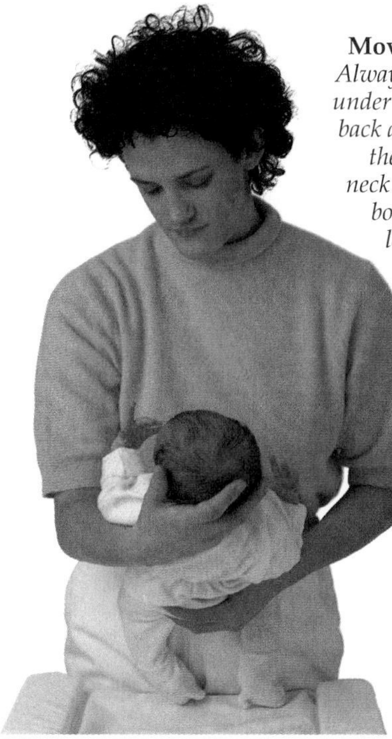

Moving your baby
Always have one hand under the baby's lower back and buttocks and the other under the neck and head so that both the upper and lower parts of the baby's body have equal support.

UMBILICAL CORD CARE

After birth, a doctor or nurse painlessly cuts your baby's umbilical cord about 3 or 4 inches from the abdomen. The doctor places a clamp on the cord stump and applies antibiotic ointment. The stump dries and falls off in 10 to 14 days. Your doctor may tell you to wipe the stump with alcohol swabs to help it dry. Keep the cord dry until the stump falls off.

BATHING YOUR BABY

Your baby does not need complete bathing in the first few weeks of life. When you decide to give your baby his or her first full bath, gather all the items you need before you begin. You will need a baby bathtub, a changing mat, towels, cottonballs, liquid baby soap, diaper-changing items (see page 30), and clean clothes. Make sure the room you use is warm.

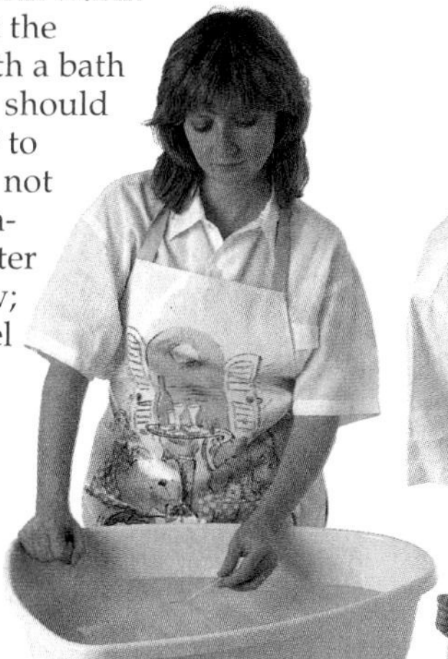

1 Fill the tub with warm water. Check the temperature with a bath thermometer. It should range from 98°F to 100°F. If you do not have a thermometer, test the water with your elbow; it should not feel hot. Add liquid baby soap.

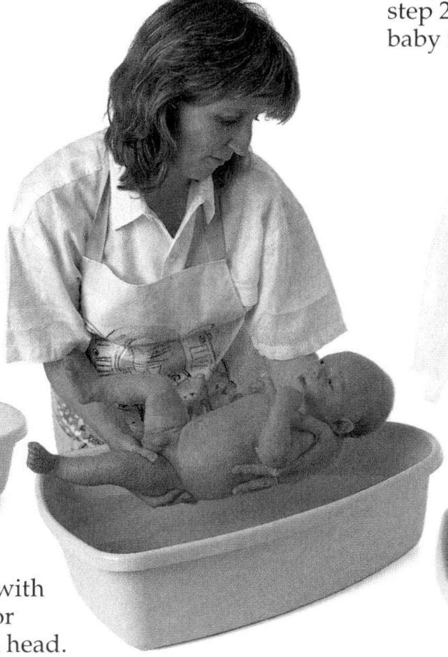

2 Hold your baby securely with one hand supporting his or her shoulder, upper arm, and head. Use your other hand to support the baby's legs and buttocks by holding one thigh, as shown. Keep the baby's head and neck out of the water.

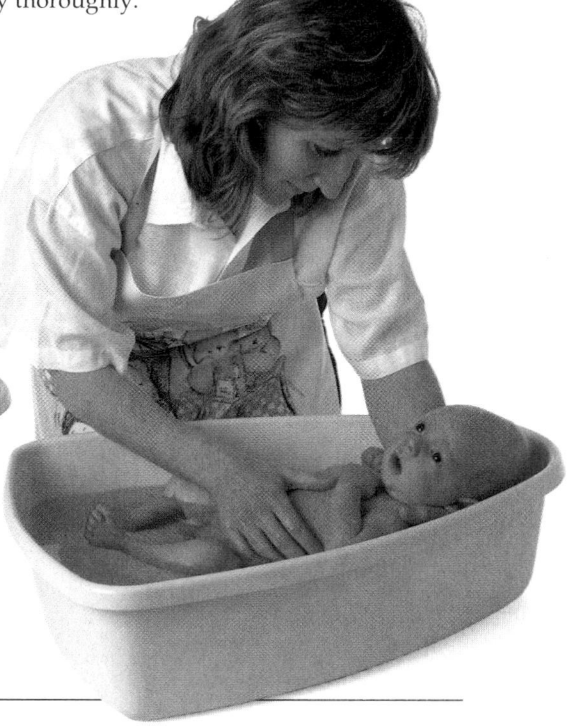

3 When the tub supports your baby's weight, remove your hand from under the baby's thigh and splash water over his or her body. Use a washcloth to gently cleanse the baby's skin. To wash your baby's hair, use a baby shampoo and carefully avoid getting it in your baby's eyes. Rinse the shampoo off with a wet washcloth. Lift your baby out of the tub by supporting the body as in step 2. Always dry your baby thoroughly.

CHANGING DIAPERS

You must change your baby's diapers often to keep him or her comfortable and to prevent diaper rash. To minimize the possibility of diaper rash, always clean the diaper area thoroughly. If you notice irritation or rash, use a diaper rash cream to provide a protective layer over the skin. Never leave your baby unattended while changing his or her diaper. He or she could fall off the changing table.

Choosing diapers
Since the introduction of disposable diapers, square cotton cloth diapers with rubber pants have become less popular. Disposable diapers eliminate the need for laundering and contain an absorbent layer that reduces leakage. Many cloth diapers combine outer layers of waterproof fabric with cloth inserts, making them similar to disposable diapers. Diaper services are also available to clean and deliver diapers.

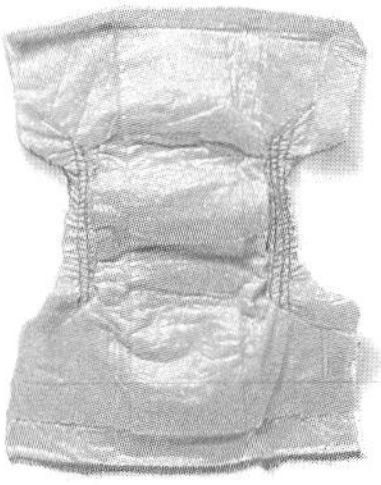

Disposable diaper

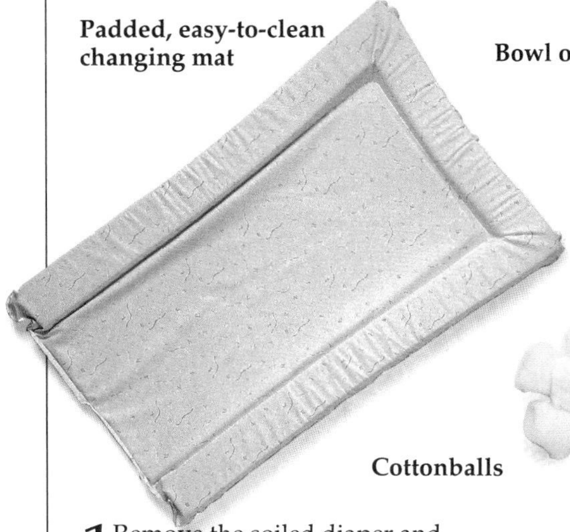

Padded, easy-to-clean changing mat

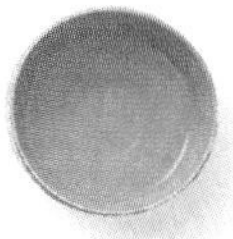

Bowl of warm water

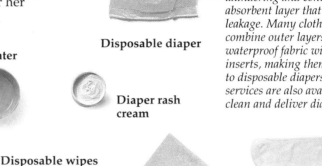

Diaper rash cream

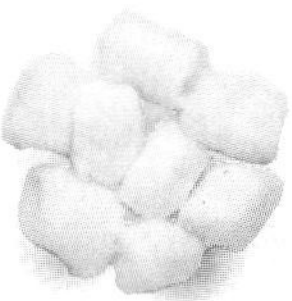

Cottonballs

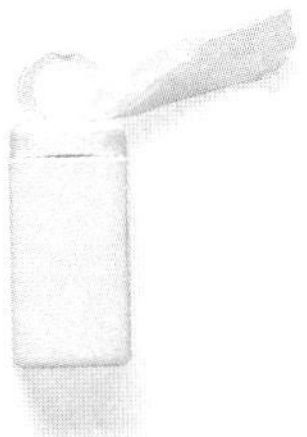

Disposable wipes

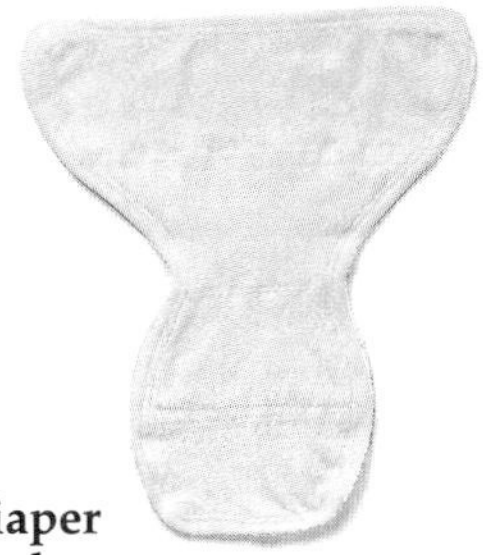

Cloth diaper insert and cover

1 Remove the soiled diaper and clean any feces off your baby with disposable wipes. Wipe the baby's genitals and the surrounding skin with another disposable diaper wipe to remove urine.

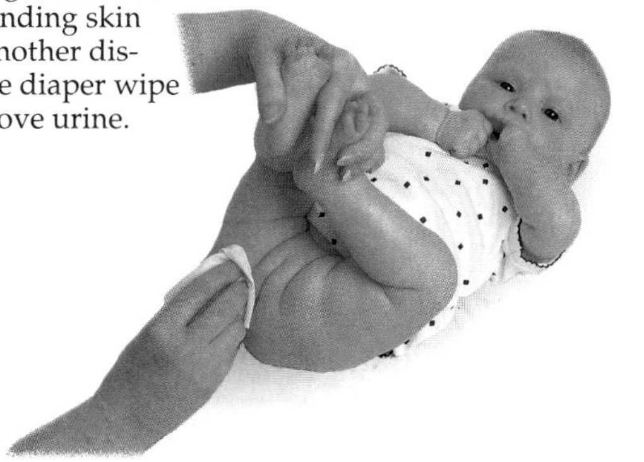

2 Dry your baby thoroughly. Apply diaper rash cream if your baby has a diaper rash.

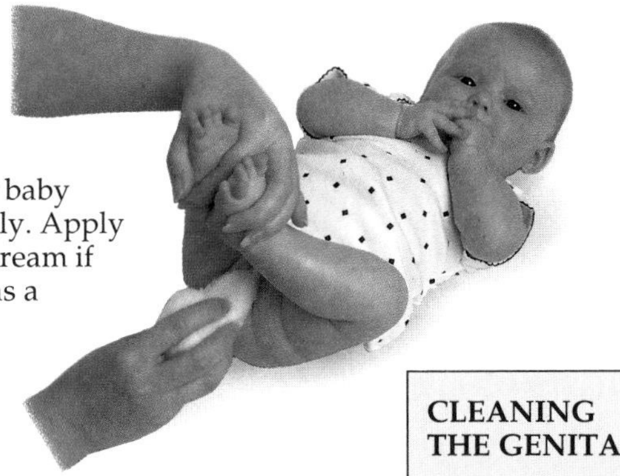

3 Open a new diaper with the tape at the top. Lift up your baby's buttocks as shown, keeping a finger between the baby's ankles. Align the top of the diaper with your baby's waist.

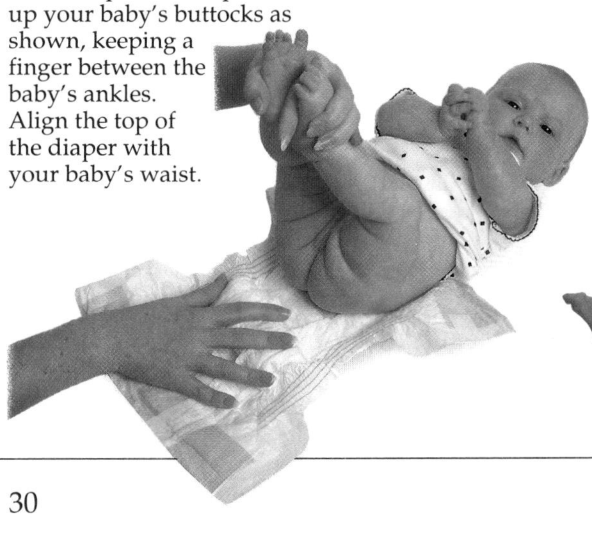

4 Bring the front of the diaper up, positioning a boy's penis downward. Hold one corner of the diaper in position and unpeel the adhesive tab. Pull the tab firmly over the front flap. Repeat the process on the other side. If you are using a cloth diaper, pin each side to secure it.

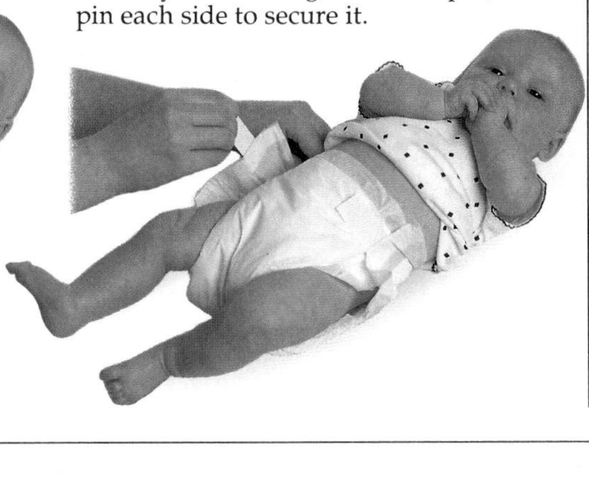

CLEANING THE GENITALS

Every time you change your baby's diaper, clean the genitals and buttocks. For girls, always wipe from front to back so bacteria from the anus do not enter the urinary tract. Clean the vaginal lips but not inside the vagina. For boys, work from the leg creases toward the penis. Do not pull the foreskin back. Clean the penis thoroughly.

DENTAL CARE

Your baby will show the first signs of teething at around 6 months of age. The emergence of first teeth may cause irritability and drooling but seldom causes serious problems. If your baby seems cranky when teething, do not use teething gels. Instead, give the baby acetaminophen or try gently rubbing your baby's gums with a clean finger to comfort him or her. It is never too early to start caring for your child's teeth. Clean your baby's teeth and gums by rubbing them gently with a dry washcloth. When your baby is about 12 months old, you can use a baby-sized toothbrush.

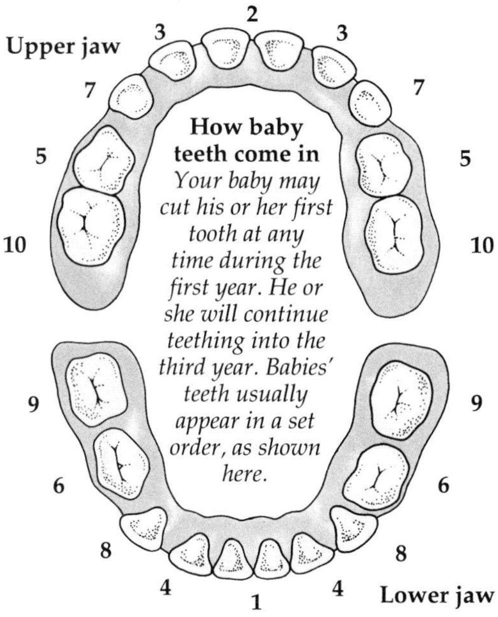

How baby teeth come in
Your baby may cut his or her first tooth at any time during the first year. He or she will continue teething into the third year. Babies' teeth usually appear in a set order, as shown here.

SUDDEN INFANT DEATH SYNDROME

Sudden infant death syndrome occurs when a baby inexplicably stops breathing during sleep and dies. This syndrome strikes two in every 1,000 babies worldwide. It usually occurs between 1 and 12 months of age, with the peak incidence at around 3 months. The cause is unknown, but current research is seeking an explanation for this terrible phenomenon. Placing an infant on his or her stomach to sleep has been implicated. Doctors recommend that babies be placed on their backs while sleeping. Do not use pillows, and make sure the mattress is firm.

TIPS FOR TIRED PARENTS

A newborn baby sleeps most of the time – about 16 hours a day – but the baby's periods of sleep may not last longer than a few hours, even at night. You can do several things to encourage your baby to sleep for longer periods at night.

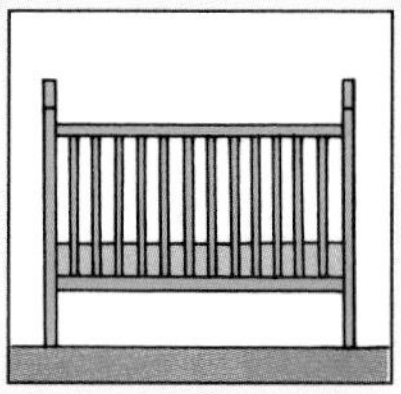

Put the crib in a quiet room but do not worry about background noise. Although sudden noises may frighten your baby, he or she will soon get used to sleeping through the normal sounds in your house. Keep the room at a constant temperature of about 75°F because your baby can lose body heat easily.

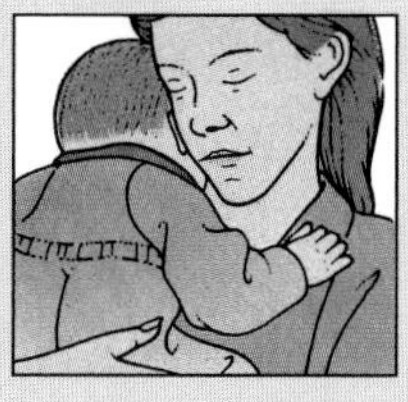

Keep nighttime feedings quiet and brief to reinforce the idea that night is the time for sleeping. Always stay with your baby for a moment or two to give him or her some time to settle down before you finally leave. Some babies need burping (see page 33) after every feeding, especially at night.

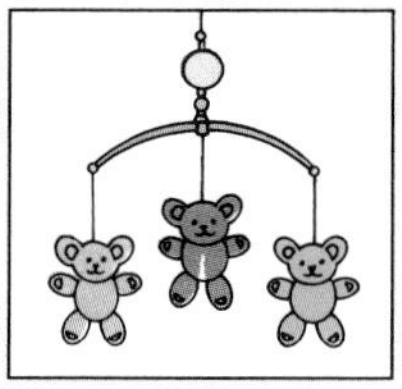

Give your baby plenty to look at, such as brightly colored mobiles, when he or she is awake in bed. A very young baby clearly sees only those objects that are close to him or her, so hang objects a few inches above your baby's head in the immediate field of vision. Make sure objects are out of reach for safety.

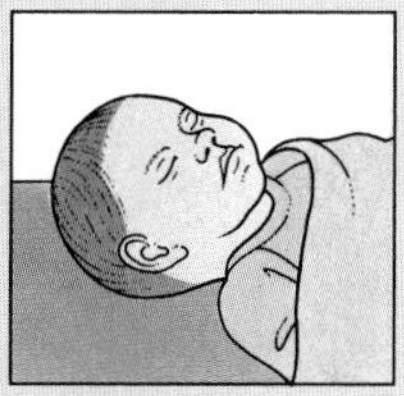

Use a firm mattress that fits the crib. Attach side padding firmly so the baby cannot get stuck in it. Padding should be low so you can see your baby. Do not use a pillow or a water bed; breathing could be obstructed. Never use electric blankets or plastic mattress covers, which have caused infant deaths.

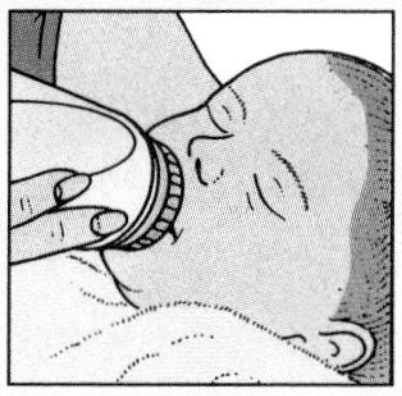

Share the responsibility of attending to your crying baby with your partner. For example, you and your partner can plan alternate nights "on duty" so that at least one of you can sleep through the night. If the mother is breastfeeding, she can express some milk for her partner to use when feeding the baby.

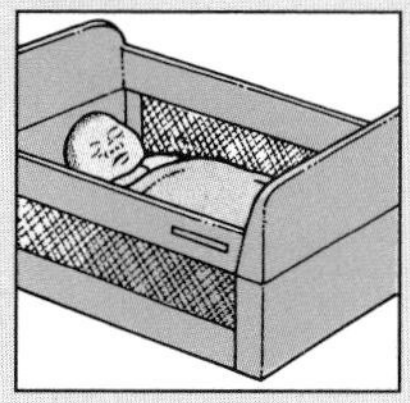

Keep the baby in a bassinet in your bedroom for the first 4 to 6 weeks, so that you can reassure your baby when he or she starts to cry. Having the baby in your room also makes it easier to nurse during the night. If you are constantly tired and depressed after the baby arrives, talk to your doctor or seek counseling.

FEEDING YOUR BABY

Should you breast-feed or bottle-feed your baby? The choice is entirely up to you. Both methods have advantages and disadvantages. Breast milk is easier for your baby to digest and contains antibodies that help protect your baby against disease, especially in the first few days. But fatigue, illness, or stress can reduce a mother's supply of breast milk, and some women are uncomfortable with the idea of breast-feeding. Bottle-feeding allows both parents to take turns feeding the baby, and the mother's state of health has no effect on bottle-feeding.

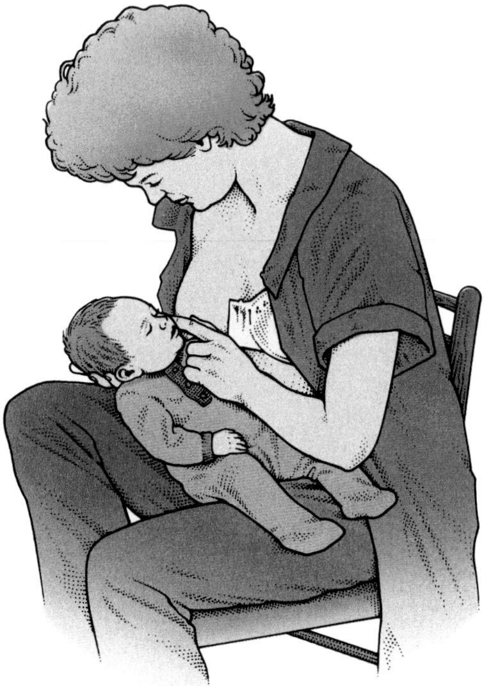

BREAST-FEEDING

Breast-feeding can be emotionally rewarding for you and your baby. It also enables you to provide the best and most natural nourishment for your baby. But you need to make sure that you produce enough milk for your baby by eating a healthy diet containing plenty of calcium and protein. Drinking fluids and avoiding excessive stress and fatigue also promote breast milk production. Breast milk flows on a "supply-and-demand" basis – the more milk the baby consumes, the more your body produces.

1 Sit comfortably in an upright position with your back supported, or try lying on your side. Bring your baby's head close to your breast and stroke the baby's cheek nearest to you so that your baby turns toward your breast.

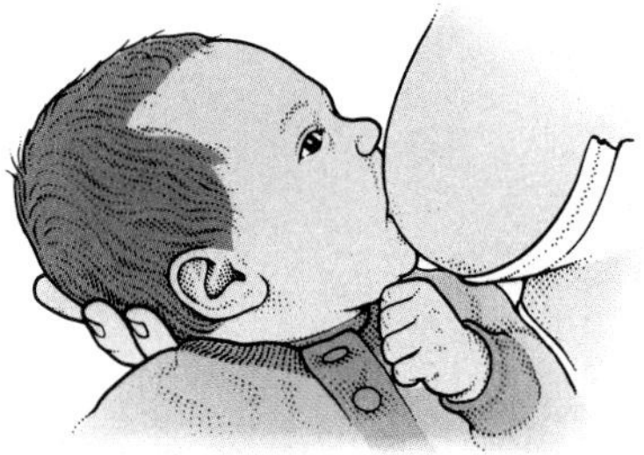

2 Guide your nipple into your baby's mouth. Make sure that the entire pigmented area surrounding the nipple is in the baby's mouth. When the baby presses his or her mouth against the milk reservoirs at the base of this area, your breast releases its milk.

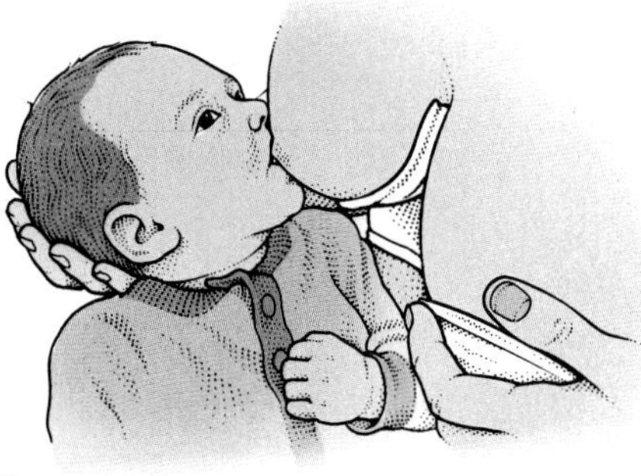

3 As your baby starts to feed, both breasts may release milk. Press your hand against your other breast to prevent leakage.

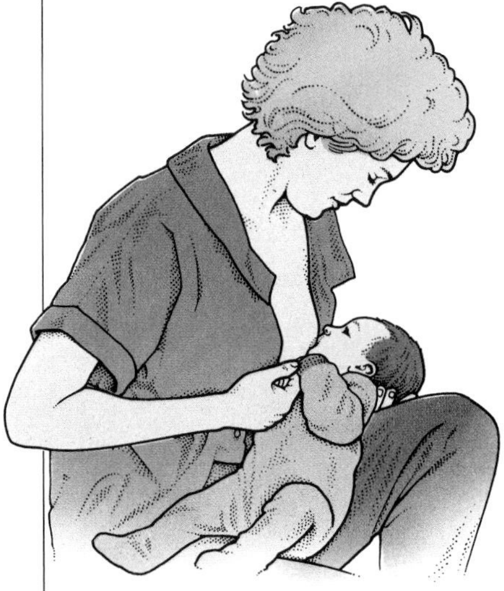

4 After your baby has nursed for 10 to 20 minutes on the first breast, transfer him or her to your other breast. Alternate the breast you start with at each feeding, because a baby often takes more from the first breast.

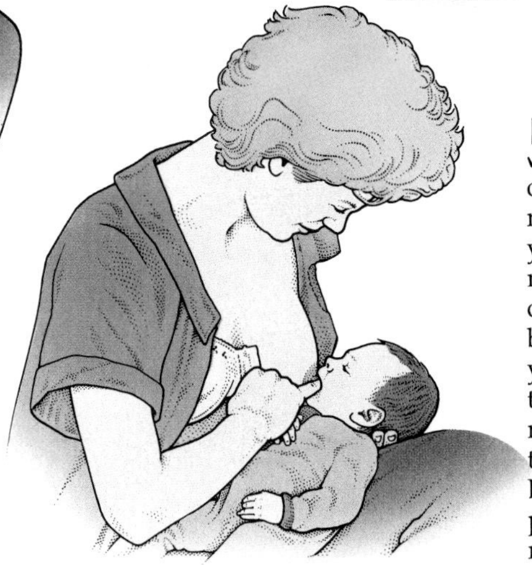

5 When your baby has had enough, he or she stops taking milk and just sucks on your breast for several minutes. Remove him or her from your breast by slipping your finger between the baby's gums. Do not let your baby suck to the point of pain. Burp your baby (see page 33) and let your nipples air dry.

GIVING MEDICINES

Measure the medicine according to your doctor's instructions. If you are using a medicine spoon, let it rest on your baby's lower lip so that he or she can suck the medicine off. If you are giving the medicine through a dropper, support the baby's head, put the dropper into the corner of the mouth, and squeeze slowly. Never give an infant, child, or teenager aspirin because it can cause Reye's syndrome, a rare but sometimes fatal disorder.

BOTTLE-FEEDING

Once you decide to bottle-feed, do not agonize over your decision. Choosing to bottle-feed does not imply that you are depriving your baby of love, attention, and cuddling, because you can still give your baby all of these things at feeding times. Only specially prepared infant formula is suitable for babies less than a year old. Do not introduce cow's milk into your baby's diet before 8 months of age.

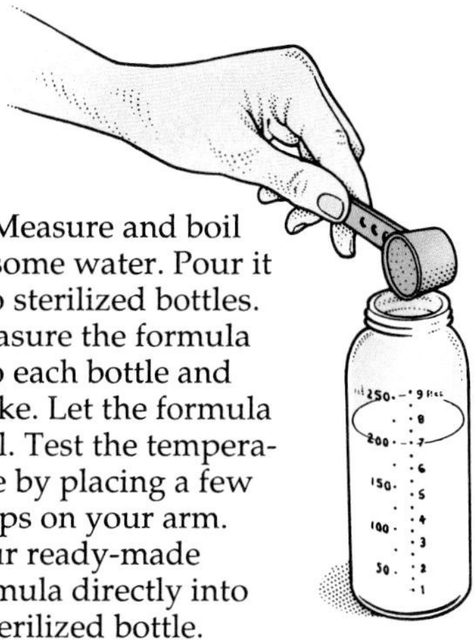

1 Measure and boil some water. Pour it into sterilized bottles. Measure the formula into each bottle and shake. Let the formula cool. Test the temperature by placing a few drops on your arm. Pour ready-made formula directly into a sterilized bottle.

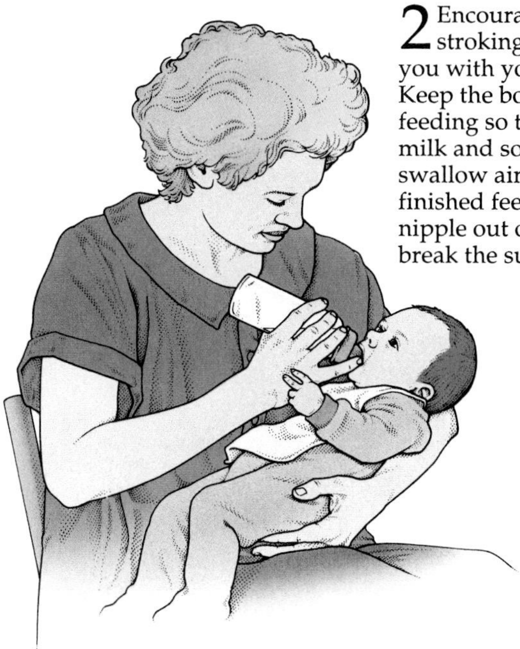

2 Encourage your baby to suck by stroking the cheek nearest to you with your finger or the nipple. Keep the bottle tilted when you are feeding so that the nipple is full of milk and so your baby does not swallow air. When your baby has finished feeding, gently pull the nipple out of his or her mouth or break the suction with your finger.

PREVENTING INFECTION

A bottle-fed baby is more at risk than a breast-fed baby of exposure to the microorganisms that cause diarrhea and vomiting, because these organisms breed very rapidly in formula, especially at room temperature. Prepare formula exactly according to the manufacturer's instructions. Sterilize bottle-feeding equipment every day. Store prepared bottles of formula in the refrigerator for no longer than 24 hours and warm them just before use. Discard any formula left at room temperature for more than 4 hours.

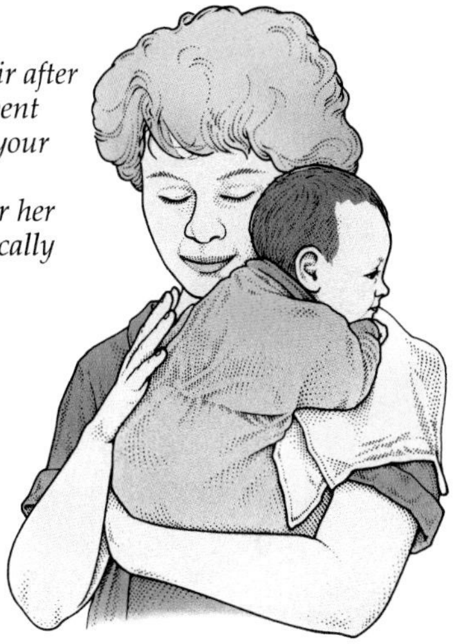

Burping
Your baby needs to release swallowed air after each feeding to prevent discomfort. Cradle your baby against your shoulder. Pat him or her gently and rhythmically several times on the back until he or she burps.

WEANING ONTO SOLID FOOD

Babies need only breast milk or formula until they are about 6 months old. At this age, you can try feeding your baby solid foods. Start with a taste of baby cereal. Your baby can eat commercial baby food or foods your family eats – fruits, vegetables, and meats – as long as they are pureed. Do not add salt or spices. Introduce foods one at a time to make sure your baby can tolerate them. Do not give a baby under 1 year of age honey because it may contain bacteria that could cause food poisoning.

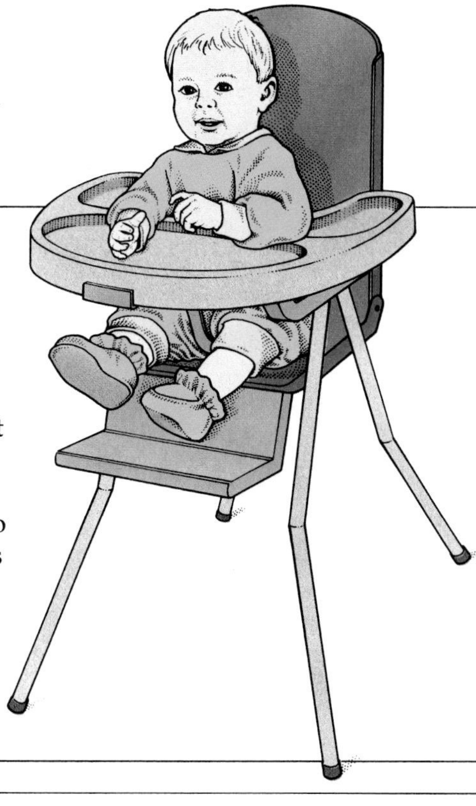

Mealtime can be fun
By about 1 year, your baby will be able to make a reasonably successful, although messy, attempt at feeding himself or herself. Pour drinks into a closed cup with a spout so the baby can half suck and half drink its contents. A plastic bib with a crumb catcher will protect against spilled food. Make sure your baby's high chair has a wide base and conforms to product safety standards. Fasten your child securely into the high chair.

CHILD CARE

More women are working outside the home than ever before, and child care services have rapidly proliferated in the last 20 years. Choosing some type of child care is one of the most important decisions a parent makes. Sometimes a family member or close friend can care for your child while you work, but many parents rely on professional care givers. The best care giver for your child is the one who can satisfy the needs of your particular household – and especially of your particular child.

Adapting to child care

To help your child adapt to and accept care from another person, visit the day care center or care giver's home that you have chosen with your child before the first day of care. Make it obvious to the child that you like and trust the care giver, and be careful to explain to an older child why you cannot stay at home.

Do not feel guilty about leaving your child with a care giver. It does not mean that you love your child any less than parents who stay at home. Good child care offers vital support to working parents and can help children grow socially, mentally, and emotionally. If you choose the care giver carefully, your child should be able to accept the new person.

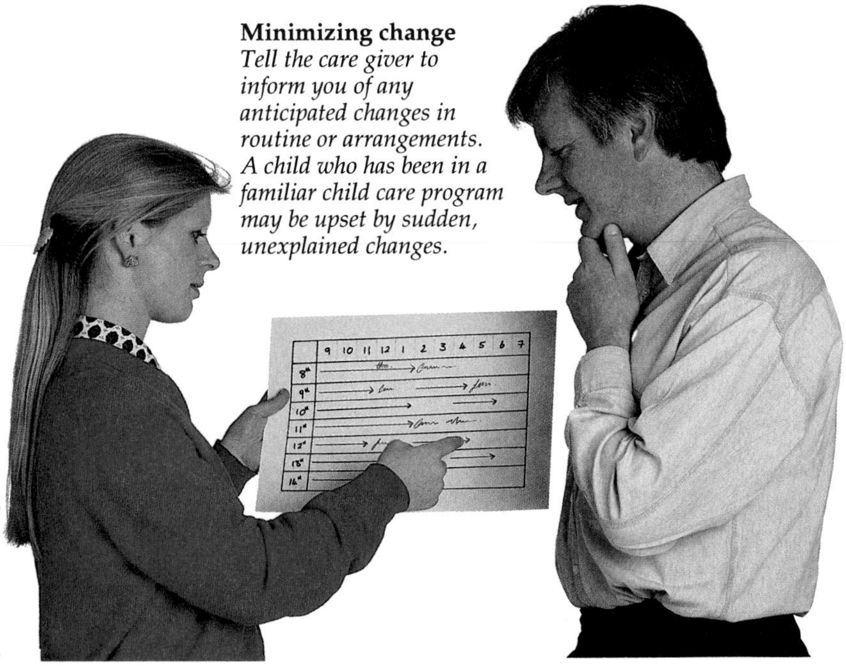

Minimizing change
Tell the care giver to inform you of any anticipated changes in routine or arrangements. A child who has been in a familiar child care program may be upset by sudden, unexplained changes.

TYPES OF CHILD CARE

Three basic types of child care are currently available in the US. In-home care describes the type in which the care giver works or lives in your home. Family day care is offered to a small group of children in the care giver's home. Day care centers link larger groups of young children with a staff of trained care givers in a facility outside the home. After-school programs often supplement these child care options for school-age children. Whichever type of care you choose, make sure that the location is convenient. Fully discuss the hours of care with the

CHECKLIST FOR DAY OR FAMILY CHILD CARE

When searching for the best child care setting for your child, consider the following factors:

- ◆ Is the facility licensed and inspected by the state?
- ◆ Are enough care givers present at all times?
- ◆ Do the children look happy and safe?
- ◆ Is there a written contract spelling out costs and policies?
- ◆ Is the care giver trained in first aid and management of infectious diseases?
- ◆ Are the bathroom facilities adequate?
- ◆ Is the environment clean?
- ◆ Is the food age-appropriate and nutritious?
- ◆ Do care givers have references?

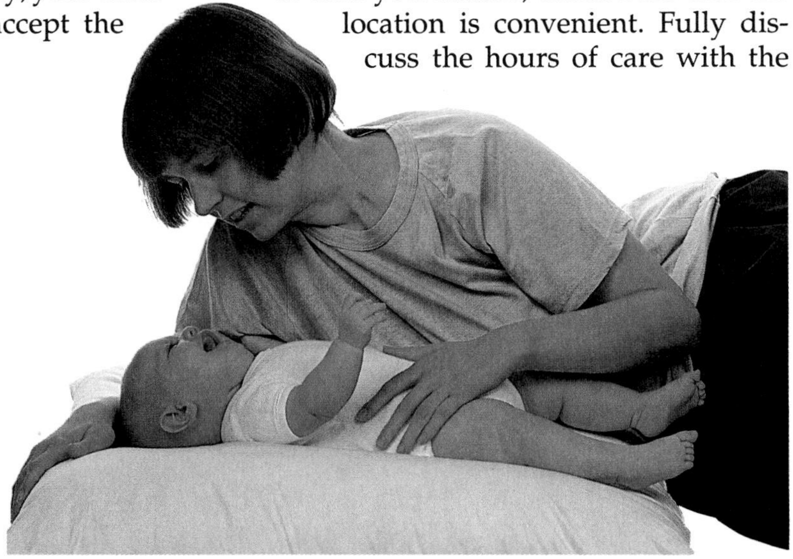

Your baby's needs
Infants need a care giver who is always close at hand. To make your child feel secure, care should always be provided by the same person or by a few consistent care givers responsible for only a few babies. Close human contact helps your baby develop socially and emotionally. Care givers should spend as much time as possible playing with and talking to infants.

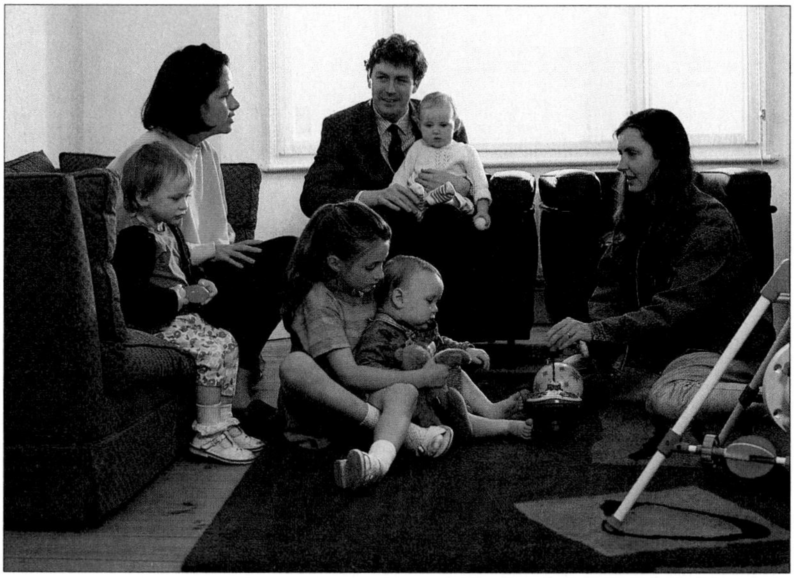

Visiting the care giver's home
Family day care can provide a homelike atmosphere. But, before choosing a family day care provider, visit his or her home to evaluate its suitability. Is the house clean and safe? Do the care giver's children seem happy and healthy?

care giver, including how to cover the times when you are delayed in the evening. Tell the care giver how you can be reached in an emergency.

In-home care

In-home care can be very comfortable because the care giver comes to your home and your child does not have to adapt to a new setting. Your child will probably receive more attention at home than in a day care setting and will be less frequently exposed to communicable diseases from other children. But in-home care can be expensive, and other arrangements have to be made when the care giver becomes ill or goes on vacation. Also, no government laws regulate home care, so you must be the sole judge of the care giver's character and attitude. Interview the prospective care giver to find out how he or she approaches such issues as discipline. Ask yourself if the care giver seems patient and attentive. Be sure to check the care giver's references.

Family day care

Many parents choose family day care because it provides care for the child in a home environment where there are other children with whom to play. But make sure that the care giver does not have responsibility for more than six children. When they are ill or on vacation, family day care providers should have a back-up care giver available to take care of your child. Family day care is not always licensed by the state, and states set varying standards for licensed care givers. So you must base your choice of care giver on your best judgment.

Day care centers

Many day care centers are profit-making businesses. Others are run by parent co-operatives or social service agencies. Make sure that the one you choose is licensed. Licensure ensures that the center meets the state's standards for safety, cleanliness, staffing, and program content. Day care centers provide stimulating activities and give your child the chance to interact with different people.

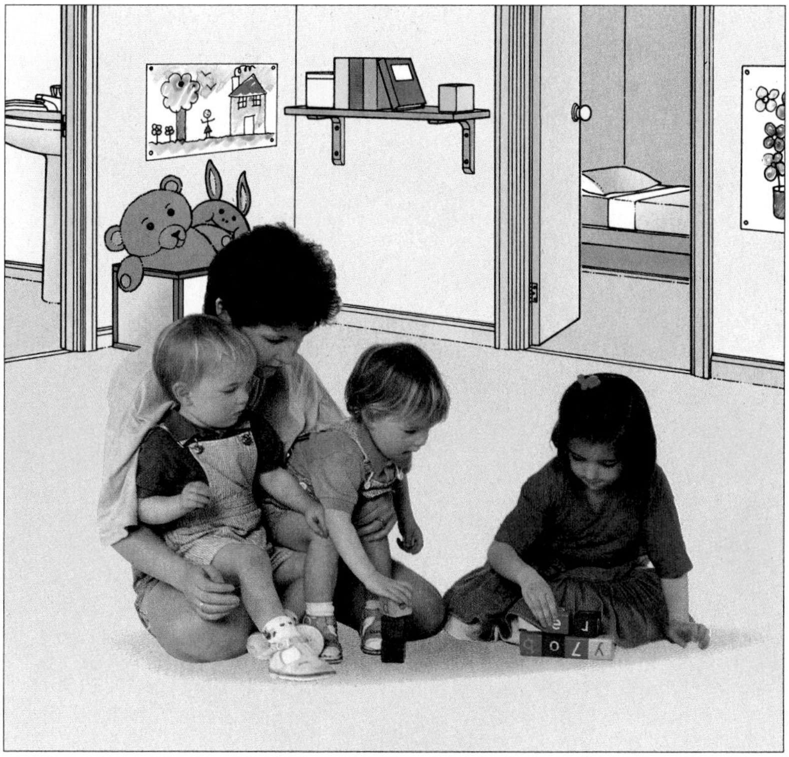

Choosing day care
When choosing a day care center, make sure that the care givers have basic training and experience in child care and development. A well-run center should appear clean and have safety equipment, such as gates and electrical outlet covers, in place. Separate areas should be available for eating, diapering, and napping.

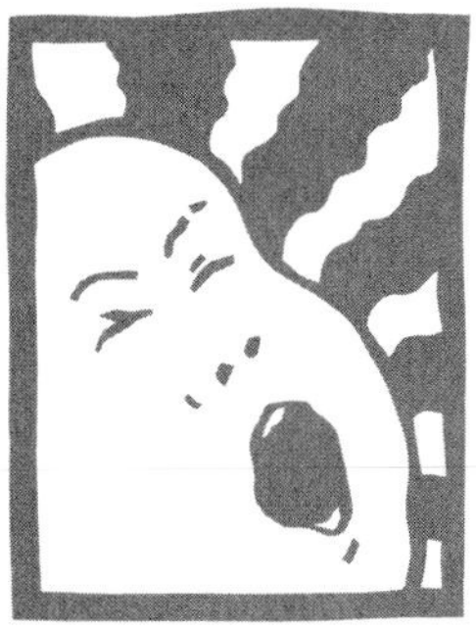

COMMON PROBLEMS IN BABIES

THE FIRST TIME your baby gets sick, you may feel overwhelmed by anxiety. How serious is the illness? Should you call the doctor? What if the symptoms get worse? As you become familiar with your baby's reactions to the rashes, fevers, and stuffy noses that he or she will inevitably get, you'll be able to tell the difference between a minor problem and a possible emergency.

Babies receive protective antibodies from their mother's blood before birth (by way of the placenta) and from their mother's milk after birth. These antibodies temporarily protect babies against many common disease-causing organisms. In spite of this natural protection, most babies often have rashes and minor infections during the first year of life.

SKIN DISORDERS

A baby's soft and sensitive skin is easily irritated. Harmless rashes may often appear and disappear on your baby's skin after the slightest irritation.

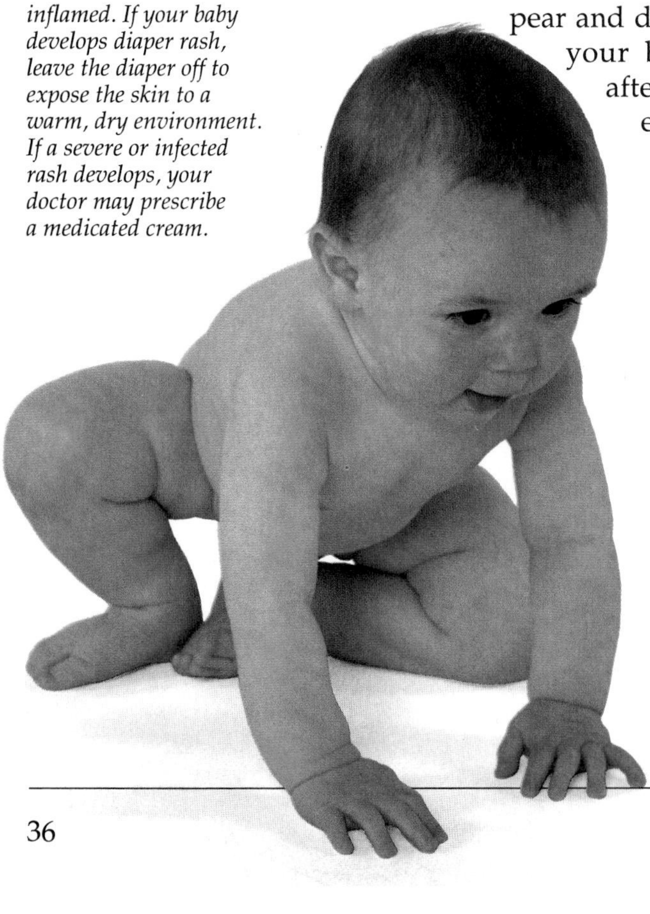

Diaper rash
Wet or abrasive diapers can cause the skin on your baby's buttocks, inner thighs, and genital area to become red and inflamed. If your baby develops diaper rash, leave the diaper off to expose the skin to a warm, dry environment. If a severe or infected rash develops, your doctor may prescribe a medicated cream.

Diaper rash

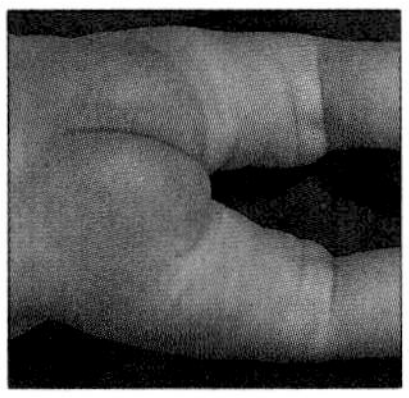

Rashes caused by wet or abrasive diapers are common in babies. Diaper rash can vary in severity from simple redness to severe ulceration caused by infection of the skin. To prevent diaper rash, or to alleviate an existing rash, change your baby's diaper frequently – experience will tell you how often to do so. Wash the diaper area with mild soap or disposable wipes and carefully dry it each time you change your baby's diaper. If a rash has started, use a diaper rash cream containing zinc oxide before putting on the clean diaper. With cloth diapers, use a liner to help keep your infant dry. Do not use plastic pants, because they create a warm, damp environment inside the diaper that promotes the development of a rash. Avoid scented fabric softeners, harsh detergents, and strong bleaches when laundering your baby's diapers and clothes, because they can further irritate the skin.

Yeast infection

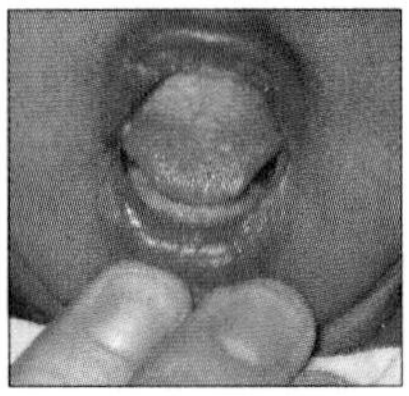

If a baby's immunity is lowered by infection, medication, or malnutrition, the yeast organisms that normally inhabit the baby's mouth can grow excessively, spread through the digestive tract, and cause persistent, sometimes severe diarrhea. The yeast infection can also produce white patches inside the baby's mouth (thrush) or a red, pimplelike rash around the anus, genitals, and inner thighs.

Yeast infections are rarely serious and usually clear up on their own. Your doctor can prescribe a medicine to speed up this process. If you are breast-feeding, your doctor may check to see whether the infection has spread to you.

Hives

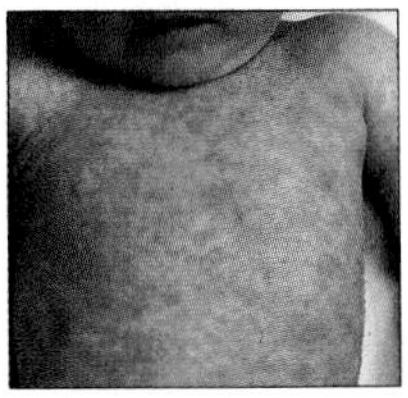

Hives (neonatal urticaria) is an uncommon rash that can appear in the first month of life. It is characterized by red blotches with pale centers. The rash can appear on any part of the baby's body and can be itchy. Hives is usually caused by an allergic reaction triggered by a particular food or medicine. Hives requires no specific treatment and usually clears up on its own a few hours after a bath and a change of clothing. Try to avoid the factors that trigger the rash. Dress your baby comfortably in natural fibers, such as cotton, and wash his or her clothes and diapers in mild detergents to prevent hives.

Cradle cap

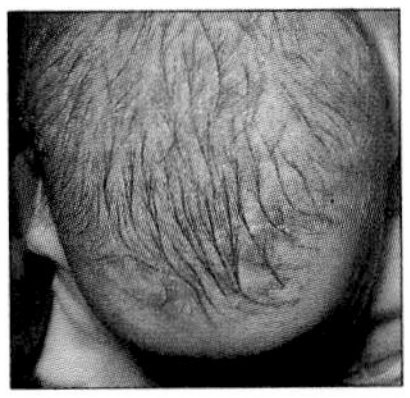

Cradle cap is a harmless, dry scalp condition that occurs in babies aged 3 to 9 months. The yellow-gray crusts of cradle cap form when the normal secretions of glands in the skin build up on the baby's scalp. You can allow cradle cap to come off on its own or rub baby oil into your baby's scalp and leave it on overnight. The oil moistens and loosens the crusts, which you can wash off the next day. Repeat this process for a few days until all the scales are removed. Moisturizing shampoos also help remove cradle cap. If the condition does not improve in 5 days and it concerns you, if it spreads to other parts of the baby's body, or if it becomes inflamed, call your doctor.

Milk spots (milia)

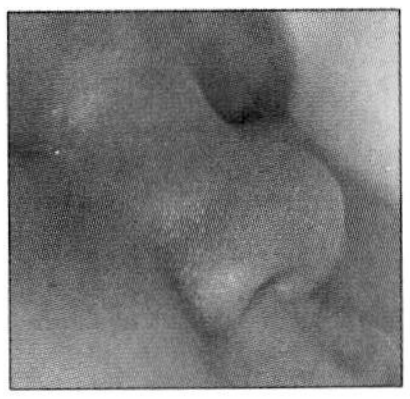

Minute, yellowish white spots, called milk spots, often appear on and around a baby's nose. Milk spots develop when sweat glands in the skin become clogged. They disappear within a few weeks.

SUCKING BLISTERS

Sucking on a bottle or your nipple can cause blisters to appear on your baby's lips. The blisters can be large and may alarm you, but they do not hurt your baby. Call your doctor if the blisters hinder feeding or spread elsewhere on the face or body.

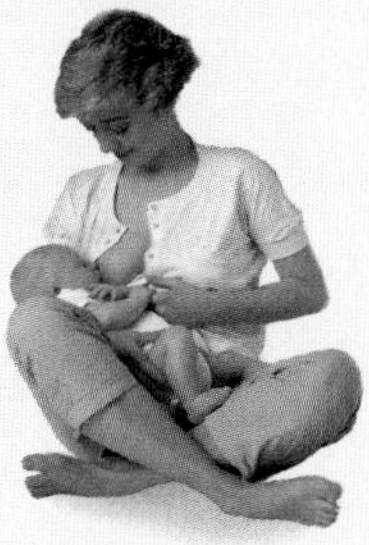

EYE INFECTIONS

During delivery, fluid and blood can enter your baby's eyes, causing an eye inflammation called conjunctivitis. This inflammation often causes the eyelashes of a newborn baby to stick together during sleep. Eyedrops given at birth can also cause a chemical inflammation that clears up in the first few days of life. But if your baby's eyes become sticky and bloodshot, he or she probably has a bacterial or viral eye infection. Your doctor can prescribe eyedrops and ointment to cure conjunctivitis caused by bacteria. No treatment exists for viral conjunctivitis, which must clear up on its own.

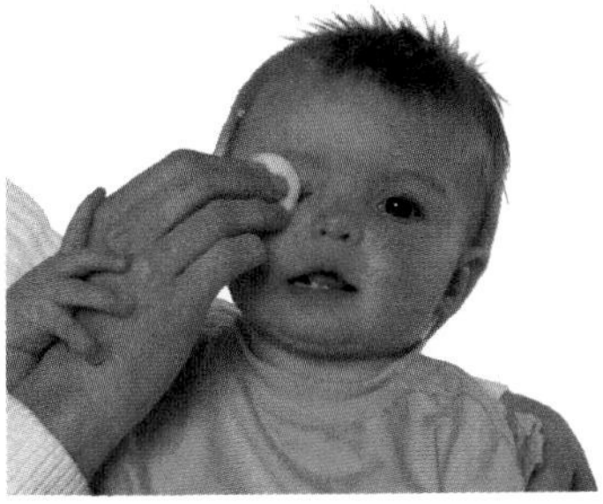

Cleaning a sticky eye
When the membrane lining the eyeball becomes inflamed, mucus can cause the baby's eyelids to stick together. Clean the eye at least four times a day with cottonballs soaked in cooled boiled water. Wipe downward away from the nose. Use a different cottonball for each eye.

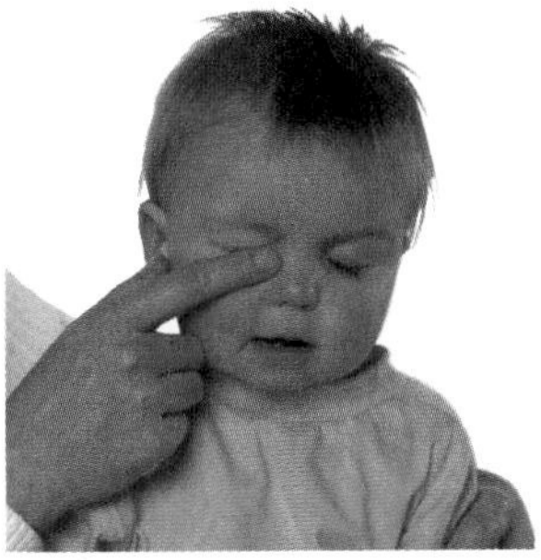

Unblocking a tear duct
Blocked tear ducts can also cause mild conjunctivitis. Massage the baby's lower eyelid five to 10 times in a circular motion to help open clogged ducts. Massage the eyelids frequently, until the eye discharge stops. Always wash your hands before touching your baby's face.

CASE HISTORY
A WORRISOME RASH

COURTNEY WAS BORN FULL-TERM and has always been healthy. She recently developed a red, raised rash on her scalp, face, and arms. The rash did not improve after her mother applied zinc oxide cream, and then a similar rash appeared on Courtney's diaper area. The rash got worse, so Courtney's mother took her to see the doctor.

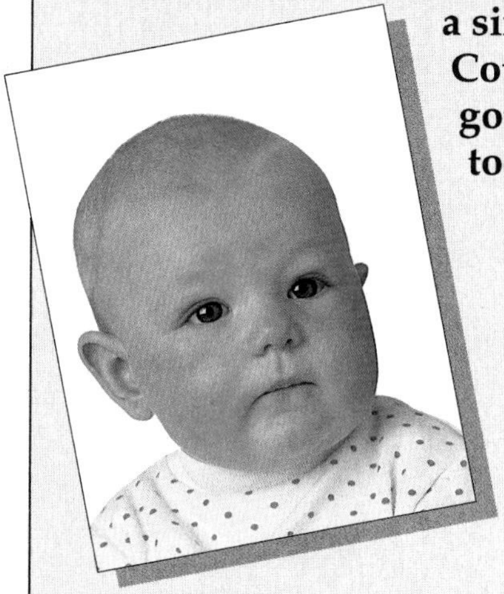

PERSONAL DETAILS
Name Courtney Hurst
Age 6 months
Family Both of Courtney's parents are in good health. Courtney has a 4-year-old brother who has asthma.

MEDICAL BACKGROUND
Until the rash appeared, Courtney was a happy, healthy baby.

THE CONSULTATION
The doctor examines Courtney's rash, which is now quite severe. The rash appears red and inflamed on Courtney's arms. On her diaper area, the rash is yellow, crusty, and oozing slightly. Some areas of Courtney's rash also appear dry and scaly.

The doctor asks Courtney's mother if anyone in the family has allergies. He also asks whether the rash got worse when Courtney's mother changed the baby's formula. Courtney's mother explains that the rash does not seem to be affected by her daughter's diet and that the only person in the family with an allergy is Courtney's brother, who has asthma. She tells the doctor that the rash seems to be very itchy because Courtney has become increasingly irritable. The discomfort is also keeping Courtney awake at night.

THE DIAGNOSIS
The doctor tells Courtney's mother that her daughter has an allergic rash called ATOPIC ECZEMA. The doctor says this type of rash is common in infants and often runs in families with other allergies. Although eczema subsides in about 50 percent of infants by the time they are 2 years old, the doctor says that a milder form of the rash sometimes persists.

Reducing irritation
Courtney's mother checks the labels of her daughter's clothes to make sure that they are made of cotton. Cotton irritates atopic eczema (shown below) less than wool and synthetic fibers. The intense itchiness of eczema often causes the baby to scratch. The damaged skin can bleed or become infected.

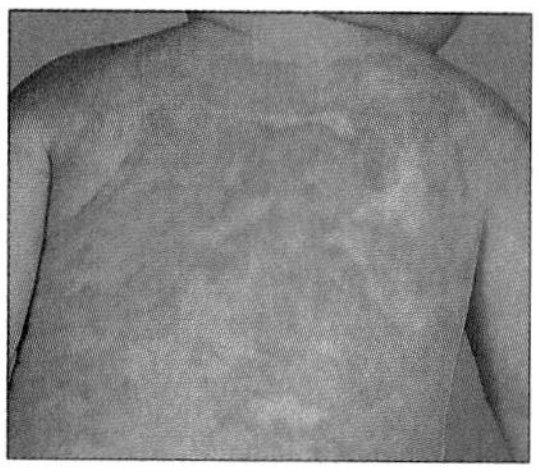

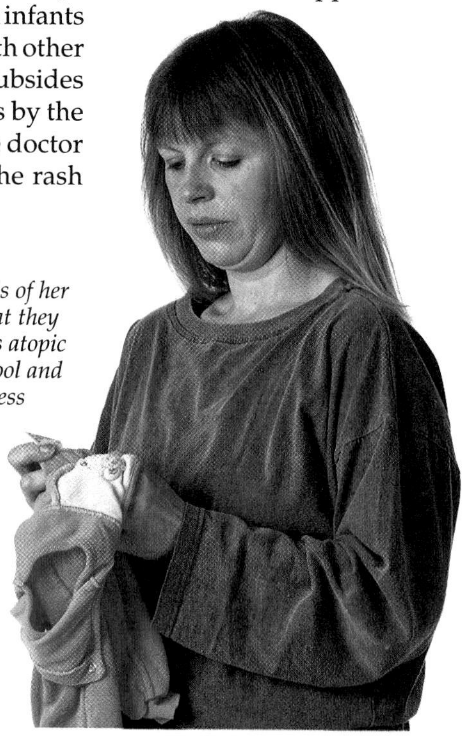

THE TREATMENT
The doctor explains to Courtney's mother that many factors can trigger the reaction that causes eczema, including some foods, soaps, detergents, and perfumes. The doctor suggests that Courtney's mother wash her clothes and bedclothes in a mild detergent. He tells her to use unscented baby soap and shampoo and to dress Courtney in cotton garments whenever possible. Fabrics such as wool and synthetic materials irritate sensitive skin and should be avoided. The doctor prescribes a mild, unscented moisture cream to use after washing Courtney. The doctor also prescribes a mild corticosteroid cream and tells Courtney's mother to apply it to the rash.

THE OUTCOME
Courtney's mother carefully follows the doctor's instructions, and the condition gradually improves. By the time she is 2 years old, Courtney's eczema has disappeared.

VOMITING

All babies spit up a small amount of milk when feeding. This process is called gastric reflux and it is often mistaken for vomiting. Gastric reflux is not a symptom of an illness and requires no treatment. Babies rarely vomit, but when it happens they forcefully bring up most of the last feeding. Repeated vomiting may mean that your baby has an inflammation of the lining of the stomach and intestines caused by infection. Gastrointestinal obstruction that is present at birth can also cause persistent vomiting. The excessive loss of fluid and minerals caused by vomiting can rapidly lead to dehydration, which requires immediate medical attention in an infant.

DIARRHEA

Infants usually pass loose yellow or tan stools a few times a day. But if your baby passes very watery stools more than six times a day, then he or she has diarrhea, which is a serious condition because it can dehydrate a small infant very quickly. Dehydration can be life-threatening. Stop formula feeding and give your baby rehydration solution (available from drugstores) to drink. You may continue frequent breast-feeding during episodes of diarrhea. Call your doctor if diarrhea persists for more than 6 hours.

CONGESTED NOSE

Some babies often seem to have a congested nose. These babies have sensitive mucous membranes in the nose that react to changes in temperature and humidity. During feeding, a baby with a stuffy nose may have to periodically release the nipple to breathe in through the mouth. Your doctor can prescribe drops to help loosen nasal secretions and may tell you to use a bulb syringe to remove the mucus. Doctors do not prescribe decongestants for young infants.

SIGNS OF A SERIOUS EMERGENCY IN THE FIRST YEAR

Babies can get sick very quickly. During the first year of life, certain symptoms, listed below, signal a need for prompt medical attention. If your baby has any symptom that seriously concerns you, call your doctor. It is always best to err on the side of caution.

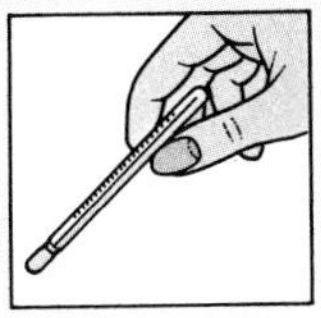

A high fever
Call your doctor if your baby has a temperature over 101.5°F. To reduce the temperature, remove the outer layer of clothes and sponge the baby down with lukewarm water. Give your baby acetaminophen – never aspirin – to reduce the fever.

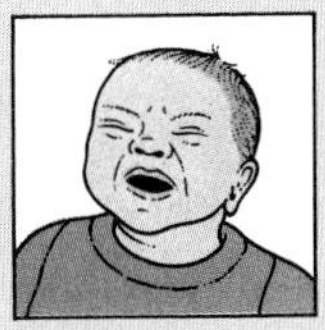

Uncontrollable crying
Uncontrollable screaming or crying that persists for an hour may indicate that your baby is in pain. The pain could be caused by colic or could indicate something more serious. Call your doctor if your baby cries violently for more than an hour.

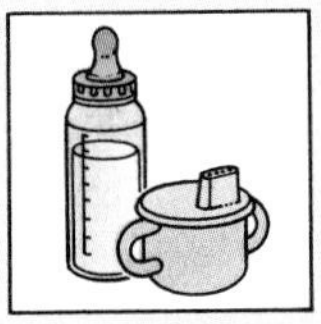

Persistent vomiting or diarrhea
Vomiting or diarrhea that continues for up to 6 hours can cause rapid dehydration. Call your doctor and stop bottle-feeding your baby. For diarrhea, replace feedings with small, frequent drinks of rehydration solutions (see page 88).

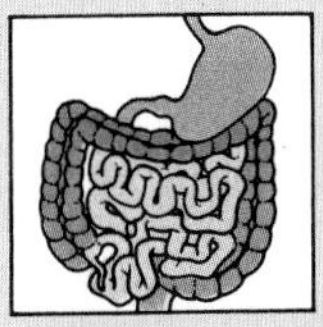

Forceful vomiting or blood in stools
Green vomit, forceful vomiting, or stools that contain blood and mucus and that resemble red currant jam may indicate an intestinal obstruction. Call your doctor, and do not feed your baby. Give the doctor a sample of the stool or vomit.

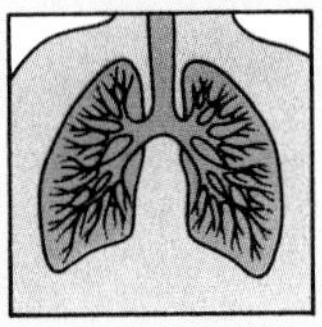

Rapid breathing
Noisy and rapid breathing may signal a chest infection. Call your doctor, calm your baby as much as possible, and hold him or her in a position that makes breathing easier. If your baby has a fever, try to keep him or her cool.

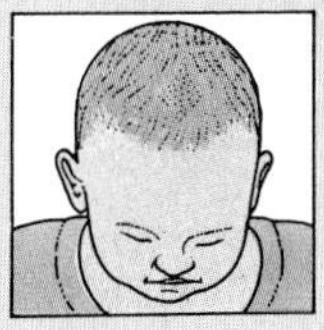

Bulging or sunken soft spot
A baby's soft spot (fontanelle) usually bulges when he or she is crying. A soft spot that bulges when the baby is not crying can indicate a buildup of fluid inside the skull. A sunken soft spot could indicate that your baby is severely dehydrated.

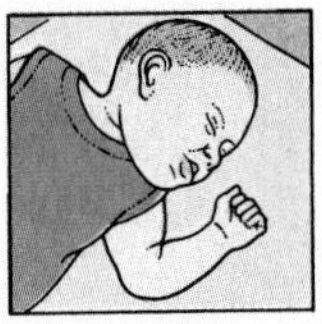

Unusual drowsiness
A baby who does not wake up for his or her usual feeding and is reluctant to suck may have an infection. Infections can rapidly become serious in babies. Call your doctor if your baby seems unusually drowsy or is difficult to arouse.

WHY IS YOUR BABY CRYING?

Many babies cry a lot during their first year. Crying is a baby's only way of communicating discomfort or a need for attention. It can be difficult to pinpoint the exact cause of a newborn baby's crying, but by the time the baby is about 3 months old, parents usually have become much better able to interpret their baby's cries. When you cannot tell what is making your baby cry, check the most likely causes, such as hunger, a dirty diaper, or a need for sleep. Then see whether the crying persists.

Too hot or too cold
Babies cannot control their own body temperature and may quickly become too hot or too cold. A baby is too hot if his or her neck feels warm and moist. Loosen or remove some of the baby's clothing or pull down the bed-clothes. If your baby's neck feels cold, take him or her into a warm room and offer a feeding. The temperature of a baby's room should not be lower than 68°F to 70°F.

Insecurity
Crying may simply signal that your baby is feeling insecure and needs to be picked up and hugged by a familiar adult.

Teething
Babies often cry and need more attention when their teeth are coming in. Some babies have a fever when teething. You may need to sponge down your baby to lower the temperature.

Hunger
Babies begin to cry when they get hungry. Feed your baby if a reasonable period has elapsed since the last feeding.

Wet diaper
Babies can become very uncomfortable when their diapers are wet or dirty, especially if they have diaper rash.

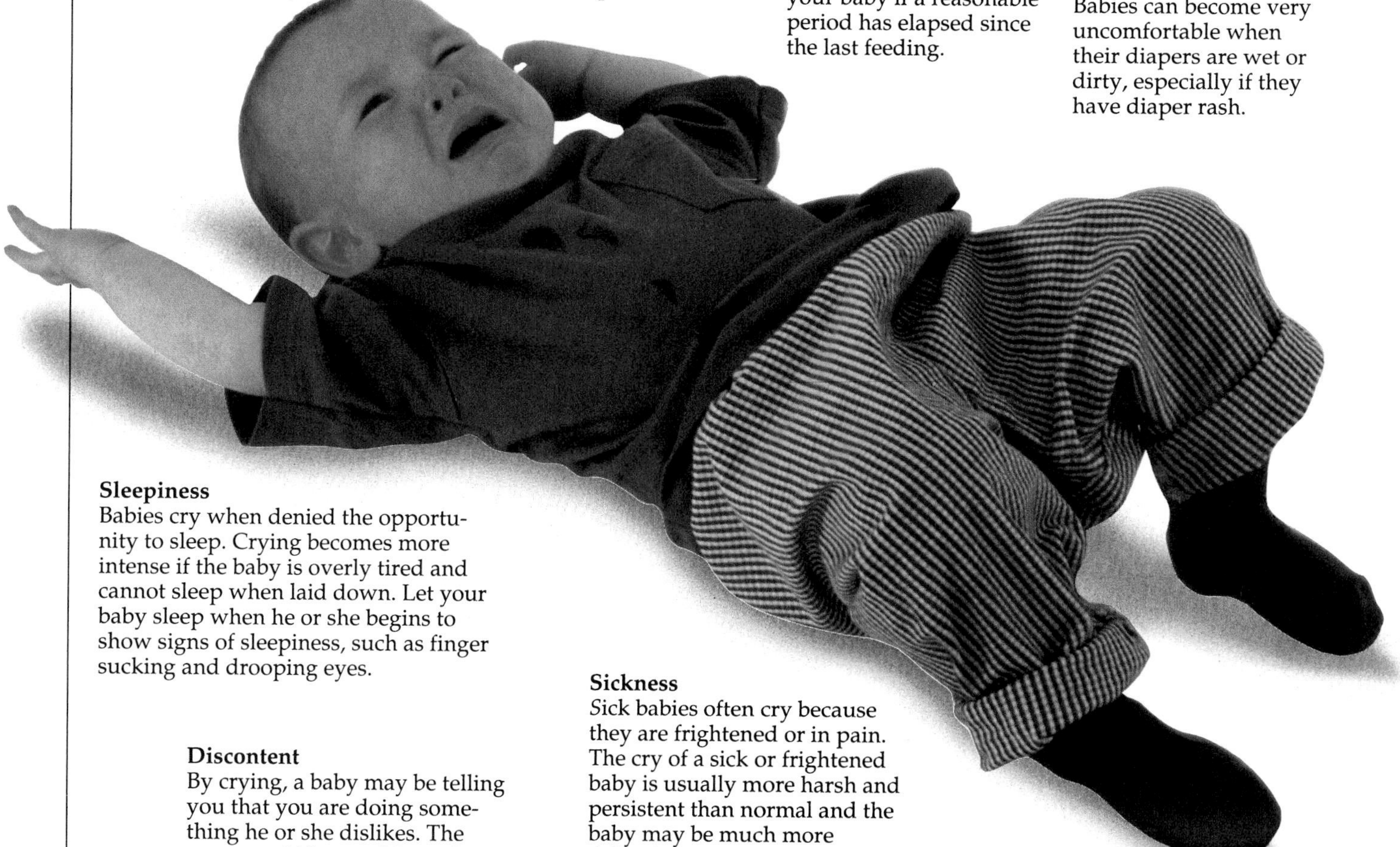

Sleepiness
Babies cry when denied the opportunity to sleep. Crying becomes more intense if the baby is overly tired and cannot sleep when laid down. Let your baby sleep when he or she begins to show signs of sleepiness, such as finger sucking and drooping eyes.

Sickness
Sick babies often cry because they are frightened or in pain. The cry of a sick or frightened baby is usually more harsh and persistent than normal and the baby may be much more difficult to calm. If you think your child is sick, call your doctor immediately.

Discontent
By crying, a baby may be telling you that you are doing something he or she dislikes. The cause could be anything – from diaper changing to lights that are too bright. In many cases, you must finish what you are doing despite the crying, but sometimes you can adapt your technique to avoid unnecessary discomfort for the baby.

Gas
Babies have small digestive tracts. Even a small amount of trapped air can cause pain. To help your baby expel the gas, hold him or her upright against your shoulder and pat or rub his or her back rhythmically until you hear the gas being expelled.

SOOTHING A CRYING BABY

Babies who have been fed and changed may still cry for no apparent reason. Infants who cannot sleep should never be left to cry indefinitely. A touch or a soothing remark may be enough to settle them.

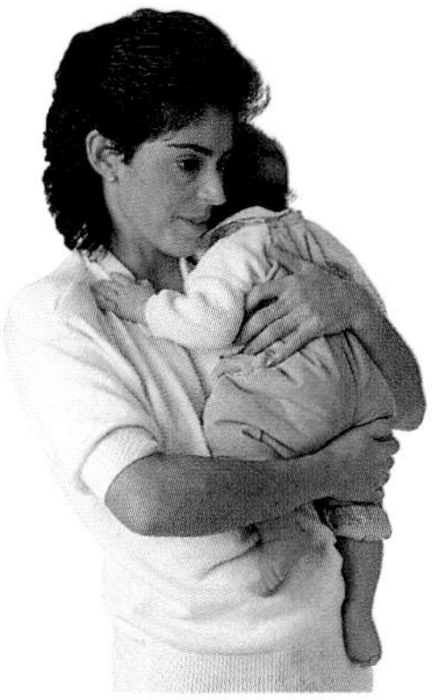

Cuddle your baby
Loving contact with a familiar adult very often has a calming effect that soothes a crying baby and allows him or her to drop off to sleep. Keep lighting subdued; bright lights will keep your baby awake.

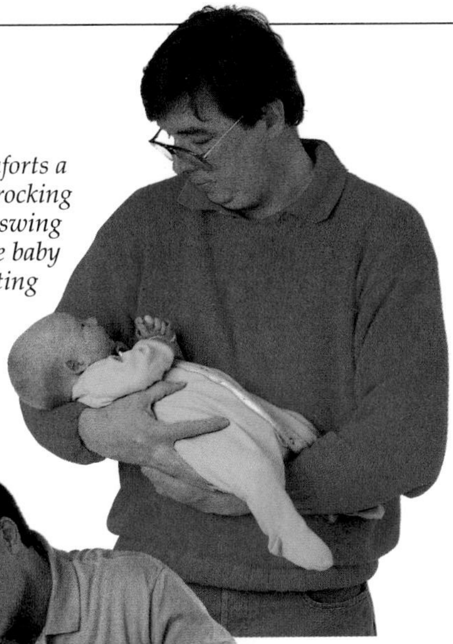

Rocking
Movement often comforts a crying baby. Gentle rocking in your arms or in a swing or simply moving the baby up and down by shifting from one foot to the other can have a soothing effect.

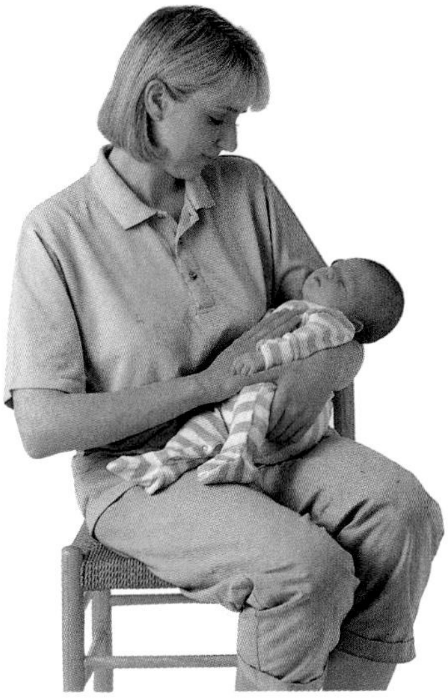

Rhythmic patting
Rhythmically patting or rubbing your baby's back or belly has a calming effect that may stop his or her crying or help the baby sleep. Patting can also help to expel any gas that may be making your baby uncomfortable.

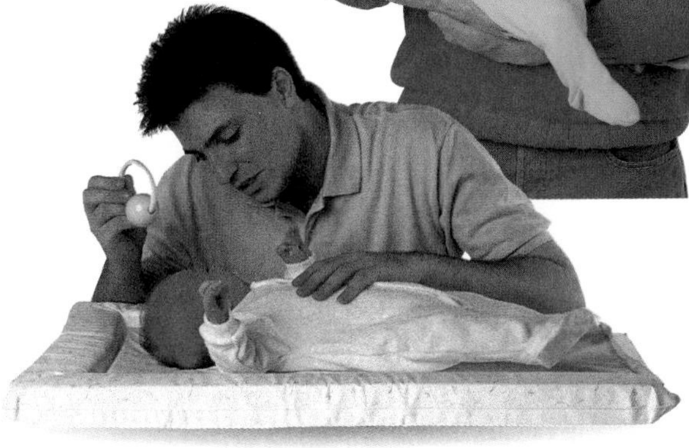

Distract your baby
Bright, colorful, but simple patterns, toys, or mirrors can help distract your baby and make him or her stop crying for a while. Try carrying your baby around your home while speaking consolingly to stop the crying.

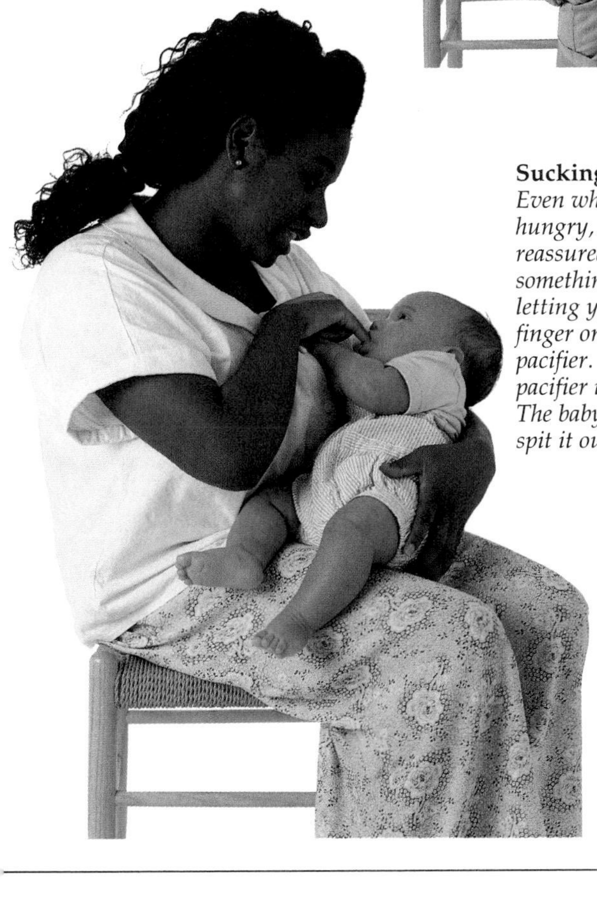

Sucking
Even when your baby is not hungry, he or she may feel reassured by simply having something to suck on. Try letting your baby suck your finger or give him or her a pacifier. Do not hold the pacifier in the infant's mouth. The baby should be able to spit it out of his or her mouth.

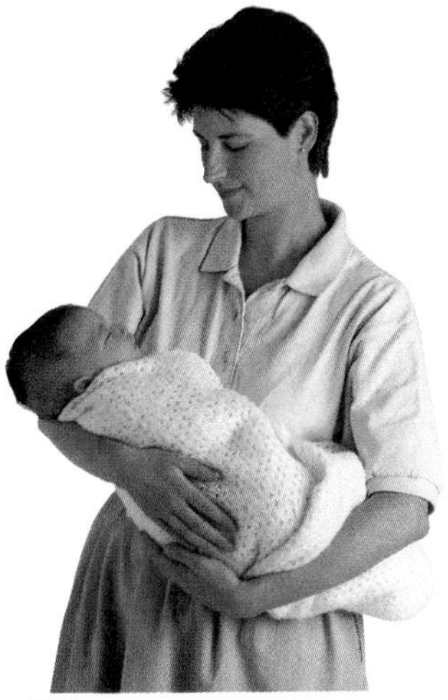

Swaddling
Wrapping and holding your baby in a shawl or blanket can be calming and may help reduce the crying. But do not swaddle your newborn while he or she is asleep in a crib because a newborn needs to be able to move. Swaddling can also cause overheating during sleep.

COPING WITH COLIC

Colic is a sporadic intestinal pain that commonly occurs in babies aged 3 weeks to 3 months. Some doctors think that the pain is caused by a spasm in the intestines, although this theory has not been proven. Colic causes periods of intense crying, usually in the evening. Rocking, patting, or walking with your infant may soothe him or her. Colic is not harmful, although the baby may be uncomfortable. Colic rarely lasts beyond the first 3 months of life. Doctors do not recommend any medication. Never give an infant any medicine that contains alcohol.

CHAPTER THREE

CHILDHOOD

Childhood, the years between infancy and adolescence, builds the physical, mental, and emotional foundation for adult life. Between birth and age 5, children acquire the basic skills that determine how well they will walk, talk, and solve problems. During these years, children begin to understand how they interact with their surroundings and learn to exert control over their environment. Young children begin to recognize themselves as separate individuals and then learn how to form relationships with other people.

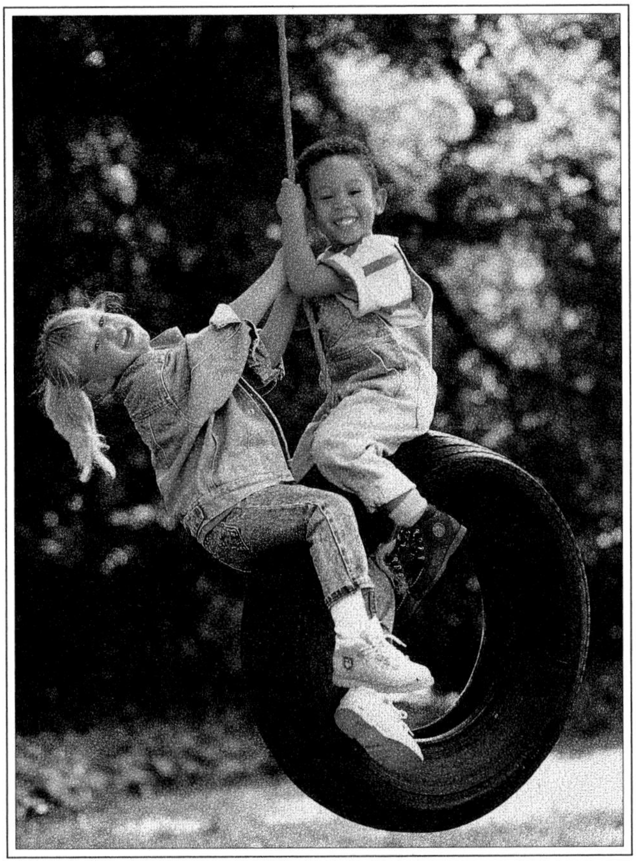

During the later stages of childhood, after mastering the basic developmental skills, children assimilate a vast amount of information. They develop intellectually at a much faster rate than adults. The focus of their personal relationships shifts increasingly from parents to peers. Older children begin to see themselves as members of a social group. This socialization process accelerates during adolescence.

Throughout childhood, growth and development are closely linked with physical health and emotional well-being. Children are greatly influenced by their home environment and their family relationships. A stable, caring home provides the emotional security a child needs to explore his or her potential. Parental consistency may be the most important factor in encouraging a child's healthy emotional development. Every child needs close relationships, initially with parents and later with a group of people – usually close family and other care givers – on whom the child can rely for his or her basic physical needs and for security, guidance, and understanding.

This chapter describes the predictable patterns of physical growth and the important developmental milestones that occur during childhood. It also shows how you can be more sensitive to your child's physical, mental, and emotional needs, so you can give your child what he or she requires at each stage of development. The chapter discusses developmental delay and explains how doctors test and treat children for it. The importance of diet and nutrition, exercise, and safety are also covered in this chapter, along with methods of discipline. Because every child occasionally contracts one of the common childhood illnesses, such as a cold or a sore throat, this chapter provides practical advice about the best way to care for your child when he or she is sick. This chapter also presents up-to-date information about current immunization recommendations and shows you what to expect when you take your child to your doctor's office for regular checkups.

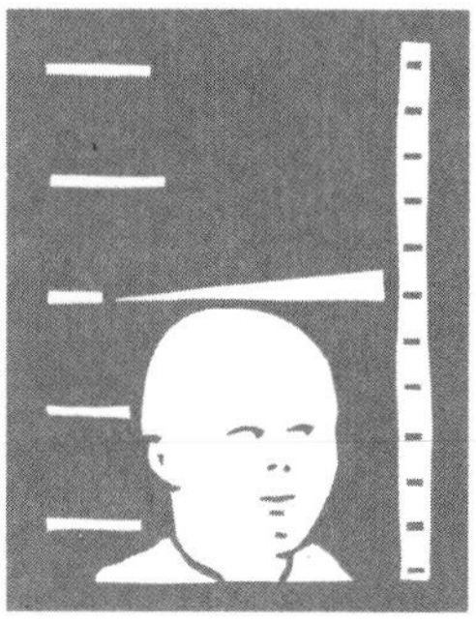

CHILD GROWTH AND DEVELOPMENT

GROWTH AND DEVELOPMENT follow similar recognizable patterns in all children, but individuals vary widely. Although most children develop a particular skill, such as walking, by a certain age, the precise age at which your child begins to walk could be earlier or later than the norm. By 1 year of age, a baby triples his or her birth weight and grows as much as 12 inches. Between ages 1 and 2, a child grows about 5 inches and gains 5 to 6 pounds.

After they reach 2 years of age, most children grow steadily at a rate of just over 2 inches a year. A child's weight increases at a rate of 5 to 10 pounds a year. But different parts of a child's body grow at different rates, so the child's body proportions change as he or she gets older (see below). After the first year, the child's body grows faster than his or her head and the child's limbs grow more rapidly than the trunk. This pattern reverses at puberty. When a boy or girl reaches puberty, his or her growth rate increases rapidly, often doubling the growth rate of early childhood. The brain grows quickly during early childhood, reaching about 75 to 80 percent of its adult size by age 2 and 90 percent of its adult weight by age 5. The brain's growth slows at about this time.

CHANGING BODY PROPORTIONS

Dividing a child's body into eight equal parts shows that the proportions of the body change radically in relation to the body's overall length. For example, a newborn's head represents nearly one fourth of his or her height. Throughout childhood, the head-to-body ratio changes until, at adolescence, the head comprises only about one eighth of total height. A newborn's legs comprise three eighths of total height, while an adolescent's account for one half.

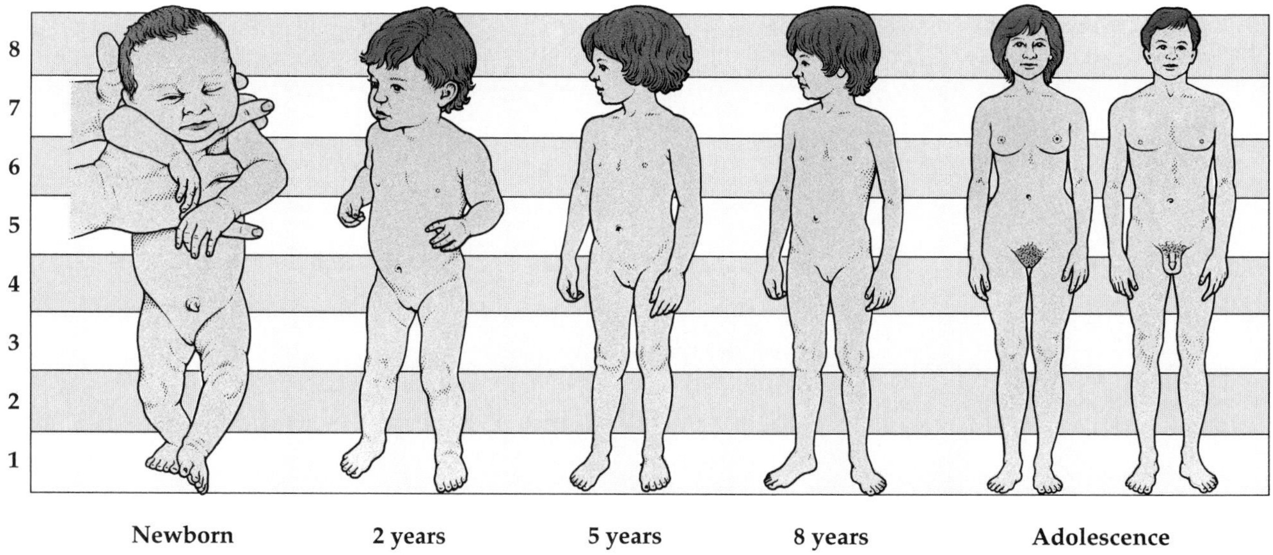

PHYSICAL GROWTH

Girls and boys grow at the same rate during childhood, although boys are generally slightly larger than girls. Boys usually become taller than girls as adults because they start puberty later and therefore have more time to grow in childhood before the final growth spurt occurs at puberty. This growth spurt happens between the ages of 13 and 16 in boys (with peak growth at age 14) and between the ages of 11 and 14 in girls (with peak growth at age 12). During the growth spurt, the child reaches most of his or her adult height. Final adult height is attained by 18 years of age (see right). The growth spurt is the body's response to an increased output of sex and growth hormones. Bone growth accelerates for a year or so – for example, a boy may grow 4 inches in 12 months – but the diminished output of growth hormone eventually stops bone growth at about 18 years of age, on average.

Predicting height

You can predict fairly accurately the final height that your child will reach by calculating the midpoint between the height measurements of you and your partner, then adding $2\frac{1}{2}$ inches for a boy and subtracting $2\frac{1}{2}$ inches for a girl. A child reaches about half of his or her adult height at the age of 2. But a child's final height depends not only on parental height but also on ethnic background, the socioeconomic status of the family, and age at the onset of puberty.

Height differences

Pediatricians become concerned about a child's height only if it is far below the normal lower limit or far above the normal upper limit for the child's age.

Short stature may be apparent at birth or may become evident later in childhood. Most short children are normal in every other way. They may become short

Growth charts

Doctors monitor a child's growth by regularly measuring height and weight. Doctors plot these measurements on growth charts to find out whether a child's height and weight are within the normal range for his or her age. Doctors also use growth charts to determine the child's growth rate (the amount grown over a given period of time).

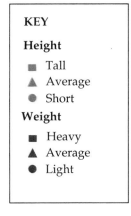

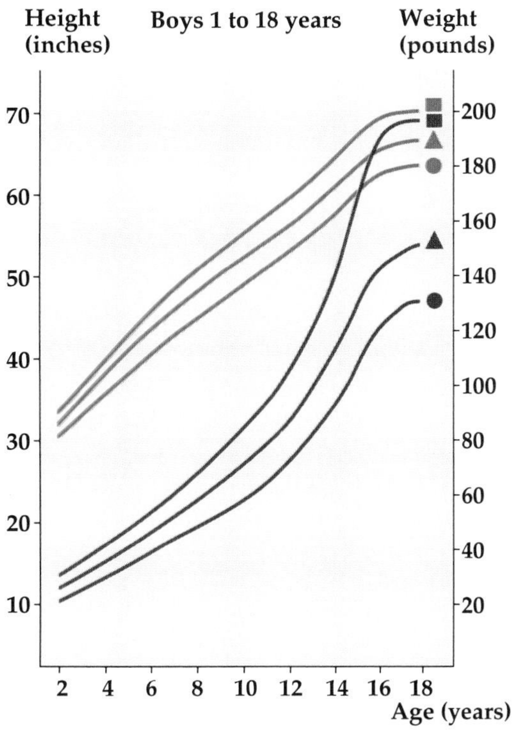

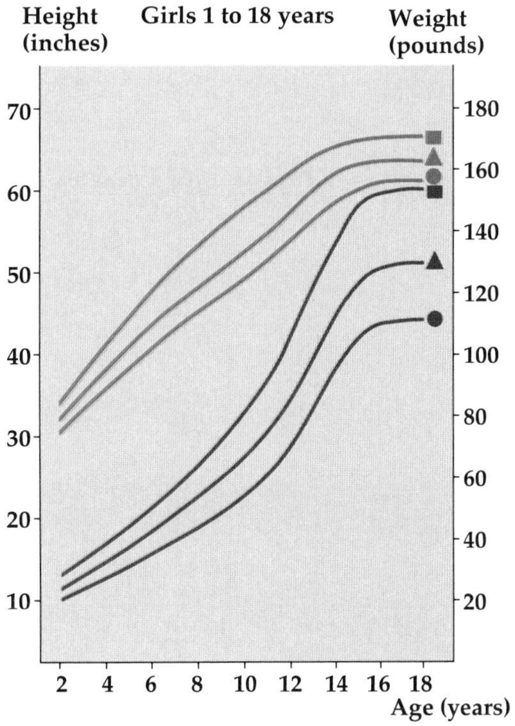

HORMONES AND GROWTH

A number of hormones regulate growth during childhood. For example, growth hormone, which is secreted by the pituitary gland, stimulates the production of protein in muscle cells and promotes the release of energy during the breakdown of fats. Thyroid hormone stimulates body metabolism. Both of these hormones are essential for normal childhood growth; a deficiency of either hormone can cause short stature. A complex interaction between growth hormone, thyroid hormone, and the sex hormones regulates the growth spurt at puberty.

KEY

Height

- ■ Tall
- ▲ Average
- ● Short

Weight

- ■ Heavy
- ▲ Average
- ● Light

and be very small at birth because their parents are short. Sometimes hereditary factors delay growth. In children who possess such factors, the pubertal growth spurt occurs later than usual, but the growth rate eventually speeds up so that the child attains a normal height when he or she reaches adulthood. Another cause of short stature is inadequate nutrition. Less commonly, short stature may signal an underlying disorder, such as growth hormone or thyroid hormone deficiency, cystic fibrosis (see page 96), or celiac sprue (see page 87).

Most tall children have tall parents. Very rarely, children become abnormally tall because of a medical disorder, such as Marfan's syndrome (a rare genetic disorder) or oversecretion of growth hormone that causes a condition known as gigantism, in which children can grow as tall as 7 feet. Some children who go through puberty very early (before age 8) are tall for their age as children but become fairly short adults. The abnormally early surge of hormones causes the growth centers in the bones to close early, producing short stature.

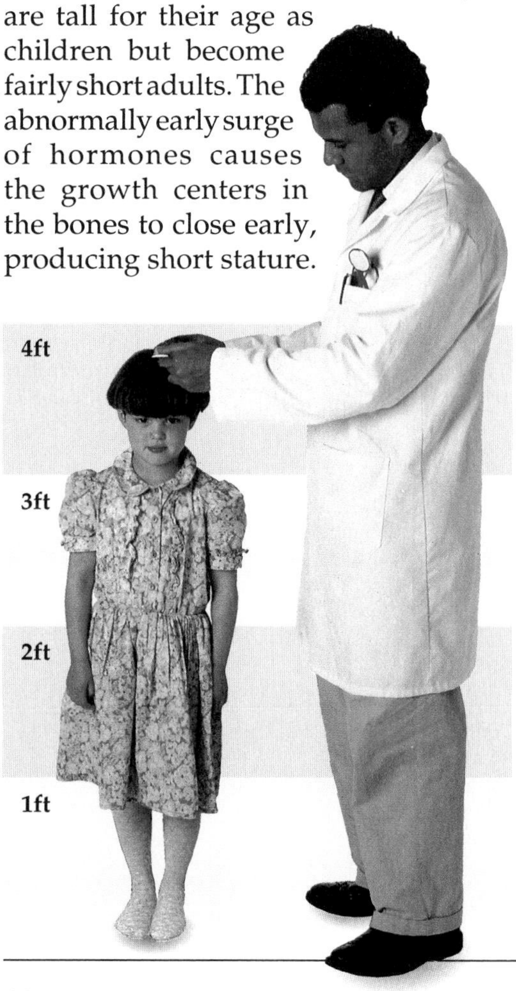

Your child's growth
Do not worry if your child looks shorter or taller than other children of the same age. Children grow at markedly different rates. Talk to your doctor if your child seems dissatisfied or emotionally upset by his or her height.

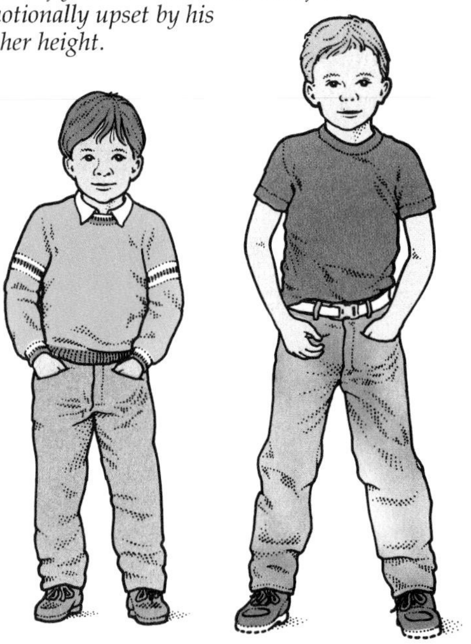

Investigating growth patterns

If a child appears to be much shorter or taller than average, the pediatrician will take a medical history and perform a complete physical examination to identify any medical problems that may be contributing to the condition. The pediatrician calculates the rate at which the child is growing and, if the rate is abnormally high or low, investigates further. Tests may include X-rays to examine the child's bones and blood tests to determine growth and thyroid hormone levels. Treatment depends on the findings. Because height is almost always determined by heredity, encourage your child to accept his or her stature as it is. Build self-confidence by reminding your child of his or her other good qualities.

Assessing growth rate
If you are seriously concerned about your child's growth, your doctor can perform a series of preliminary tests to find out whether your child is growing normally. During a period of 6 to 12 months, your doctor will regularly measure your child's height and weight to determine the rate at which he or she is growing. In most cases, doctors find that the growth rate is normal and no further action is needed.

HUMAN GROWTH HORMONE

Doctors use injections of human growth hormone to treat children who are exceptionally short because of a deficiency of growth hormone. Researchers are also investigating the use of growth hormone to treat diseases, such as kidney failure, that can cause short stature. Some doctors have aroused controversy by using growth hormone to treat children who are short but are not deficient in growth hormone and who are otherwise healthy. Injections of growth hormone do not seem to produce a consistent increase in the growth rate of these children, and doctors cannot accurately predict final height. The treatment requires daily injections of the hormone. Treatment with human growth hormone is very expensive and carries a small risk of accelerating coronary heart disease (hardening of the arteries) and the formation of tumors.

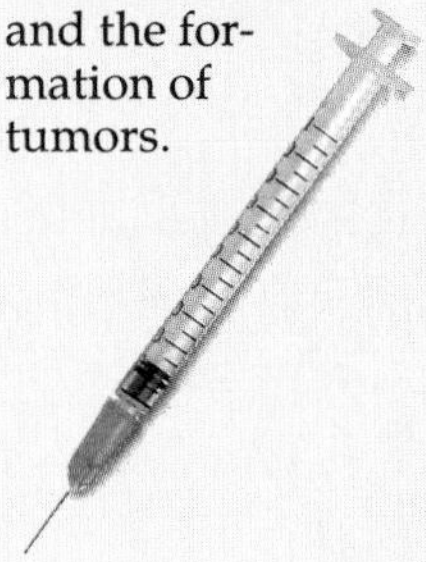

CHILDHOOD DEVELOPMENT

Child development refers to a child's physical, mental, and social progression. Children do not develop at an even rate. A child's progress may seem to stop for several weeks or months, only to leap forward as the child masters a new skill. It is possible to determine the average ages at which a child will acquire certain abilities. Doctors use these averages to assess how well a particular child is developing (see page 48).

Encouraging your child's development

Along with abundant love and security, your child needs intelligent and positive guidance from you. Giving your child too little of your attention can hinder his or her development. Conversely, some parents push their children to attain certain skills before the children are ready. Forcing children to learn beyond their capabilities or against their interests can cause insecurity, depression, and resentment. A child can develop new abilities only when his or her nervous system is mature enough to handle them. Children learn mainly by imitating others, so they need to have consistent role models.

Chances to learn

To develop fully, a child must have plenty of opportunities to practice and learn. For example, children need chances to feed and dress themselves and use the toilet without help if they are to become more independent. Children generally like to try out new skills. As they get older, they need the opportunity to find things out for themselves. But the desire to try out new activities will diminish if you scold your child for making mistakes and causing accidents.

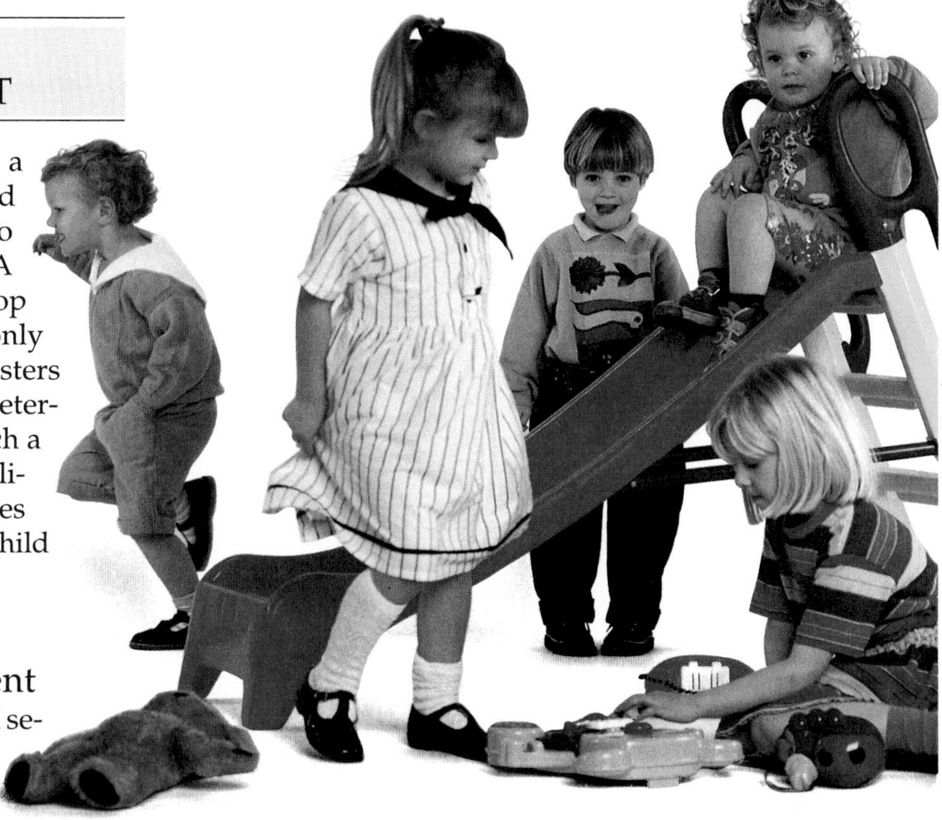

Interacting with other people
To encourage social development, make sure that your young child interacts with other people – not only within your family but also with other adults and children. Socializing provides vital opportunities to practice new physical and language skills.

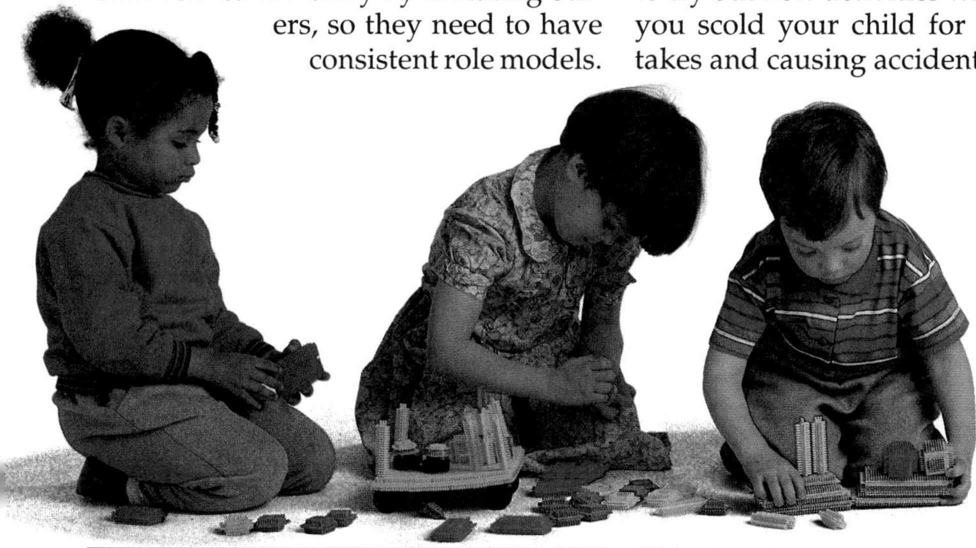

Stimulating activities
A stimulating environment encourages a child to investigate and learn. For example, children learn the meaning of words before they can say them. The more you talk to your child, the quicker he or she will learn to speak. Toys increase coordination and stimulate the ability to manipulate objects.

DEVELOPMENTAL MILESTONES IN CHILDHOOD

Child development specialists identify four main areas of development: movement and coordination, vision and manipulation, hearing and speech, and play and social skills. Children acquire these skills in predictable steps described as developmental milestones. The chart at right lists these milestones up to age 5 (see pages 50 and 51 for more information on language skills). By the age of 5, most children have gained enough skills to be fairly independent, but children develop at different rates. After age 5, specialists gauge development mainly by school performance. Writing, mathematical ability, and drawing skills improve, and comprehension and the ability to think in abstract terms increase. Older children develop their physical skills through athletics and games.

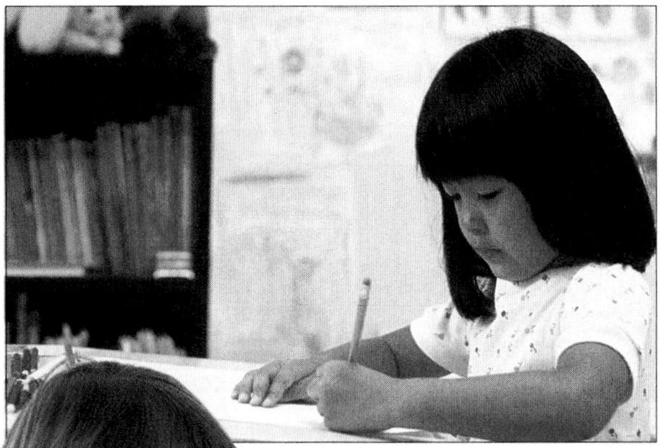

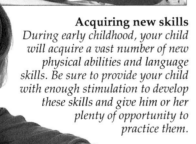

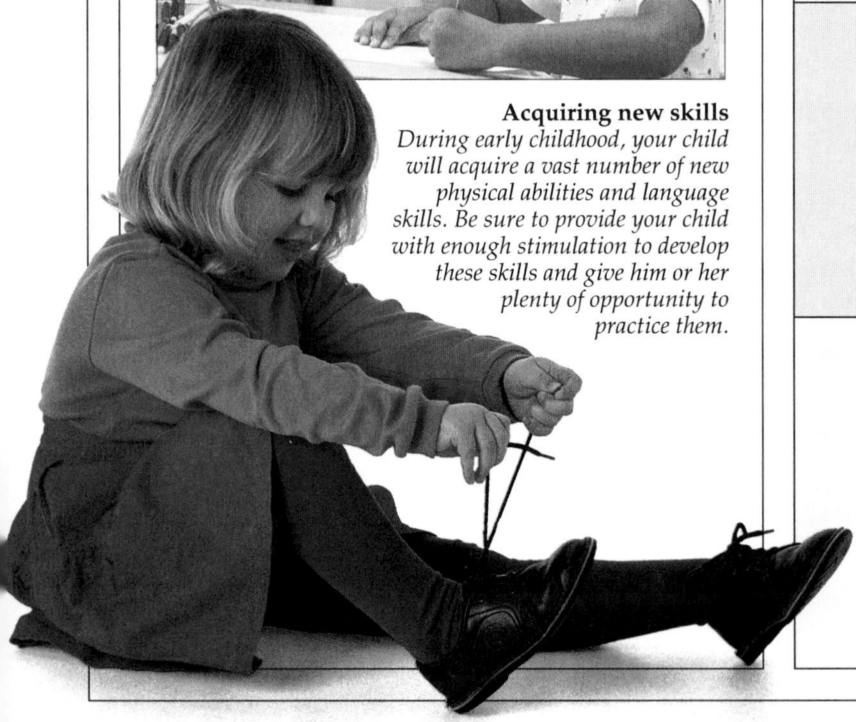

Acquiring new skills
During early childhood, your child will acquire a vast number of new physical abilities and language skills. Be sure to provide your child with enough stimulation to develop these skills and give him or her plenty of opportunity to practice them.

	MOVEMENT AND COORDINATION
18 MONTHS	Your child can walk up and down stairs holding onto your hand or a rail, can sit in a chair without help, and can throw a ball overhand. 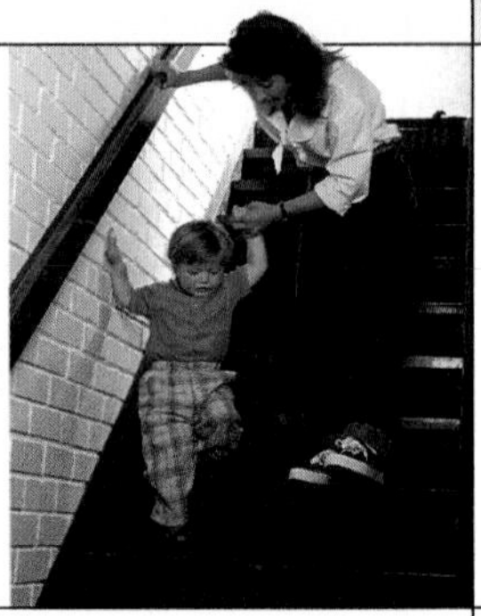
2 YEARS	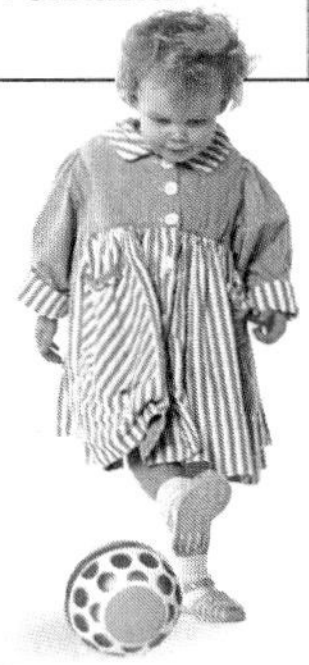 Your child runs well, kicks a ball without falling, and knows how to jump.
3 YEARS	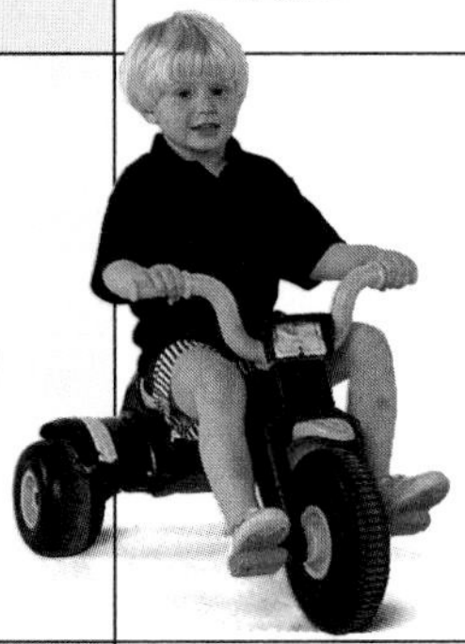 Your child can ride a tricycle, can walk up and down stairs without help one foot per step, and can balance on one foot for several seconds.
4 YEARS	Your child can balance on one foot for at least 10 seconds and can hop on one foot. He or she can run and turn without losing balance. 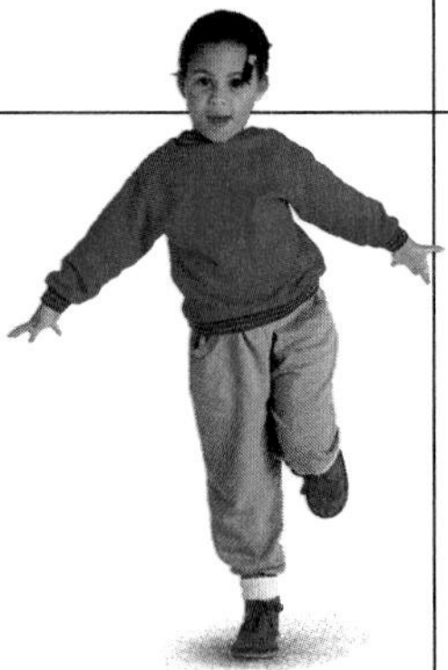
5 YEARS	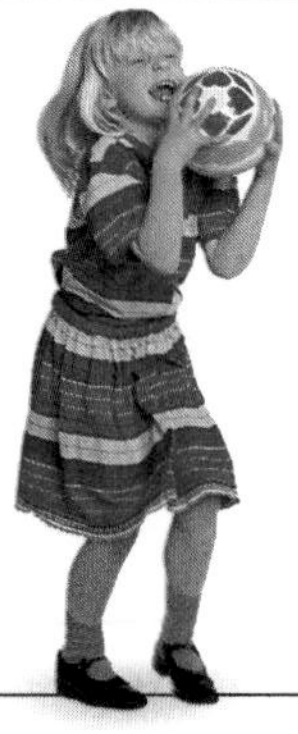 Your child can stand and hop on one foot, catch a ball, and skip with both feet. He or she can easily walk a narrow line and can move rhythmically to music.

VISION AND MANIPULATION	HEARING AND SPEECH	PLAY AND SOCIAL SKILLS
Your child can stack three or four blocks, scribble on paper, and turn two or three pages at a time. 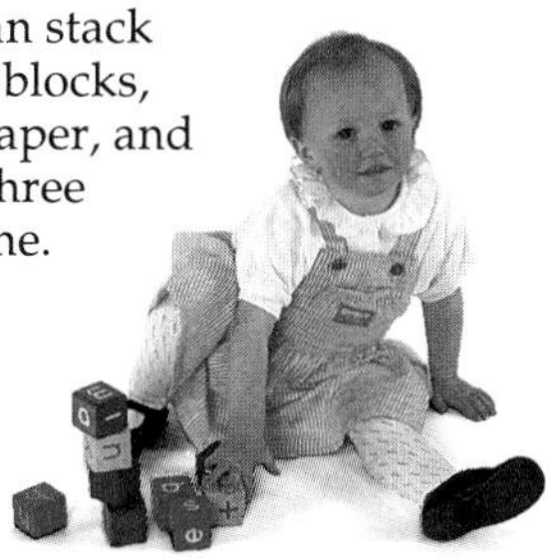	Your child obeys simple instructions, has a vocabulary of at least five words, and points to objects in pictures. 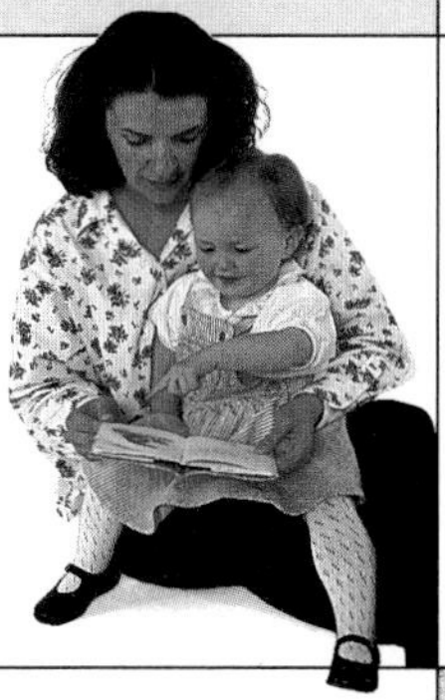	Your child plays alone with toys contentedly but likes to be near familiar adults. He or she can use a spoon, undress, and imitate actions, such as brushing hair. 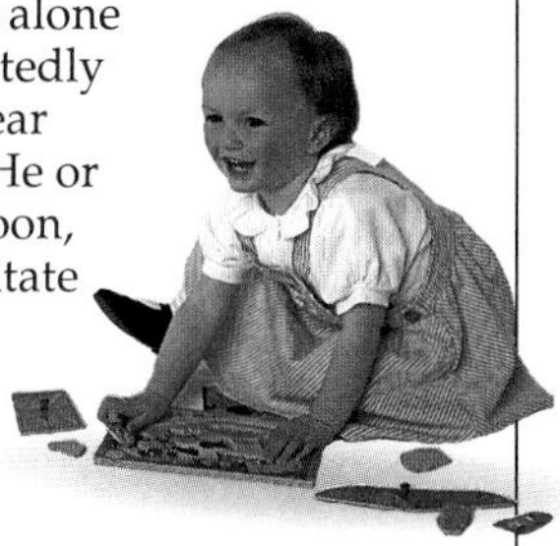
Your child can stack seven blocks, turn a doorknob, and unscrew a lid. He or she can turn pages singly and draw a vertical line. 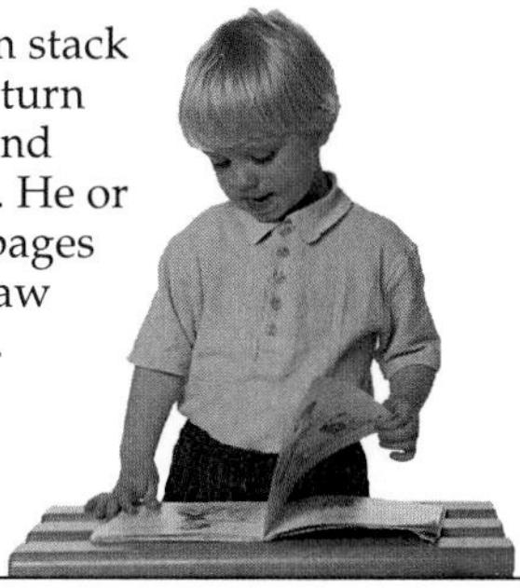	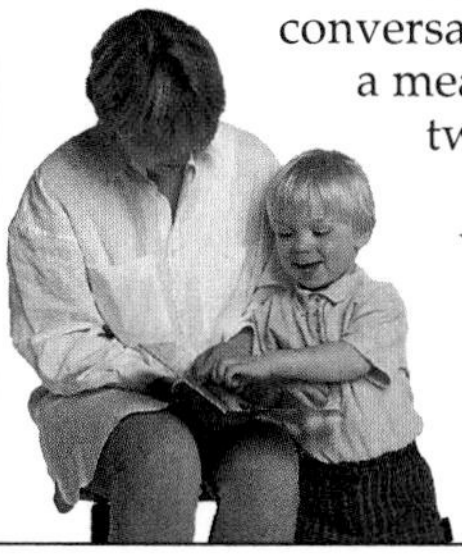 Your child listens to conversation and can form a meaningful phrase of two or more words. He or she repeats what other people say, uses plurals and pronouns, and can recite his or her full name.	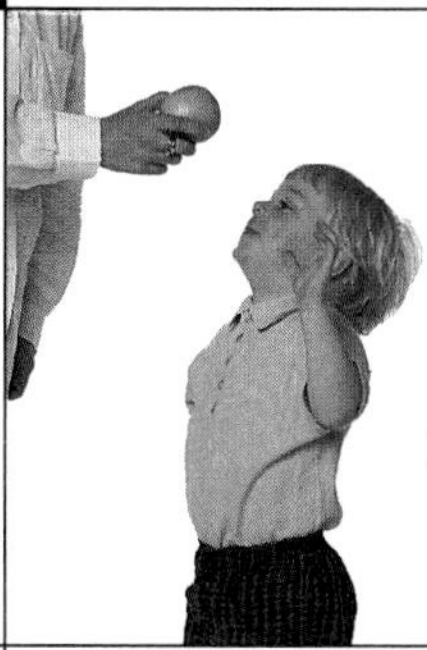 Your child asks for food and drink and can wash his or her hands without help. He or she recites nursery rhymes and sings but may not like sharing toys and may have occasional temper tantrums.
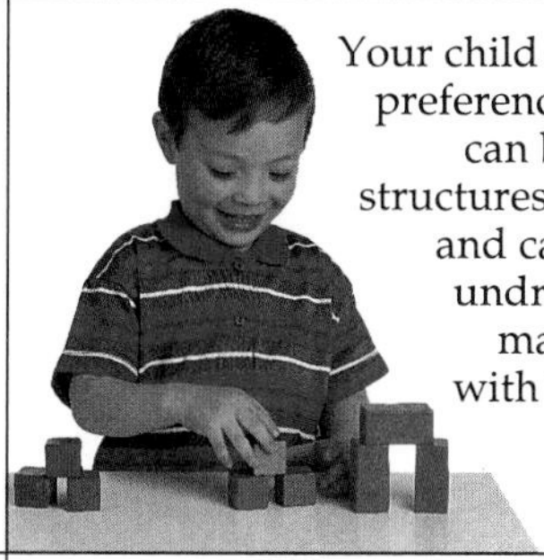 Your child shows hand preference. He or she can build simple structures with blocks and can dress and undress fully but may need help with buttons and shoelaces.	Your child knows the meaning of words such as cold and tired and can count to 10. He or she has a large vocabulary and speaks in sentences, with occasional mistakes. 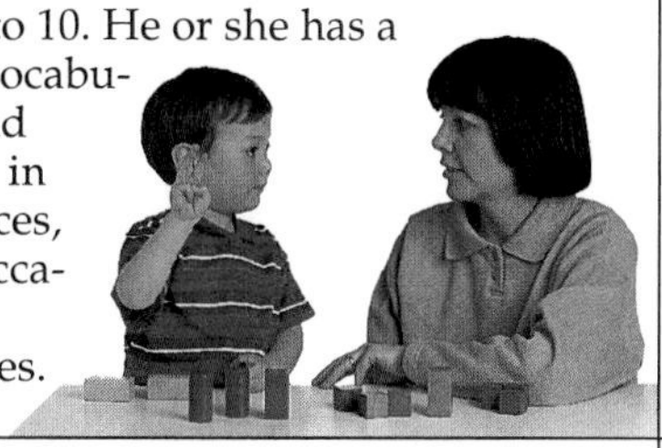	Your child plays imaginatively with other children and understands the ideas of sharing and taking turns. He or she can use the toilet without help. 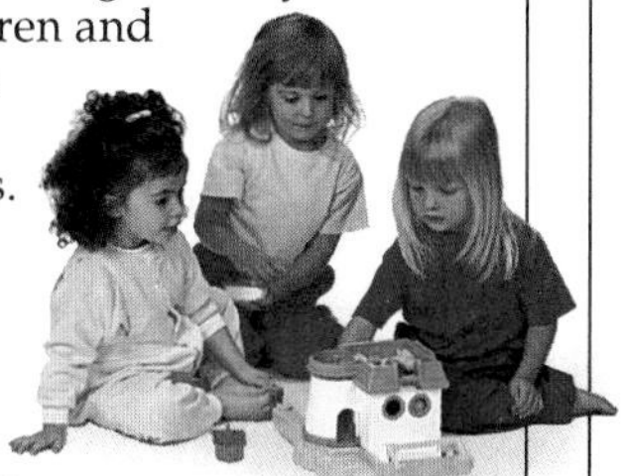
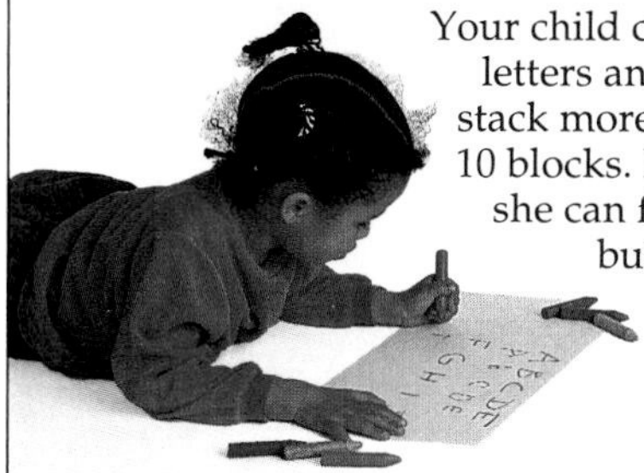 Your child copies letters and can stack more than 10 blocks. He or she can fasten buttons.	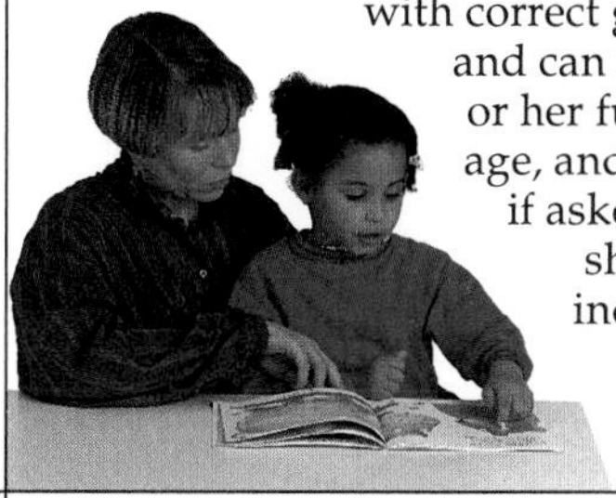 Your child speaks well with correct grammar and can recite his or her full name, age, and address if asked. He or she is very inquisitive.	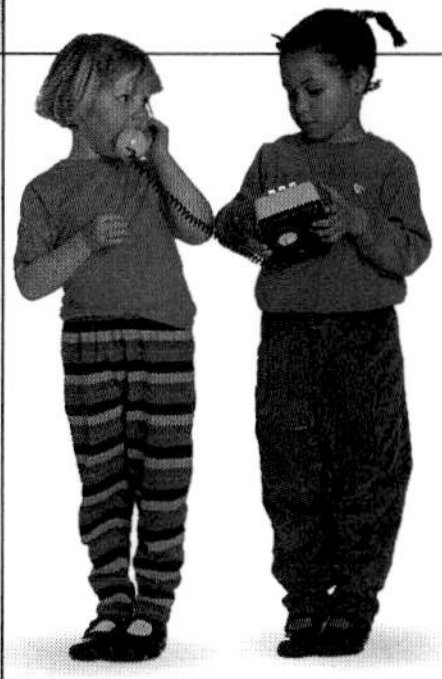 Your child has friends and enjoys companionship. He or she is very imaginative and tends to tell "tall tales" that combine fact and fantasy.
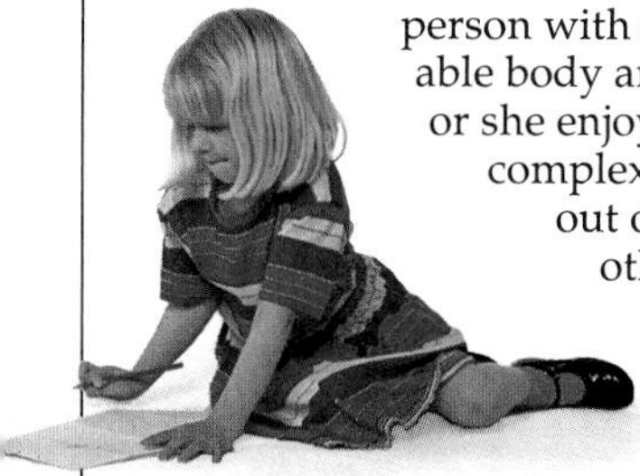 Your child can copy simple words and can draw a person with a recognizable body and face. He or she enjoys building complex structures out of blocks or other objects.	Your child can repeat stories and is able to make comparisons, such as big, bigger, and biggest. 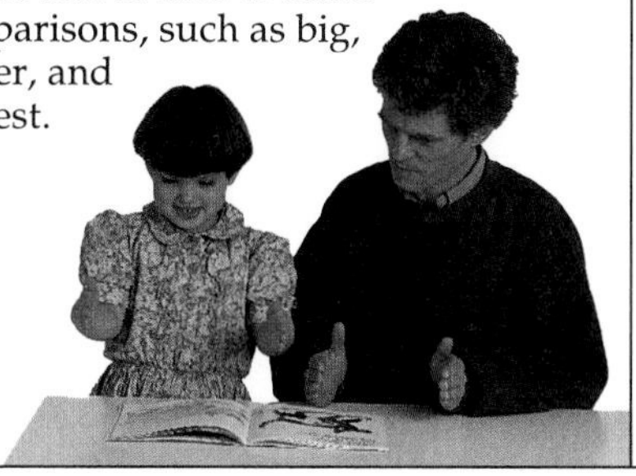	Your child distinguishes morning from afternoon, understands rules, and is affectionate and helpful to younger siblings. 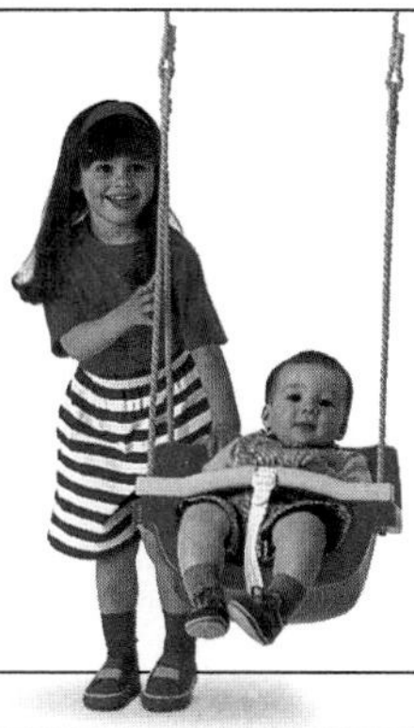

LANGUAGE AND SPEECH DEVELOPMENT

Speech is the foundation of human communication, and learning to talk is one of the most important intellectual skills that your child will ever master. By learning to use words, a child also learns about the world and the people who populate it. A child's most striking advance in language and communication skills occurs during the first 3 years of life. Developmental specialists can predict the age by which most children will acquire specific language skills.

HELPING YOUR CHILD'S LANGUAGE DEVELOPMENT

Children learn to talk most rapidly if they constantly hear the sound of other people's voices, especially those of their parents, from an early age. To give your child plenty of stimulation and encouragement to talk, follow the suggestions below. If your child does not respond, talk to your doctor.

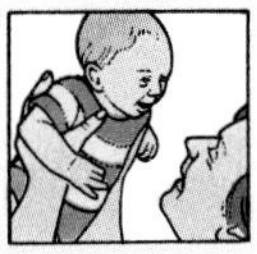

Begin talking to your child right after birth and look directly at him or her when you speak, so that your facial expressions give clues to the meaning of what you are saying. Speak clearly and distinctly.

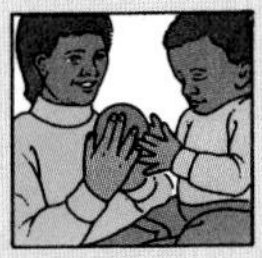

Use gestures to help your child associate particular words with objects and events. When your child understands the name of an object, he or she will look at it when you say its name.

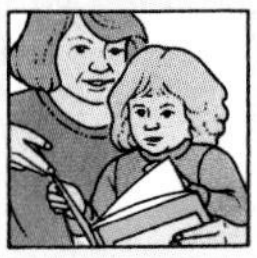

Read from simple books and repeat nursery rhymes to extend your child's vocabulary and to increase familiarity through repetition. Books also help explain complex ideas, such as colors and numbers.

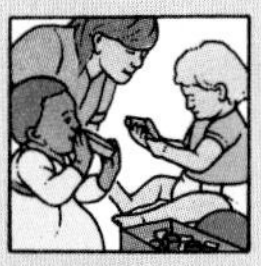

Provide plenty of opportunities for your child to interact with other children and adults.Younger children often benefit from playing with children who are 1 or 2 years older than they are.

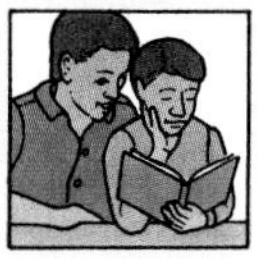

Try not to interrupt your child constantly to correct mistakes. Constant correction can undermine confidence. If you use good grammar yourself, your child will correct his or her mistakes.

The first year

Children communicate long before they are ready to talk. From birth, your child listens to the sounds of your voice and learns to associate these sounds with comfort and security. From the age of about 2 months, your baby learns how to make a variety of sounds, such as grunting, gurgling, and cooing. During the second half of the first year, these sounds develop into recognizable single syllables, such as "ma" and "da." The sounds gradually become more complex until your child begins babbling in long strings of syllables. By the end of their first year, most children can understand a few simple words and phrases and have learned to say at least one recognizable word in its proper context.

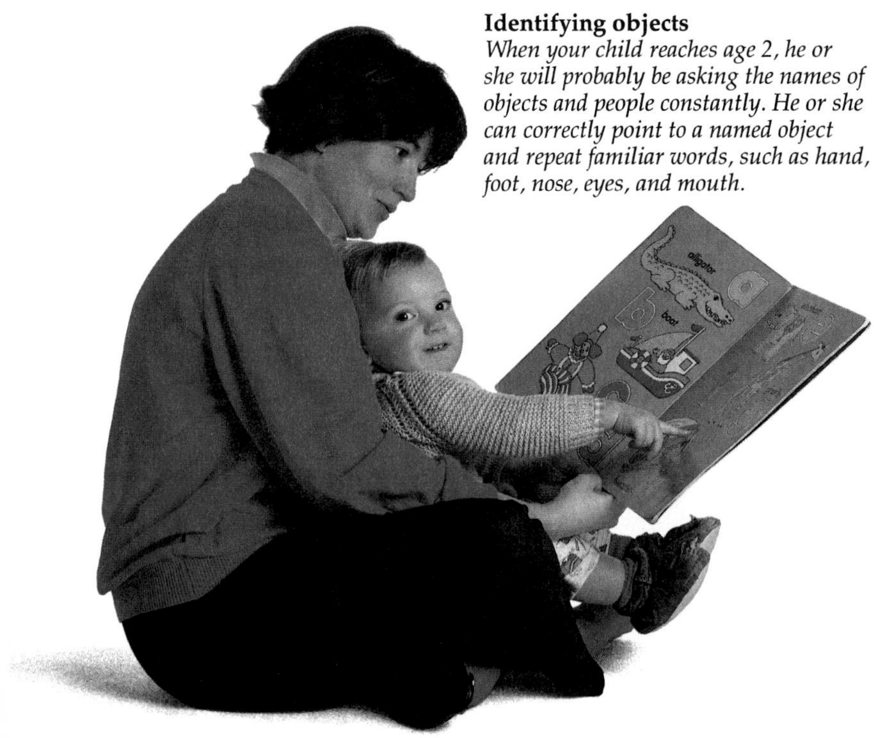

Identifying objects
When your child reaches age 2, he or she will probably be asking the names of objects and people constantly. He or she can correctly point to a named object and repeat familiar words, such as hand, foot, nose, eyes, and mouth.

The second year

During the early part of the second year, your child's vocabulary increases rapidly. He or she can usually say several words in their correct context and shows an understanding of many more. Gradually, phrases appear that link the names of people or objects with actions, such as "mommy go" or "doggy eat." At this stage, your child rapidly develops an understanding of the things you say. Although it may not be apparent in your child's speech, he or she absorbs a broad base of vocabulary and grammar.

The third year

During his or her third year, your child builds on the basic language skills that were acquired in the second year. By asking a continuous stream of questions about the names of objects and what they do, your child quickly enlarges his or her vocabulary and gains confidence in using words. Most children understand much of what an adult is saying by the end of their third year, as long as the language is simple and concrete. At this age, children can communicate their needs and thoughts clearly.

SPEECH DELAY

Do not be concerned if your child seems slow to say his or her first words. By listening to you talk, your child is building the groundwork of language. Most children who are late talkers catch up with their contemporaries very quickly once they start. If your child seems delayed in several areas, such as in general understanding and physical skills as well as in speech development, he or she may have a physical disability or a learning impairment. You should talk to your doctor if you notice such delays in development. He or she will probably order tests to reach a diagnosis and prescribe appropriate treatment.

Causes of speech delay

Speech delay in a child who is otherwise developing normally is probably not a cause for concern in the long run. But if your child is not saying words by 18 months, two-word phrases by age 2, or sentences by age 3, you should talk to your doctor. The most common cause of delayed speech is some degree of hearing impairment. Other causes include lack of stimulation (for example, when parents or other care givers do not talk to the child enough) and an inherited pattern of delayed speech, which is more common in boys than girls. In rare cases, delayed speech arises from damage to, or structural defects in, the speech muscles, larynx (voice box), or mouth. Any disorder affecting the speech area of the brain also delays speech. Bilingualism can also slow the acquisition of speech skills.

Tests and treatment

Your doctor will examine your child, especially the ears and throat, and will perform simple hearing tests in the office. If the doctor finds that your child has partial or total hearing loss or a hearing disorder, he or she will refer your child to an ear, nose, and throat specialist. Doctors can treat most forms of hearing loss with surgery or a hearing aid. If the results of your child's hearing tests are normal, a speech therapist will evaluate your child's speech. If no obvious cause for your child's speech delay can be found, your doctor will probably tell you to wait for your child to start talking on his or her own. Help your child by creating plenty of opportunities for him or her to listen to people speak.

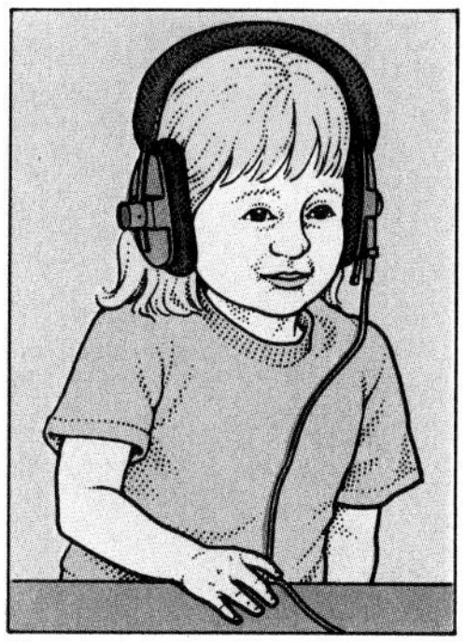

Hearing tests
If your doctor suspects that your child's hearing may be impaired, he or she will refer your child to a specialist for additional tests. These tests may include audiometry (measurement of hearing), in which a technician transmits sounds through earphones one ear at a time (above). The audiologist marks the loudness at which your child can hear each sound on a chart.

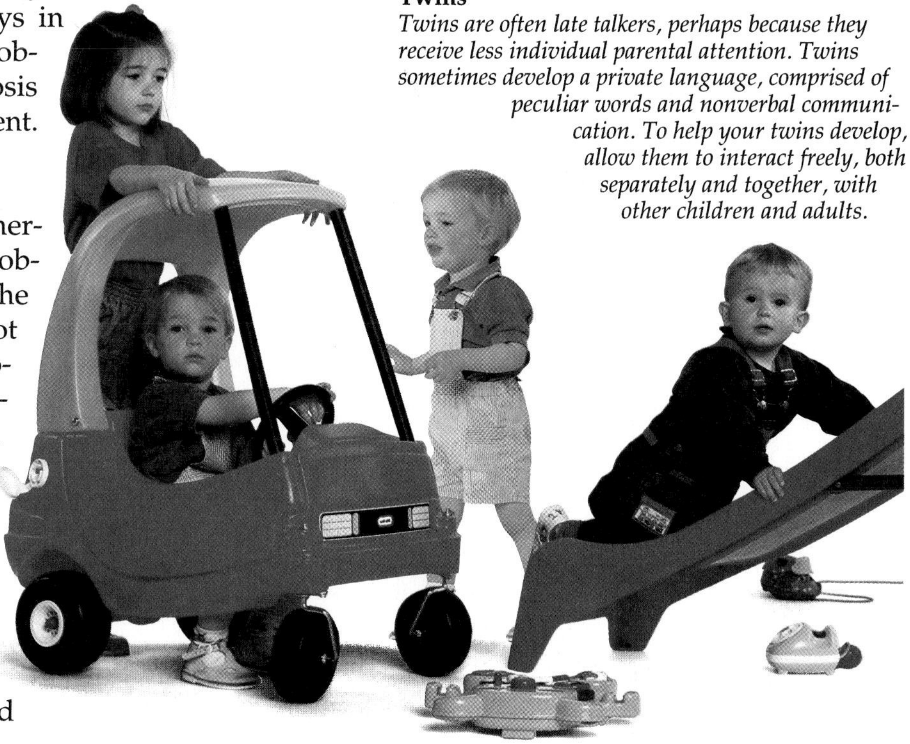

Twins
Twins are often late talkers, perhaps because they receive less individual parental attention. Twins sometimes develop a private language, comprised of peculiar words and nonverbal communication. To help your twins develop, allow them to interact freely, both separately and together, with other children and adults.

MONITOR YOUR SYMPTOMS

SPEECH DIFFICULTIES

Consult this chart if your child has any problem with his or her speech, such as delay in starting to talk, lack of clarity, defects in pronunciation, or stuttering. Most forms of speech difficulty resolve in time without treatment. But, in some cases, speech therapy can improve a child's speech.

BEGIN HERE

Some children start talking later than others.
Are you concerned because your child seems late in starting to talk?

YES → *Action* Children develop language and speech abilities at different ages and rates. Do not be overly concerned yet. See LANGUAGE AND SPEECH DEVELOPMENT on page 50 and call your doctor for an assessment if you are still concerned.

NO → *Are some of the words your child speaks unclear?*

YES → **Unclear speech may be normal for a child's age or may be a sign of a hearing abnormality.**
Has your child's hearing been tested recently?

NO → *Action* Call your doctor, who will perform a preliminary hearing test and examine your child's ears. If the doctor suspects hearing loss, he or she will refer your child to a specialist for further tests and treatment.

YES / NO → **Some children have a problem "getting words out."**
Are you concerned because your child stutters?

YES → *Is your child under 5 years old?*

YES → **Hesitancy in speaking** is normal and common in young children. It is not necessarily permanent.

Action Do not draw attention to your child's stuttering by finishing his or her sentences. This practice may create anxiety that perpetuates the stuttering. Call your doctor only if your child continues to stutter beyond age 5 or if the stuttering seriously interferes with your child's speech.

NO → **Stuttering** in children over age 5 may indicate a speech problem, which may be made worse by anxiety about speaking.

Action Consult your doctor, who may prescribe speech therapy. Children who have such therapy early usually overcome their speech difficulties.

NO → **Some children have problems pronouncing certain sounds.**
Does your child have a lisp or another type of speech defect?

YES → *Is the defect so severe that strangers cannot easily understand what your child is saying or is your child embarrassed about the problem?*

YES → **Serious defects** in pronunciation may be caused by a physical problem in the child's ears, mouth, or brain.

Action Consult your doctor, who will examine your child, paying special attention to the mouth and ears. The doctor may refer your child to a speech therapist for diagnosis and treatment. Speech therapy can correct many forms of speech defect.

NO → **Minor speech defects** are common. In most cases, children gradually overcome their difficulties with various sounds as they grow older.

Action Consult your doctor only if the speech defect starts to embarrass your child or if it interferes with communication or school performance.

NO → *Action* Consult your doctor if you are unable to identify your child's problem from this chart.

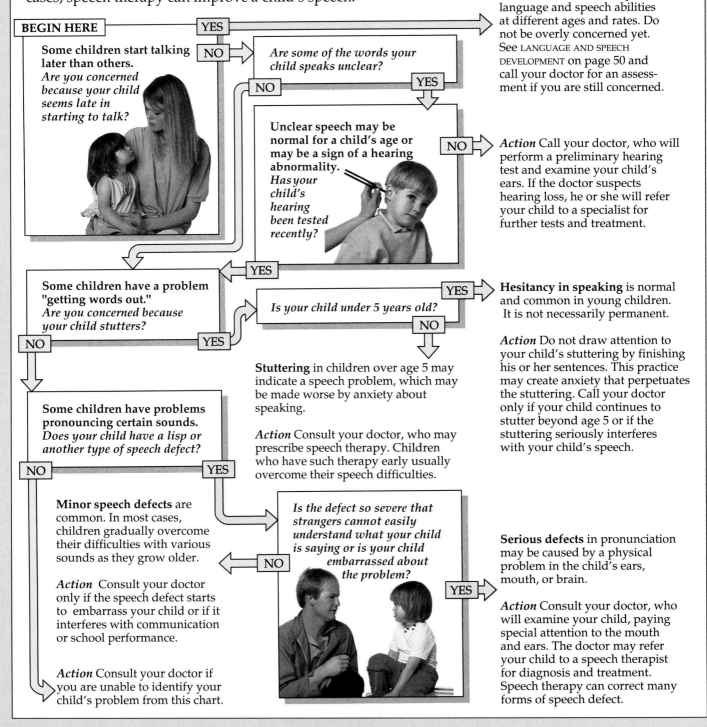

TESTING DEVELOPMENT

In the US, a pediatrician checks every child's development at periodic intervals to identify and treat any delay in development at an early stage. During developmental checkups, the pediatrician finds out whether a child has acquired the understanding, speech, and skills that are appropriate for his or her age. Doctors use various tests to check development, depending mainly on the child's age and ability. During the tests, the pediatrician observes the child's behavior and ability to perform certain tasks, such as following a set of simple instructions or drawing certain shapes. The doctor also tests hearing and vision because children learn by listening and watching and are stimulated to improve their skills through what they see and hear.

If the doctor identifies or suspects any problem during a routine developmental check, he or she may refer your child to a specialist in speech therapy, physical therapy, neurology, or developmental psychology, or to an ear, nose, and throat specialist for more detailed investigation of the problem.

COULD YOUR CHILD NEED A HEARING OR VISION TEST?

Doctors perform tests before a child is 1 year old to detect hearing and visual problems at the earliest possible stage. Then, during routine office visits throughout childhood, doctors perform simple tests to ensure that hearing and vision are developing normally. Check whether your child needs hearing or vision tests by asking yourself the following questions.

AGE	HEARING	AGE	VISION
1 year	Does your child respond to a voice $1\frac{1}{2}$ feet away at ear level? 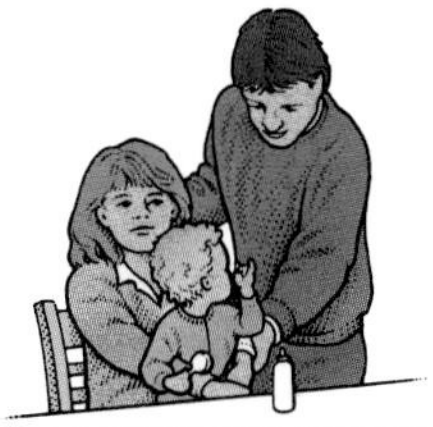	**1 to 2 years**	Can your child focus and concentrate on small objects? 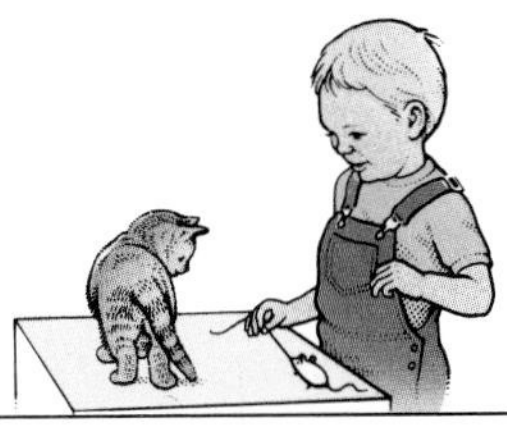
2 to 4 years	Can your child respond to and repeat softly spoken words? 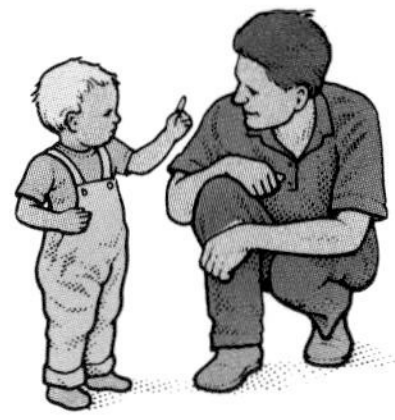	**3 years**	Can your child match letters using single-letter cards? 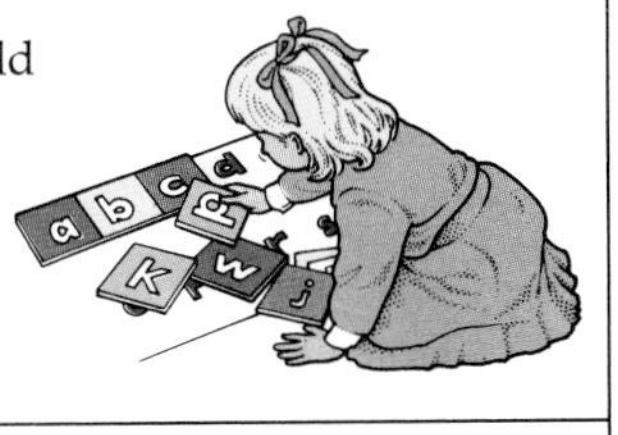
4 to 5 years	Can your child discriminate between similar-sounding words? 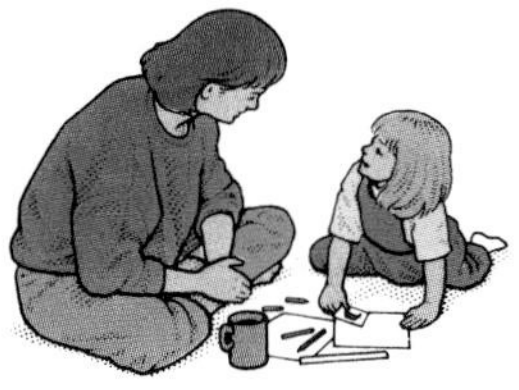	**4 to 6 years**	Does your child squint or seem to use only one eye? 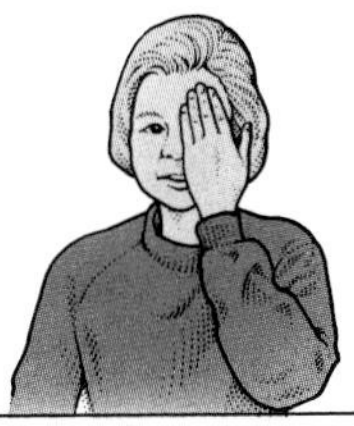
5 to 12 years	Does your child have trouble hearing the teacher, even if he or she sits in the front row? 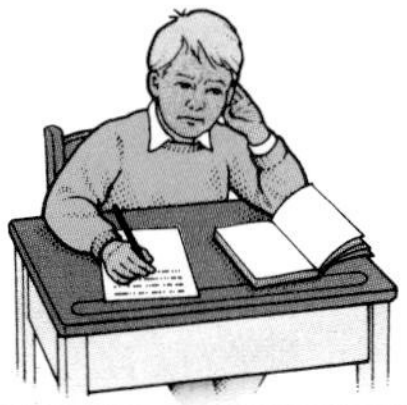	**7 to 12 years**	Does your child report trouble seeing distant objects clearly? Does he or she sit close to the TV or dislike reading? 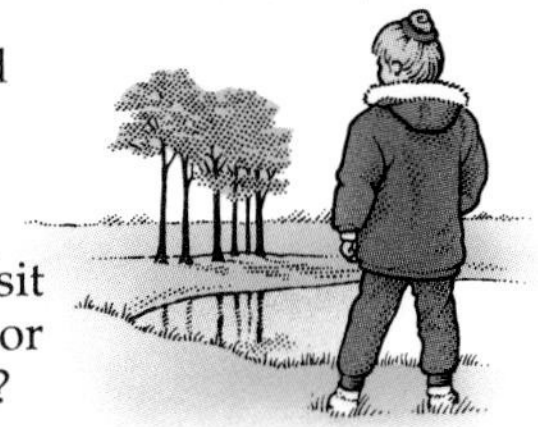

DEVELOPMENTAL DELAY

Doctors describe a young child as developmentally delayed if he or she has not attained certain abilities within the usual time range and has an inappropriate pattern of behavior for his or her age. This delay can be mild or severe and may affect one or more abilities. Seek medical advice if you are concerned that your child is not progressing as quickly as other children of a similar age. Your doctor may be able to reassure you that your young child's development falls within the normal range.

A specific disability, such as a visual impairment, can cause delay in one or two areas of development. Lack of experience from insufficient parental stimulation can also cause delay. Children showing delays in most abilities usually have a more generalized problem.

Treating developmental delay
The treatment of developmental delay depends on the underlying problem. Some children eventually catch up with their peers without treatment, although doctors may give parents advice about methods of increasing stimulation. Other children may progress rapidly after correction of a visual or hearing defect or after speech therapy, physical therapy, or family psychotherapy.

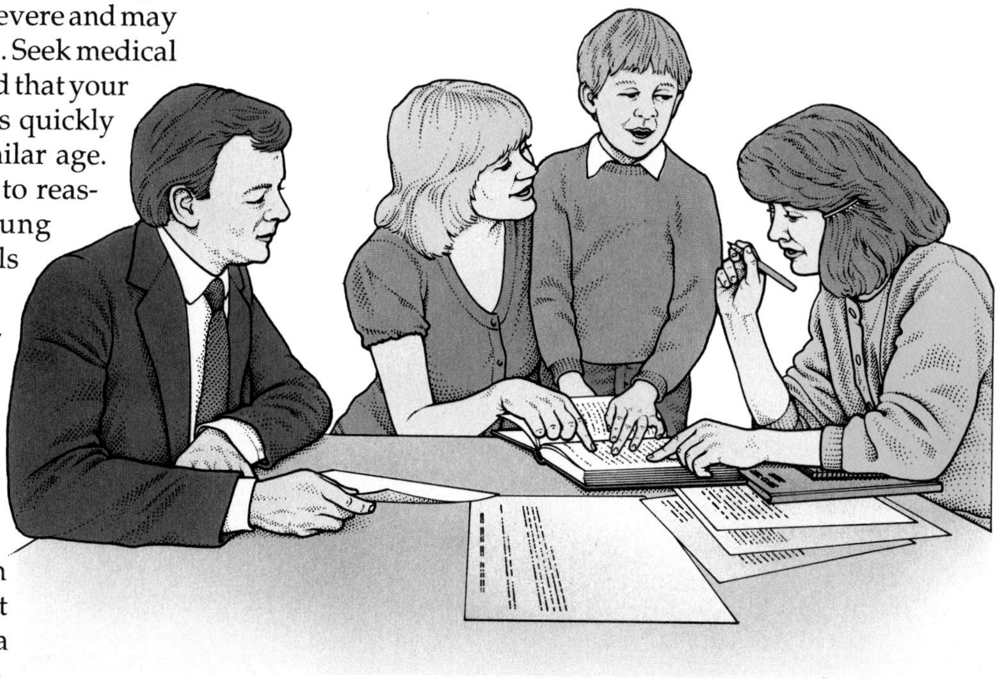

DYSLEXIA

Reading difficulties are common in older children. For some children, delayed reading ability is part of a more general problem with learning. But some otherwise intelligent children have difficulties with reading, spelling, and writing. Such children have a learning disability known as dyslexia (also called word blindness), which may be mild, moderate, or severe. A child with dyslexia may become frustrated and lose interest in learning if he or she does not receive help. Treatment consists of a program of special teaching techniques that aim to improve the child's performance and self-confidence. With appropriate guidance and support, dyslexic children usually manage to overcome their problem.

Causes and effects of dyslexia
Dyslexia often runs in families and affects boys more often than girls. Research shows that an abnormality in specific nerve pathways in the brain may cause dyslexia. Children with dyslexia have difficulty with perception and tend to reverse letters and words (below). They may also have problems with coordination, arithmetic, short-term memory, and distinguishing left from right.

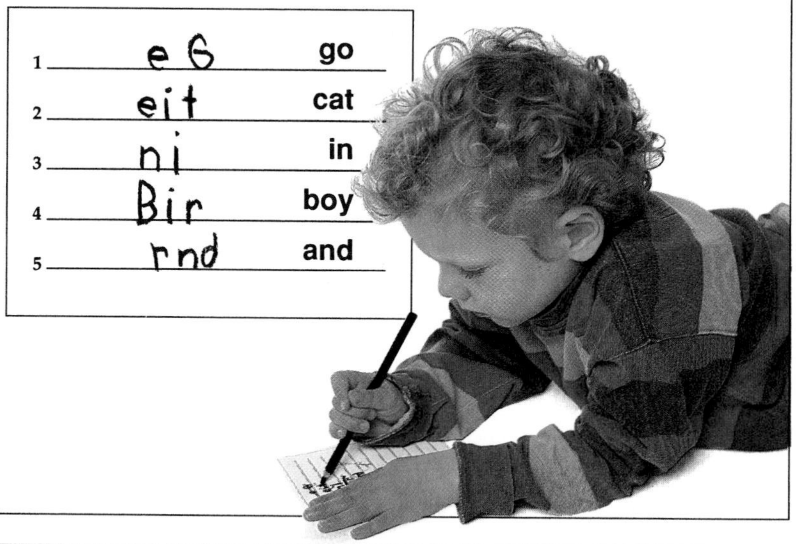
1 e6 go
2 eit cat
3 ni in
4 Bir boy
5 rnd and

SEXUAL DEVELOPMENT

By the age of 3 or 4 years, most children have a strong sense of being either a girl or a boy. Differences in behavior between the sexes usually become apparent during early childhood. For example, girls may choose to play with dolls, while boys may choose to play with cars and trucks. But a child's upbringing can greatly influence the extent to which he or she adopts the conventional gender roles.

Children have sex drives, which increase sharply during adolescence. But the intensity with which children experience sexual urges varies considerably from child to child. Fondling the genitals is common in both boys and girls, but in young children the pleasure it brings is more general than sexual. Children do not usually feel sexual excitement from engaging in masturbation until they are much older. Do not discourage fondling of the genitals, but be aware that excessive masturbation that interferes with your child's daily activities or sleep pattern may indicate an underlying problem, such as general understimulation or an emotional disturbance.

TALKING ABOUT SEXUALITY

When should you talk to your child about sex? When your child begins asking how babies are born. Do not discourage your child's questions. Talk openly and answer questions honestly. Do not use slang; teach your child the correct terminology for the subjects you are discussing. Some parents explain too much the first time a child brings up the subject. Keep your explanations simple and short. If your child wants to know more, let him or her ask.

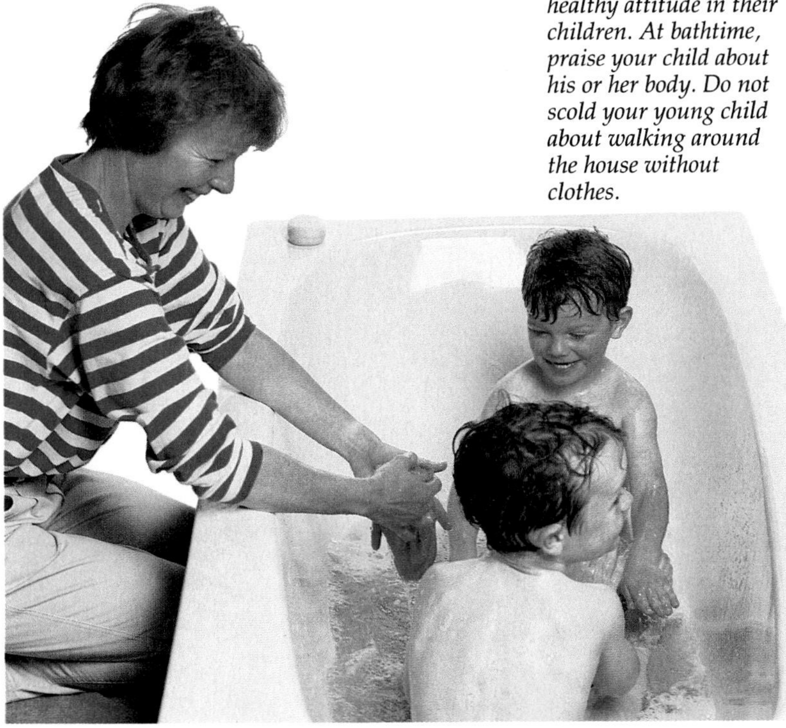

A healthy body image
Parents who have a healthy, comfortable attitude about their bodies will foster a healthy attitude in their children. At bathtime, praise your child about his or her body. Do not scold your young child about walking around the house without clothes.

ASK YOUR DOCTOR CHILD DEVELOPMENT

Q My son did not walk until he was 18 months old. Is this delay in walking abnormal ?

A The development of motor skills varies greatly. Late walking may be a family characteristic. Some children learn to walk as early as 7 months, others as late as 18 months. Most late walkers are completely normal. In rare cases, an underlying disorder may cause late walking.

Q Our 3-year-old daughter seems unable to distinguish some colors. Could she be color-blind?

A Unless color-blindness runs in your family, it is very unlikely that your daughter is color-blind. Many 3-year-old children cannot name more than three colors. By about $4^1/_2$ years of age, most children know red, blue, green, and yellow. If your daughter continues to have difficulty distinguishing colors, your doctor can check her color vision when she is 5 years old. Boys are color-blind more often than girls.

Q My 8-year-old son seems exceptionally intelligent, especially in math. Could he be a gifted child?

A Gifted children are extremely intelligent and usually score high on intelligence quotient (IQ) tests. They also possess abundant problem-solving abilities and are highly motivated to learn. Gifted children often display "genius" in a single area, such as math or chess. Your son's school can arrange to have his IQ tested, but whether or not he is gifted, you should provide plenty of encouragement and opportunities for him to explore his potential.

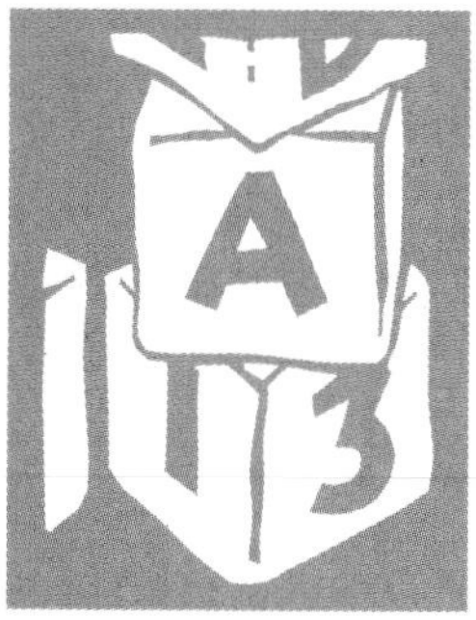

UNDERSTANDING YOUR CHILD'S NEEDS

CHILDREN HAVE physical, emotional, and intellectual needs. To develop into well-balanced individuals, children must grow up in an environment in which all these needs are met. Children also thrive in an environment that encourages them to pursue knowledge and develop their individual talents.

Many of the developing child's needs change as he or she grows older. Parents should observe their children and be ready to respond as new needs arise. But no matter what the age of your child, he or she always needs a nutritious diet.

WHAT IS A BALANCED DIET?

Carbohydrates
Carbohydrates should provide about half of the calorie content of your child's diet because they are the most healthy source of energy. Potatoes, brown rice, pasta, and whole grain bread are good, healthy sources of carbohydrates.

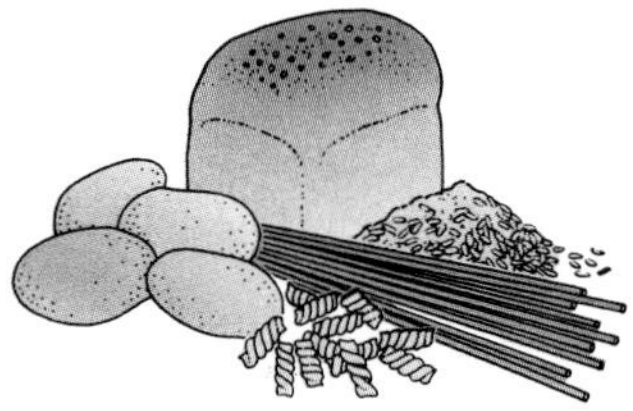

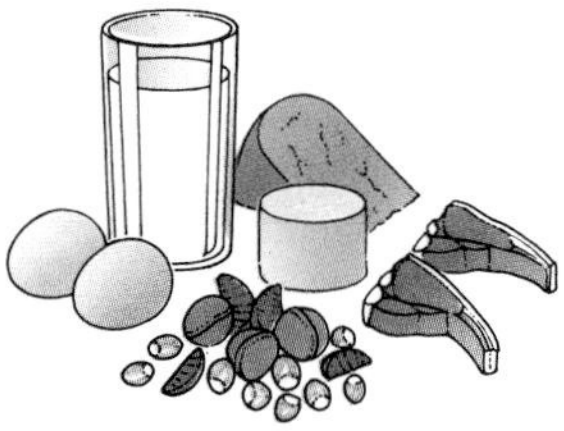

Protein
Your child's muscles, skin, and other tissues are made up mainly of protein. Protein should provide about 20 percent of the energy content of any diet. Children need protein for growth. Milk, cheese, eggs, nuts, dried peas and beans, fish, and lean meat are good sources.

Fiber
Fiber is the indigestible part of plant foods that adds bulk to the diet and prevents constipation. Fruit, raw vegetables, and cereals are good sources of fiber in your child's diet.

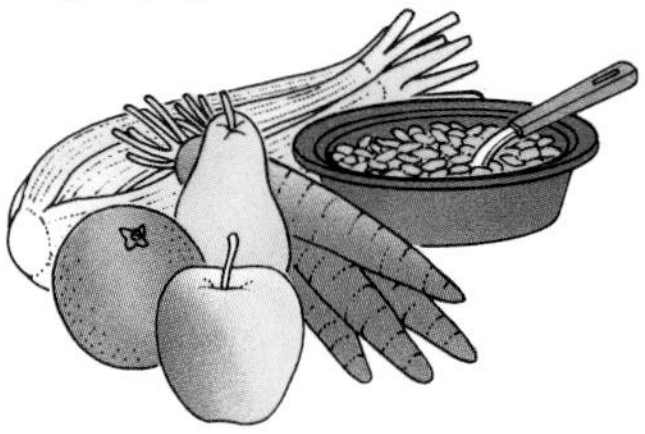

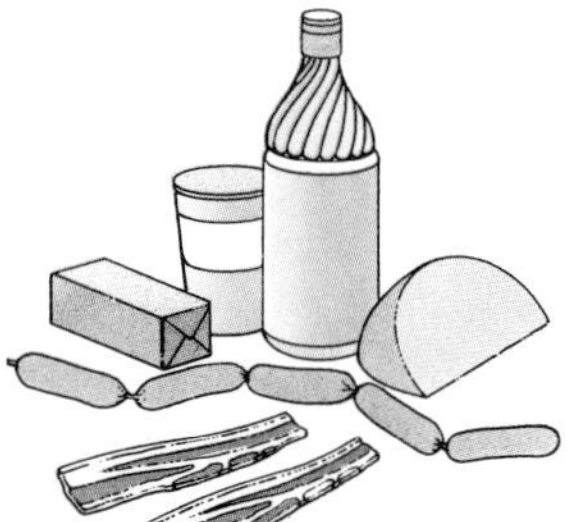

Fats
Fats are an important part of a child's diet, because they form structural components of cells and provide a source of energy. But a diet containing more than 30 percent fat is unhealthy and may lead to weight gain and obesity later in life. Dairy products and vegetable oils are sources of fats.

Vitamins and minerals
The body needs vitamins and minerals for healthy functioning. A varied diet that includes plenty of fresh, unprocessed foods will meet the body's needs. But you and your family can take vitamin supplements daily to ensure a proper vitamin intake.

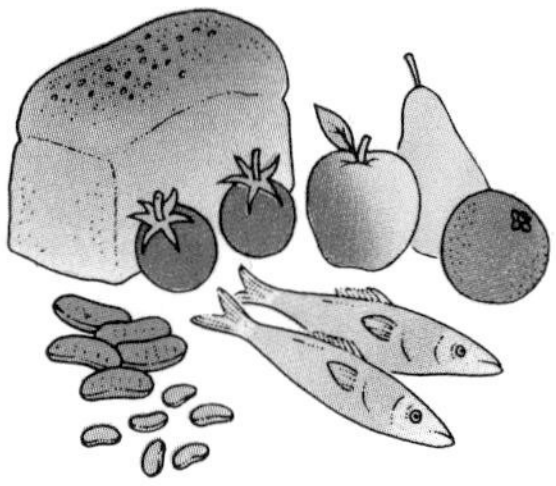

PROVIDING A HEALTHY DIET

Your children need a healthy, balanced diet that supplies all the nutrients necessary for growth and body maintenance, along with enough calories to fulfill energy requirements. A well-balanced diet should contain carbohydrates, proteins, fiber, and fats in balanced proportions, along with the recommended amounts of vitamins and minerals. Be sure to include unprocessed foods, such as grains, fruit, and vegetables, in your child's diet every day. Instill healthy eating habits at an early age to help your child reap lifelong health benefits.

Eating between meals

Because young children expend large amounts of energy, they often need between-meal snacks in addition to their regular meals. Offer your children nutritious snacks, such as fruit, raw vegetables, or slices of whole grain bread. Healthy snacks provide needed nutrition when your child is not hungry at meal time.

Picky eaters

Parents often worry that their children do not consume a balanced diet if they refuse to eat what they are given. But children will resist all the more if you try to force them to eat something they do not want. If you offer a reward for eating vegetables, for example, you may just reinforce the idea that vegetables are

Energy requirements
In proportion to their size, children eat more food than adults, because they tend to be more active and need additional nutrients for proper growth. Children's calorie requirements vary depending on their age, size, and activity level.

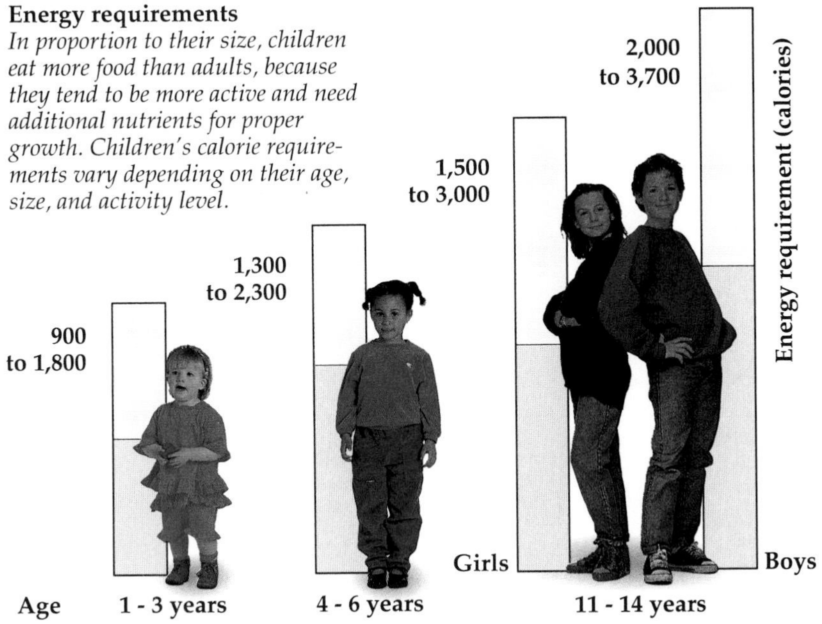

undesirable. Children usually eat some vegetables and fruit and receive adequate nutrition if you provide them with many different foods throughout the week. Children's tastes change on their own as they get older. What is unacceptable to a child at a certain age often becomes acceptable later.

Most children like sugary foods, such as candy. While it might be unfair to forbid such items completely, you should keep the amount of sweet foods you buy to a minimum. To encourage healthy eating habits, give your child sweet foods as a rare treat, only after meals and not between meals. To help protect your children's teeth, encourage them to avoid sweets. Provide healthy snacks with a high nutritional value, such as raw vegetables or cheese and crackers.

School lunches

Lunches prepared at schools follow recommended nutritional guidelines and usually include a glass of milk. If your child prefers a home-packed lunch, try to make it as nourishing as possible. Provide sandwiches made with whole grain bread filled with low-fat meats, cheese, or peanut butter, along with fresh fruit and nutritious cookies for dessert.

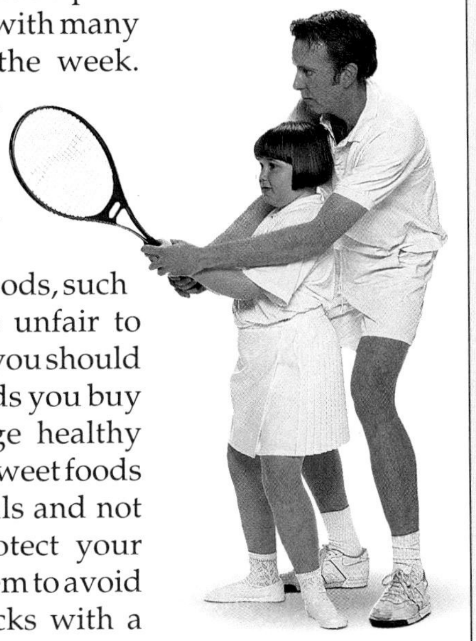

Weight problems
Children become overweight when they consume more calories in food than they burn. Your child can achieve proper weight simply by exercising more. An inappropriate weight-loss diet can compromise normal growth and can be dangerous to your child's health. Call your pediatrician before you start your child on a weight reduction diet.

ASK YOUR DOCTOR
CHILDHOOD NUTRITION

Q My children love chocolate candy. Is it all right for them to eat junk foods once in a while?

A There is no such thing as a bad food – only a bad diet. Teach your children to avoid eating too many processed or fast foods. Processed foods are generally low in fiber and contain high levels of sugar, fat, and salt. But as long as your children regularly eat nutritious meals, they will not be harmed by an occasional candy bar or bag of potato chips.

Q My daughter has recently become a vegetarian. How can I make sure she eats enough protein?

A Beans, nuts, and grains, such as wheat and rice, are all good sources of protein but, because they do not provide all the amino acids your body needs, they are called incomplete proteins. Combine certain plant foods, such as beans or nuts mixed with rice or wheat, to make sure she eats complete proteins. Eggs and dairy products, such as milk, yogurt, and cheese, provide most of the protein needed for growth.

Q I want my baby to have fresh food instead of bottled baby food. How should I prepare it?

A Fresh foods, such as meat, fruits, and vegetables, provide excellent nutrition for your baby when prepared at home. Cook the food well, then puree it in a blender or food processor. You can simply mash some foods, such as raw bananas or boiled potatoes. Do not add salt or other spices. Refrigerate the unused portion and check for signs of spoilage before feeding it to your baby.

CARING FOR YOUR CHILD'S TEETH

Although your child has "baby teeth" (primary teeth) for only a few years, it is important to keep them healthy. Primary teeth that decay not only cause pain or infection but also may interfere with the normal, regular growth of your child's permanent teeth. Encourage your children from an early age to clean their teeth as part of their daily routine to make sure that their permanent teeth will last a lifetime. Children should also visit a dentist for a checkup every 6 months from about the age of 3.

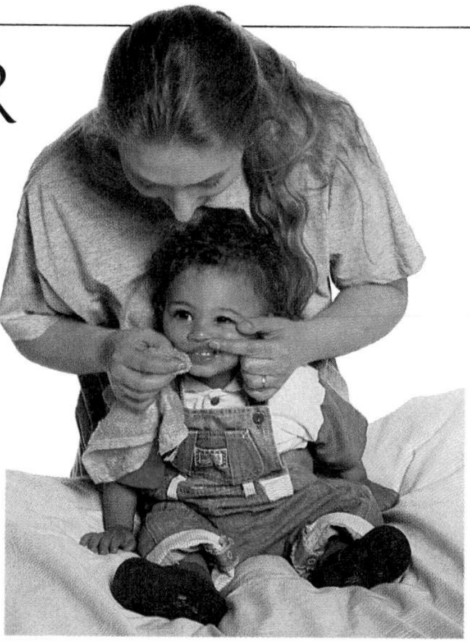

Early teeth cleaning
As soon as your child's first teeth appear, you should start cleaning them every day. Use a dry piece of gauze or a dry washcloth to wipe the teeth and gums. Do not use toothpaste for an infant. You will meet less resistance from your child if you treat toothbrushing as a game rather than as a chore.

BRUSHING AND FLOSSING TECHNIQUES

Children aged 4 or 5 can do a fairly good job of brushing their own teeth. Supervise their technique to make sure that they reach all their teeth and brush them in the right directions. Ideally, your children should clean their teeth with a fluoride toothpaste after every meal. Regular flossing removes particles of food and bacteria from between the teeth and also helps to reduce tooth decay and prevent gum disease.

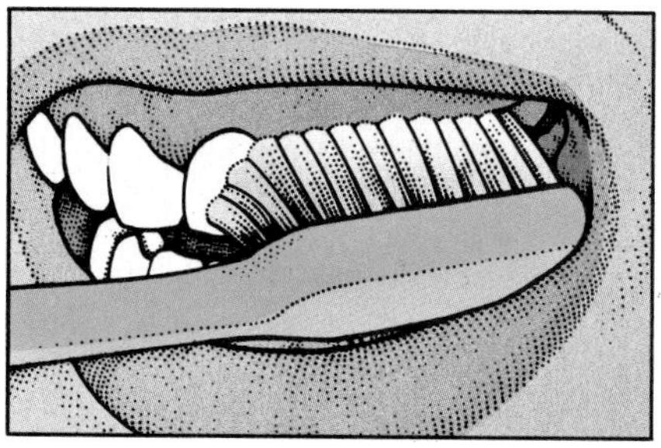

Brushing front teeth
Brush front teeth away from the gums with short back-and-forth strokes. Angle the brush toward the gum line as shown above.

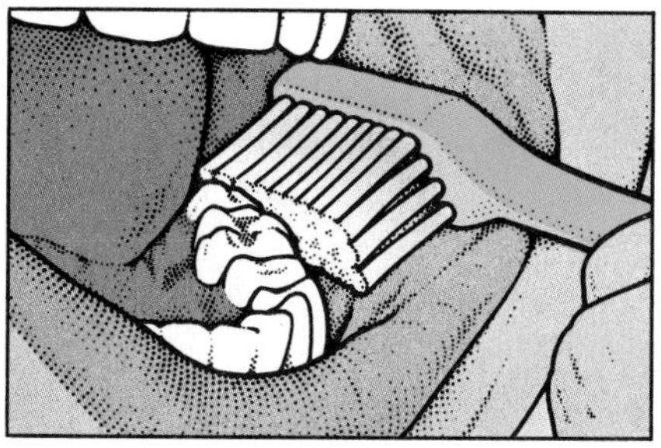

Brushing along gums
To help keep the gums healthy, encourage your child to brush along the line of the gums on the inner and outer surfaces of the teeth.

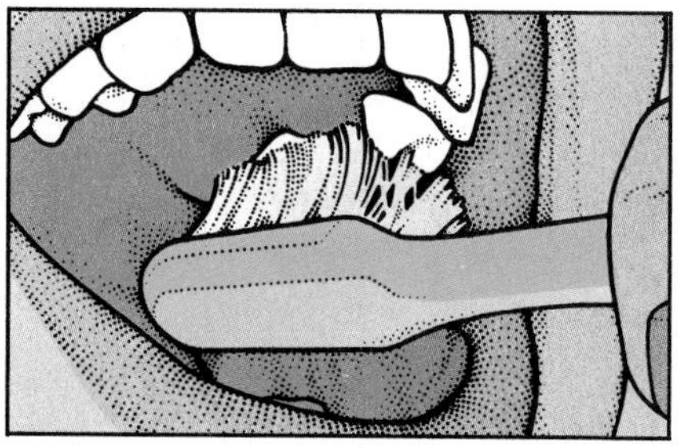

Brushing biting surfaces
All the biting surfaces, including the ones right at the back of the mouth, need to be brushed in both forward and backward directions.

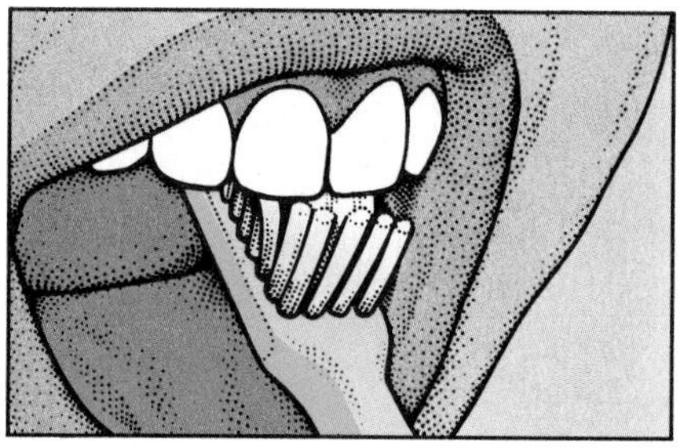

Brushing inside surfaces
Brush the inside surfaces of the front teeth with almost vertical up-and-down movements.

Flossing teeth
Your dentist can tell you when your child should start flossing; each child's ability to master such a skill is different. Incorrect flossing can damage your child's gums. Gently guide the taut floss between the child's teeth until it reaches the gum line. Using up-and-down motions, rub the sides of each tooth.

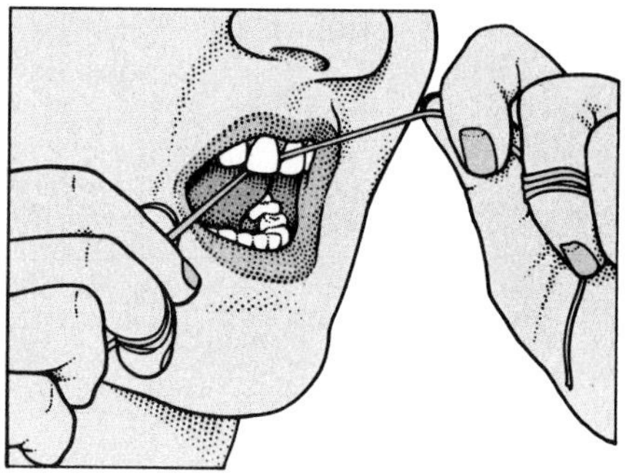

Fluoride treatment
Fluoride-containing toothpastes and mouth rinses help reduce tooth decay by strengthening the outer coating of the teeth. Fluoride is present in most water supplies. Give supplementary fluoride drops or tablets only according to a dentist's instruction. Too much fluoride can give teeth a mottled appearance.

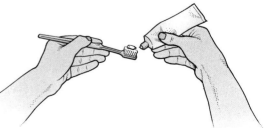

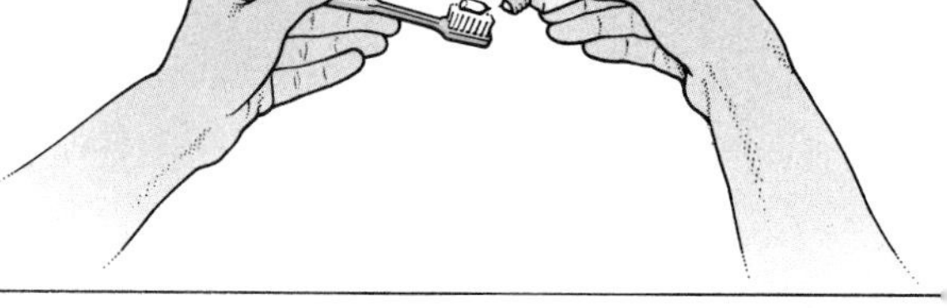

PERMANENT TEETH

Permanent teeth begin to appear at the age of 6 to 7. As the permanent teeth erupt, the primary teeth are displaced, become loose, and fall out. The full set of 32 permanent teeth usually appears in a certain order at predictable ages (shown at right).

Premolars
Premolars have two distinct ridges for grinding and chewing food. No premolars exist in the primary set of teeth.

Molars
Molars are strong, large teeth for chewing and grinding food. Third molars (wisdom teeth) sometimes need to be extracted to prevent damage to gums and other teeth. In some people, third molars never appear.

Canines
Canines are sharp, pointed teeth used to tear food. They are usually bigger than incisors and have very deep roots.

Incisors
Incisors are chisel-shaped teeth that have sharp edges for biting.

Enamel

Dentin

Pulp cavity containing nerves and blood supply

Gum

UPPER JAW

LOWER JAW

Incisors appear at 6 to 9 years

Canines appear at 9 to 12 years

Premolars appear at 10 to 12 years

First molars appear at 6 to 7 years

Second molars appear at 11 to 13 years

Third molars appear at 17 years or older

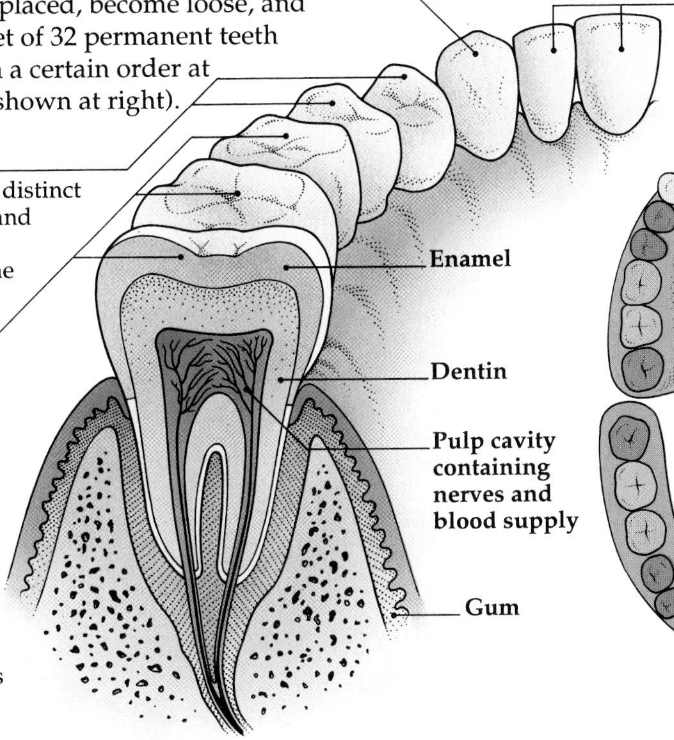

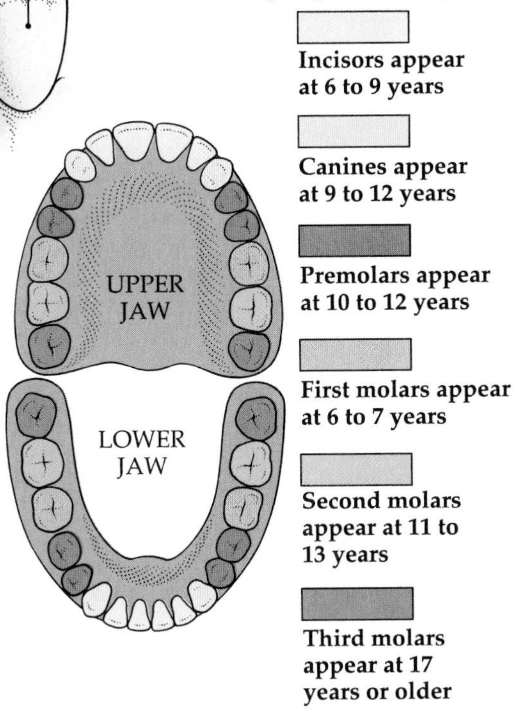

HOW DO TEETH DECAY?

The resistance of teeth to decay depends on the strength of the teeth and the quantity of protective saliva a person produces. People who frequently eat sugary foods, such as candy, and who do not clean their teeth have the most rapid rate of decay. The illustrations below show how tooth decay progresses.

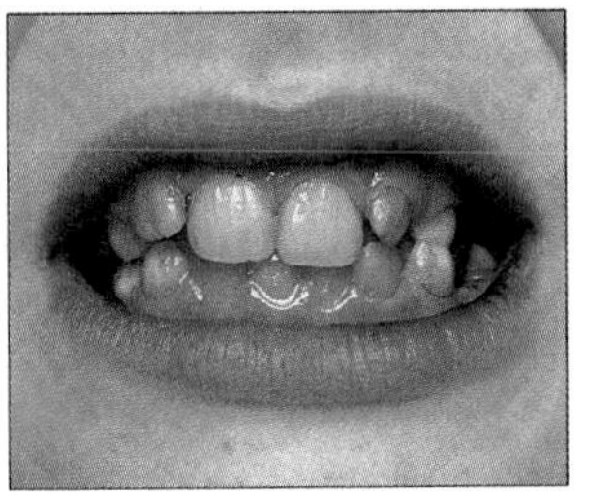

Plaque and tartar
Dentists use dyes (disclosing agents) to reveal plaque. Accumulation of plaque can lead to formation of tartar, a harder substance that causes gum damage.

SYMPTOMS OF TOOTH DECAY

Teach your child to brush his or her teeth after every meal and to floss daily to prevent tooth decay. If your child has any of the following symptoms, take him or her to the dentist promptly.

◆ Dull, white areas on the tooth where acid has destroyed the enamel.
◆ Black, decayed areas on the teeth.
◆ Persistent pain after consuming hot and cold foods and drinks.
◆ A toothache.
◆ Red, puffy gums.

Plaque Enamel

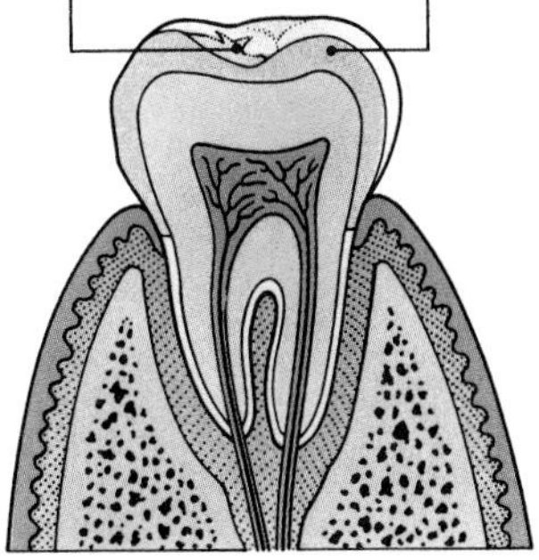

1 Inadequate cleaning allows a combination of food particles, saliva, and bacteria to form a deposit called plaque on the enamel, the hard outer coating of the teeth.

2 The bacteria in plaque react with sugar in food to form an acid that weakens and eventually destroys the enamel, exposing the dentin beneath. Dentin is the substance that forms the bulk of a tooth.

Decay

Dentin

Decay

Pulp cavity

Abscess

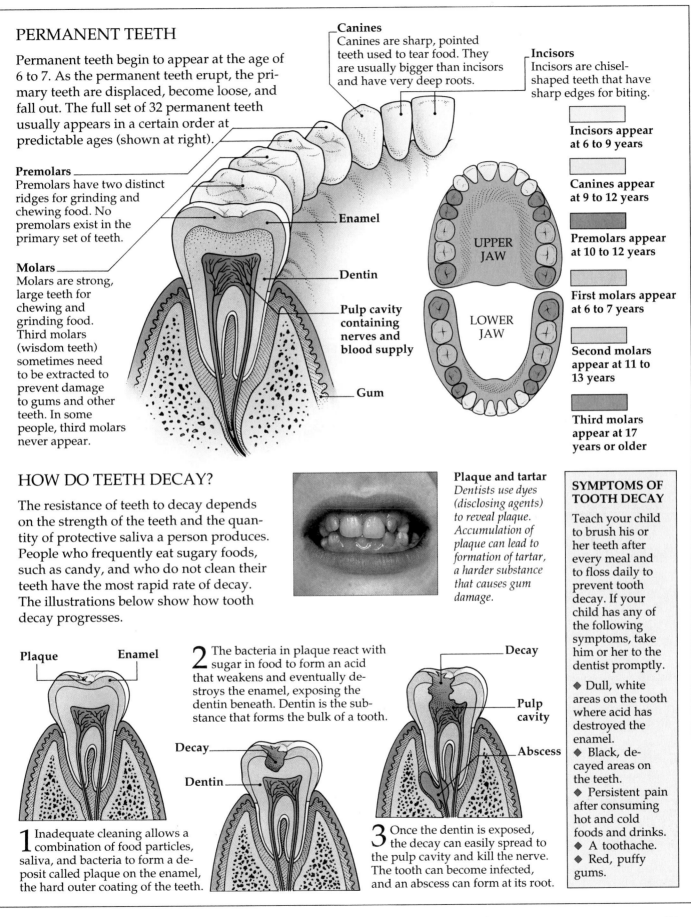

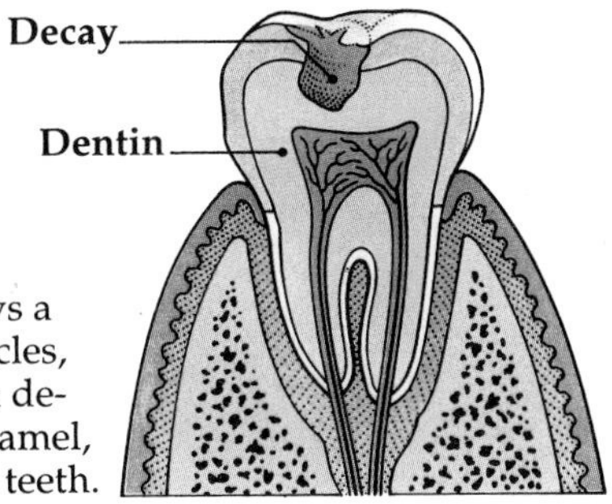

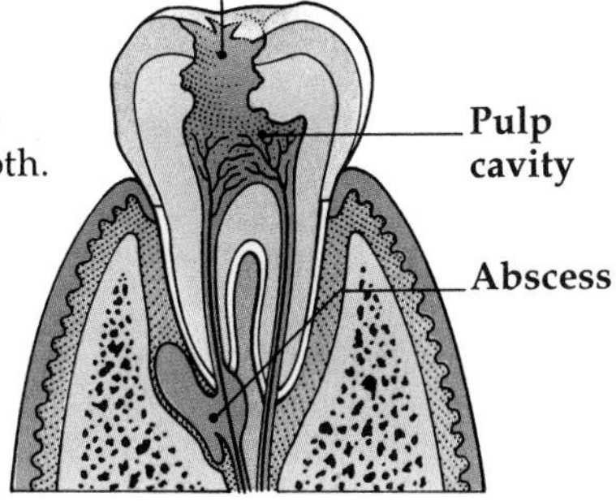

3 Once the dentin is exposed, the decay can easily spread to the pulp cavity and kill the nerve. The tooth can become infected, and an abscess can form at its root.

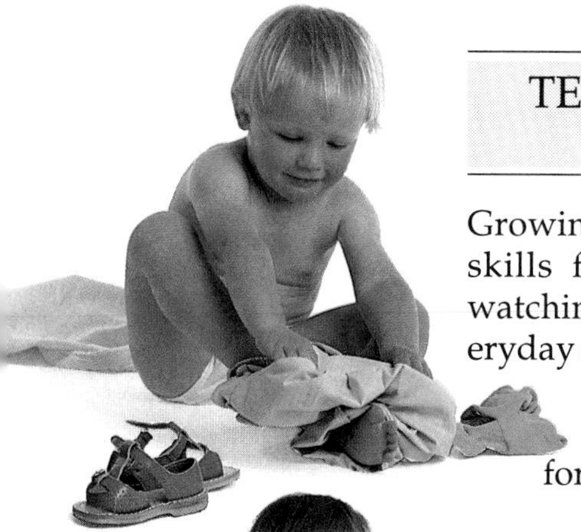

TEACHING EVERYDAY SKILLS

Growing children learn many simple skills from their parents simply by watching and mimicking them in everyday situations. But your child will not learn many of the more complex everyday skills that adults take for granted unless you explain them.

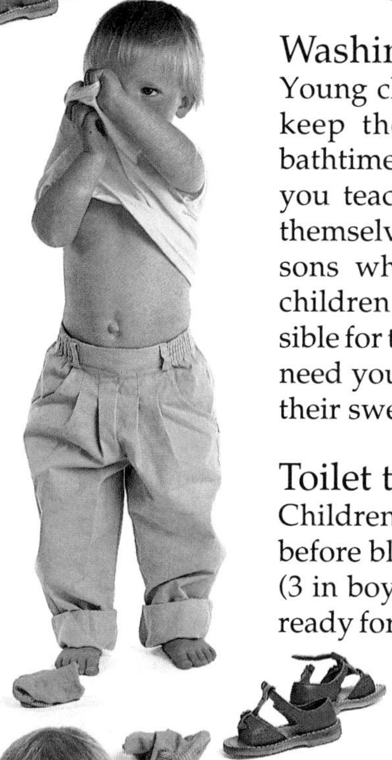

Washing

Young children rely on their parents to keep them clean and healthy. Turn bathtime into a time for fun during which you teach your children how to wash themselves and explain to them the reasons why they need to bathe. Older children become increasingly responsible for their own hygiene, but they may need your advice during puberty when their sweat glands become more active.

Toilet training

Children often achieve bowel control before bladder control. By the age of 2½ (3 in boys), your child will probably be ready for toilet training. You will need to encourage your child to use the toilet regularly, so make sure that it is always easily accessible. Always praise the child when he or she uses the toilet. Don't scold your child when accidents happen – you may not have reminded him or her to use the toilet at the right time. If, after about 2 weeks, your child shows no sign of understanding what the toilet is for, he or she is not yet ready to be trained. Try again in a few weeks.

Even after your child has achieved bladder control during the day, he or she may still wet the diaper at night. When your child's diaper has remained dry overnight for about a week, you can start leaving it off at night. Remember that lapses do occur, and you may need to start using diapers again for a while.

SLEEP

Children benefit from regular sleeping hours but tend to resist going to bed. Minimize bedtime arguments by firmly setting a fixed bedtime and by having a regular bedtime routine that includes a relaxing bath and a bedtime story.

Young children commonly experience sleep problems when they feel sick or anxious. To reassure, provide a nightlight or leave a light on outside the child's room. Sleep disturbances often follow a major change in routine, such as moving or starting nursery school. The child usually settles down within a few weeks as the new routine becomes familiar.

All children have occasional nightmares. Frequent nightmares are unusual and can signal that your child has a problem that he or she needs to talk about. Children may also experience "night terrors," during which they scream and thrash. Once awake, a child with night terrors cannot remember them and usually goes back to sleep.

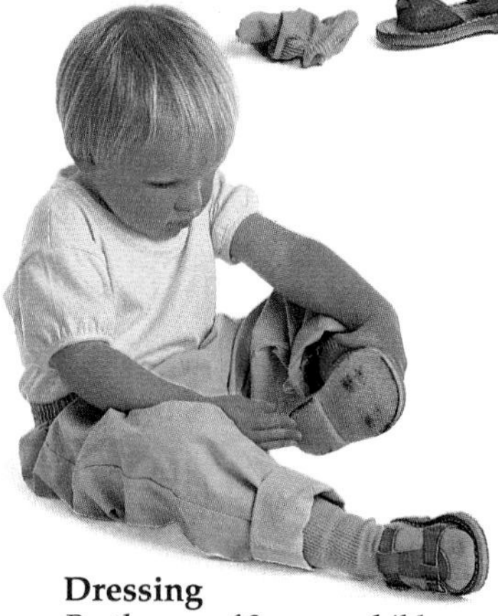

Dressing
By the age of 2, some children can undress themselves. It takes longer for them to learn to dress, but if their clothes have elastic waistbands, rather than zippers and buttons, most children can begin to dress themselves at about the age of 3. Children may find dressing easier if you lay out their clothes in the order in which they should be put on.

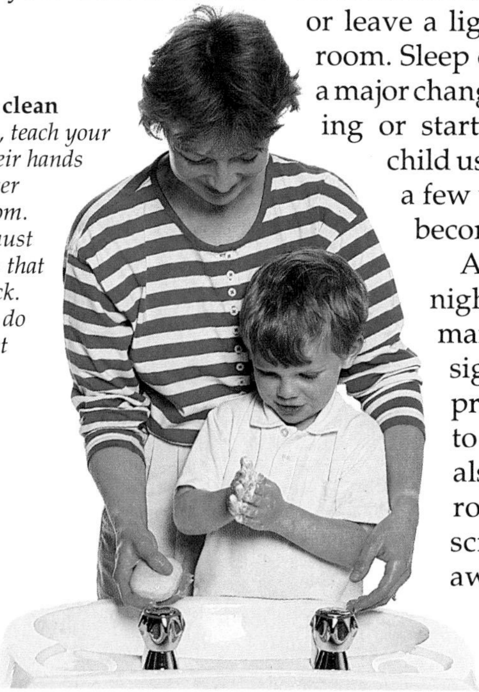

Learning to keep clean
As early as possible, teach your children to wash their hands before meals and after going to the bathroom. Explain that they must do this to kill germs that could make them sick. Make sure that you do the same thing to set a good example.

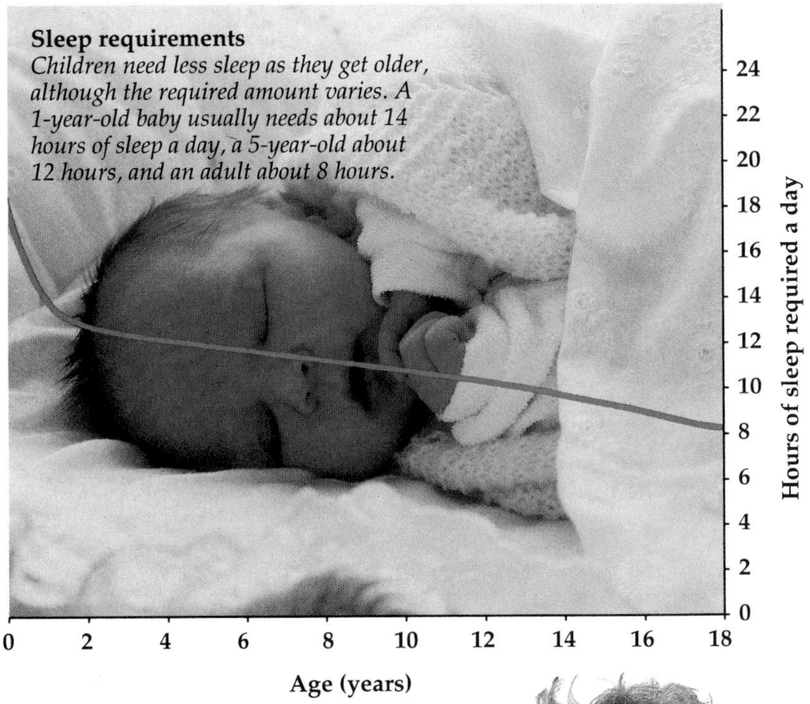

Sleep requirements
Children need less sleep as they get older, although the required amount varies. A 1-year-old baby usually needs about 14 hours of sleep a day, a 5-year-old about 12 hours, and an adult about 8 hours.

EMOTIONAL DEVELOPMENT

Children quickly learn to respond to the emotions of those around them and observe how they can influence the behavior of others by their own actions. The behavior of a child greatly depends on the way he or she has been treated. If children receive loving care, stimulation, security, and consistency, they are much more likely to develop into well-balanced individuals in adulthood.

Discipline

Children like knowing the acceptable boundaries of their behavior. Applied consistently and fairly, discipline teaches your children what you expect of them and gives them the confidence to make decisions. Do not spank or hit children. Physical punishment teaches them to solve problems with physical violence. Make sure that punishment is appropriate for the severity of the misbehavior and that it is carried out immediately after the misbehavior occurs. Explain to the child exactly what he or she has done wrong. Many doctors advocate a technique called "timeout," in which a parent sends a misbehaving child to a room or area empty of toys and distractions to sit alone for 5 minutes. Always reward good behavior with praise – sometimes withholding praise is the only discipline needed for minor misbehaving.

A death in the family

Children will grieve at the loss of a relative, care giver, and even a pet. Death is a difficult concept for young children to grasp and needs to be explained carefully and simply. Misrepresentation of death can have undesirable consequences – for example, young children may be afraid to go to bed if someone tells them that death is like never waking up.

It can take several years before children come to terms with a death in the family. Toddlers and teenagers seem to have the most difficulty. During the grieving stage, provide stability in the child's life. Encourage children to discuss their grief and explain that they should not feel guilty about enjoying their own life. Do not be afraid to express your own feelings to your child.

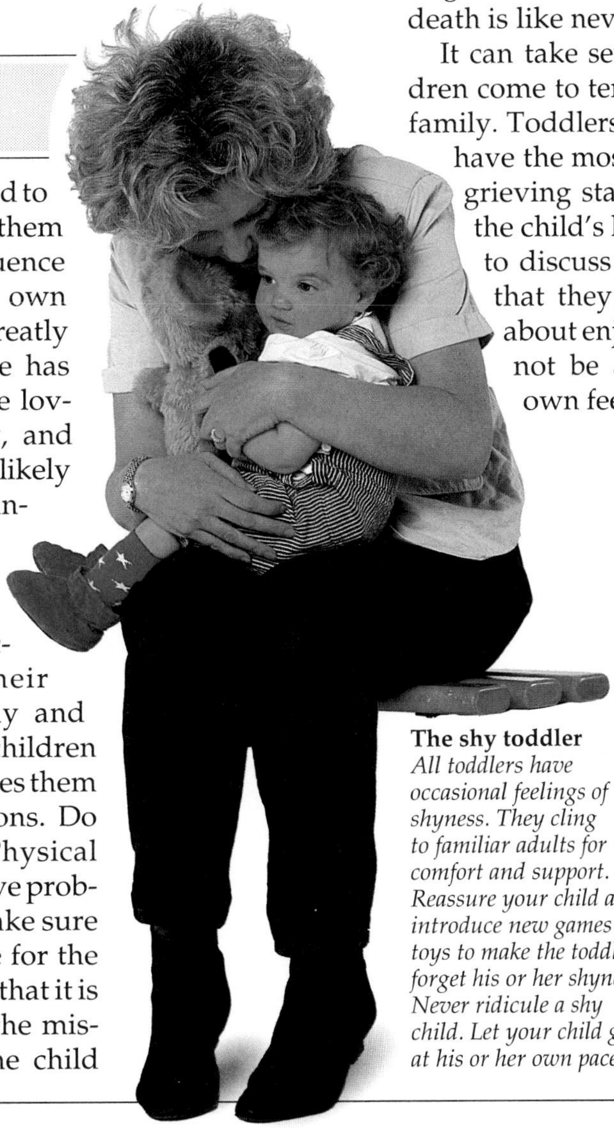

The shy toddler
All toddlers have occasional feelings of shyness. They cling to familiar adults for comfort and support. Reassure your child and introduce new games or toys to make the toddler forget his or her shyness. Never ridicule a shy child. Let your child go at his or her own pace.

SIBLING RIVALRY

Sibling rivalry is very common within families, but its intensity depends on the personalities of the children and on their parents' attitude. Avoid always supporting one child at the expense of another or giving older children too many privileges. You can minimize sibling rivalry by treating all your children equally and fairly.

MONITOR YOUR SYMPTOMS
FOOT PROBLEMS

Foot problems in children have many causes. Among the most common are infection, accidental injury, and distortion of the foot from improperly fitting shoes. Seek a doctor's advice if one or both of your children's feet become painful, swell, become infected, or develop an unusual appearance.

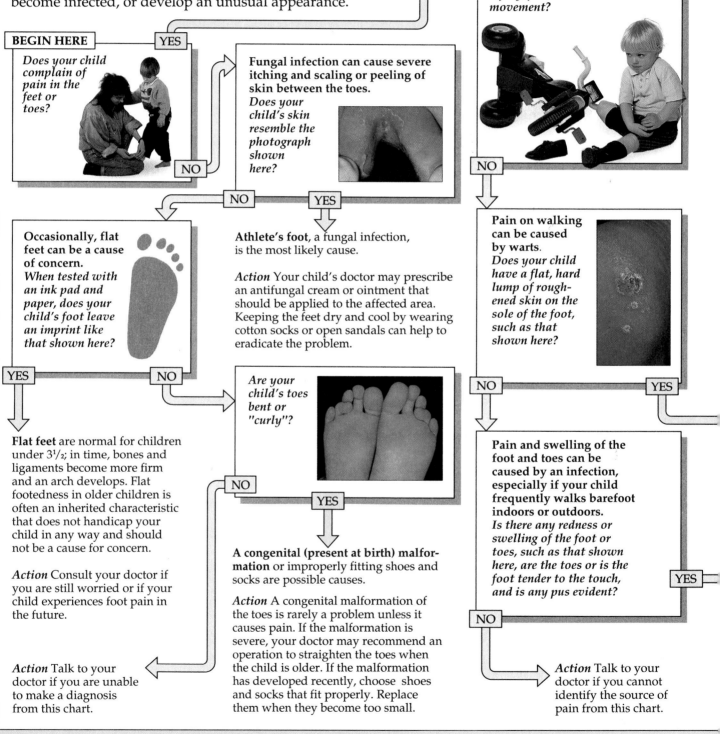

BEGIN HERE | **YES**

Does your child complain of pain in the feet or toes?

NO

Pain in the feet or toes can be caused by a variety of problems. *Did the pain follow an injury, fall, or sudden movement?* — **YES**

NO

Fungal infection can cause severe itching and scaling or peeling of skin between the toes. *Does your child's skin resemble the photograph shown here?*

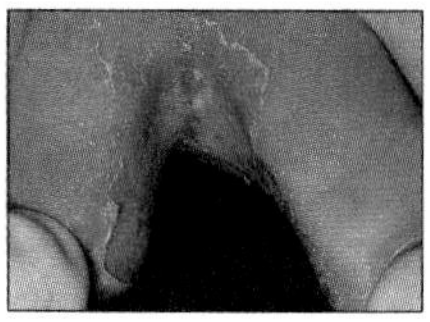

NO | **YES**

Athlete's foot, a fungal infection, is the most likely cause.

Action Your child's doctor may prescribe an antifungal cream or ointment that should be applied to the affected area. Keeping the feet dry and cool by wearing cotton socks or open sandals can help to eradicate the problem.

Occasionally, flat feet can be a cause of concern. *When tested with an ink pad and paper, does your child's foot leave an imprint like that shown here?*

YES | **NO**

Flat feet are normal for children under 3½; in time, bones and ligaments become more firm and an arch develops. Flat footedness in older children is often an inherited characteristic that does not handicap your child in any way and should not be a cause for concern.

Action Consult your doctor if you are still worried or if your child experiences foot pain in the future.

Action Talk to your doctor if you are unable to make a diagnosis from this chart.

Are your child's toes bent or "curly"?

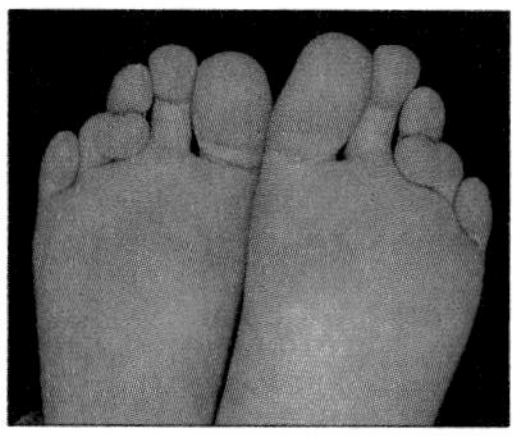

NO | **YES**

A congenital (present at birth) malformation or improperly fitting shoes and socks are possible causes.

Action A congenital malformation of the toes is rarely a problem unless it causes pain. If the malformation is severe, your doctor may recommend an operation to straighten the toes when the child is older. If the malformation has developed recently, choose shoes and socks that fit properly. Replace them when they become too small.

Pain on walking can be caused by warts. *Does your child have a flat, hard lump of roughened skin on the sole of the foot, such as that shown here?*

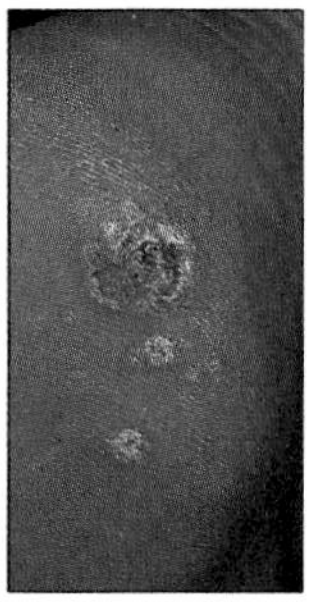

NO | **YES**

Pain and swelling of the foot and toes can be caused by an infection, especially if your child frequently walks barefoot indoors or outdoors. *Is there any redness or swelling of the foot or toes, such as that shown here, are the toes or is the foot tender to the touch, and is any pus evident?* — **YES**

NO

Action Talk to your doctor if you cannot identify the source of pain from this chart.

Accidental injury can cause dislocations and broken bones.
Is the foot or toe swollen and discolored?

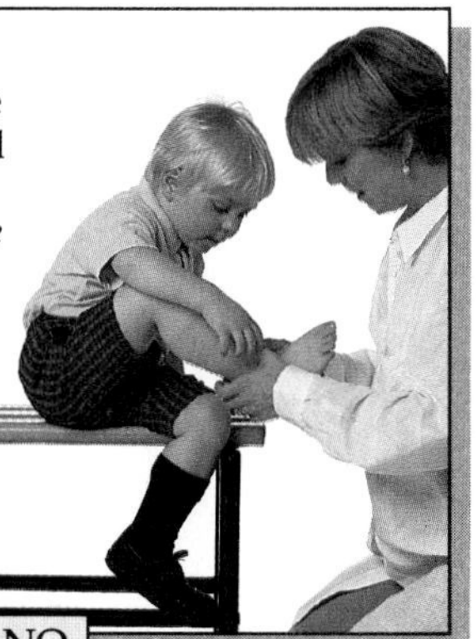

YES

NO

A minor sprain is likely.

Action Apply an ice pack to the foot and encourage your child to elevate and rest it for a few hours. If a marked limp is present or severe swelling, pain, or bruising develops, consult your doctor immediately.

SEEK MEDICAL ATTENTION IMMEDIATELY!

Dislocation or a fracture is possible.

Action Take your child to the hospital immediately. In the hospital, the foot will be X-rayed to determine the extent of the damage and may be immobilized with a bandage or plaster cast, depending on the nature of the injury.

Plantar warts (warts on the sole of the foot) are common in children.

Action Your doctor can recommend a treatment that slowly removes the wart or may decide to burn or freeze it off.

Infection from a break in the skin or the presence of an embedded object, such as a splinter, is the probable cause.

Action An embedded object can be removed by your doctor or at the hospital emergency department. If no such object is found, your child may receive an antibiotic to combat any infection. The doctor may also recommend a tetanus immunization.

CHOOSING THE RIGHT SHOES

Many foot problems in adults, such as bunions, painful corns, and crooked toes, are caused by poor foot care during childhood and adolescence. The bones of a child's foot are not fully formed until age 18. In children, especially those under age 5, bones and joints are soft and easily distorted by pressure from improperly fitting shoes and socks.

Babies' feet
Babies' feet do not need the rigid protection of shoes. Socks, booties, and one-piece suits should all provide warmth and enough room to move the toes easily. Even soft footwear that is too tight can restrict small feet.

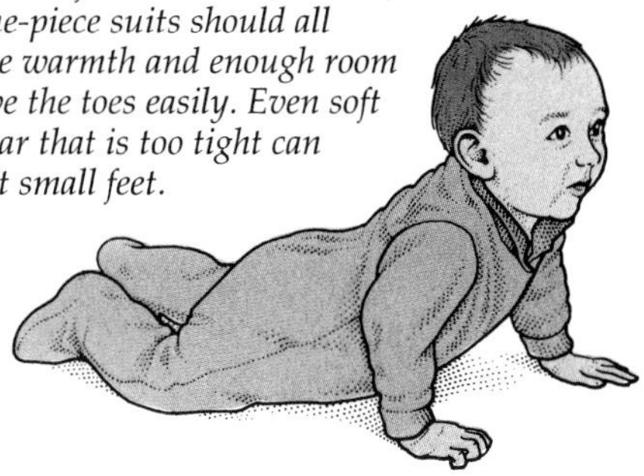

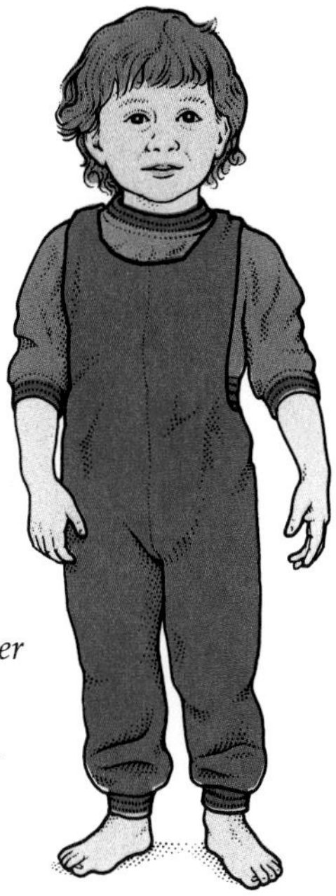

Toddlers' feet
Whenever possible, allow your toddler to walk barefoot inside your home. Delay buying shoes until your child is walking constantly and needs foot protection when walking outside.

Children's feet
Rapidly growing children should have their feet measured and refitted for shoes every 3 months. New shoes should not be too narrow and should allow a finger width of space for growth at the front of the shoe.

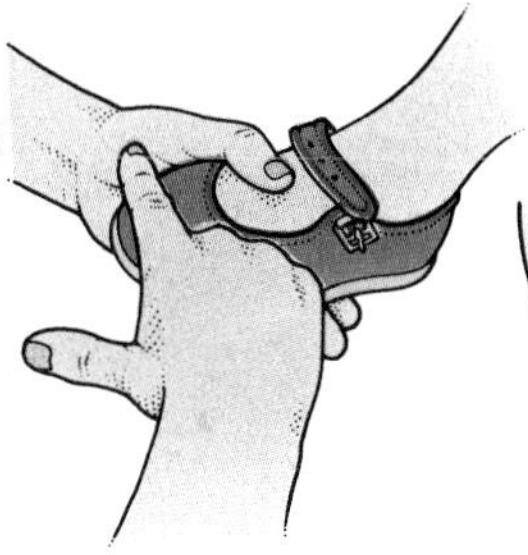

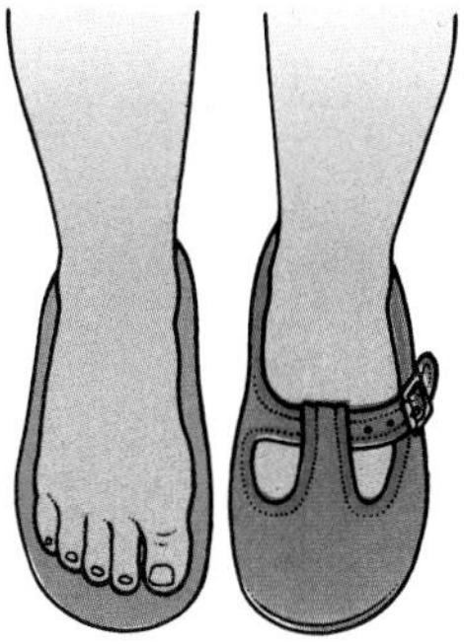

Shoe styles
Choose shoes with laces or straps that prevent the foot from slipping forward and cramping the toes. Shoes with elevated heels or pointed toes should be worn only on special occasions.

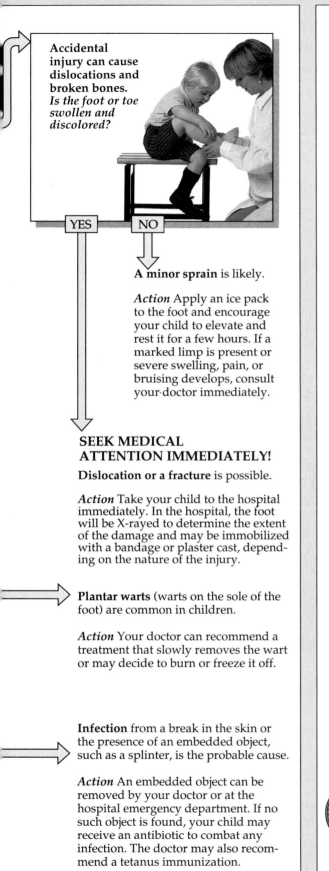

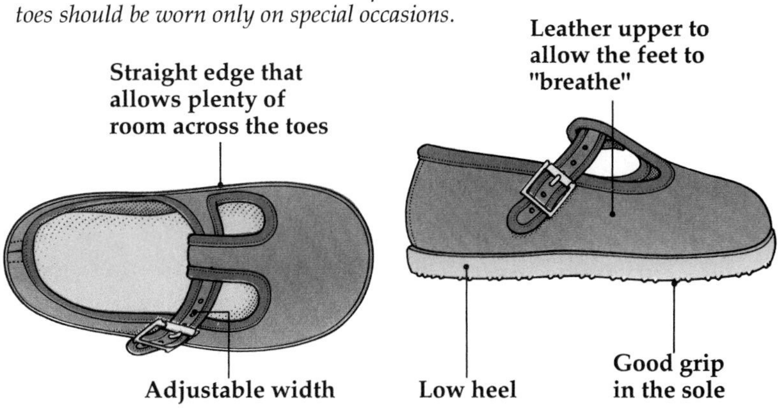

SAFEGUARDING YOUR CHILDREN

Young children must rely on adults completely to protect them. In time, they will understand the potential dangers of their environment. Because children are curious and inexperienced, minor accidents are inevitable, but you can reduce the likelihood of more serious accidents by making the child's home environment as safe as possible. Rather than simply forbidding an activity, explain the dangers so that your children can learn to anticipate hazards as they become more independent. Teach your children their full address and phone number in case they get lost and instruct them how to call 911 in an emergency.

Safety for older children

As children grow, they become more independent and spend more time away from home with their friends. Before allowing your child out on his or her own, warn against talking to strangers. You should not allow children under the age of 7 to cross busy streets alone, but you need to teach your children to look both ways before crossing the street at an early age so that it becomes a habit.

Children often enjoy activities with an element of danger, such as skate boarding. Parents should encourage responsible behavior in all activities and warn children of the risks involved. Provide your children with protective equipment, such as a bicycle helmet, and tell them to wear it at all times.

SAFETY TIPS FOR TODDLERS

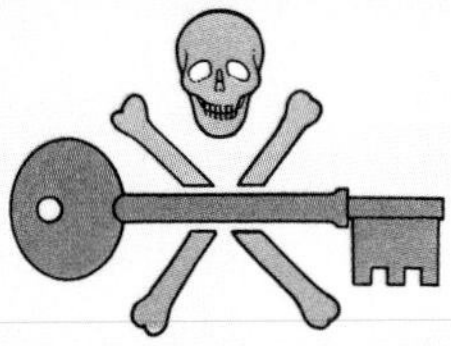

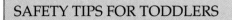

Preventing poisoning
To prevent accidental ingestion of poisons, keep all medicines, cleaning products, and gardening chemicals locked out of reach. Keep the number of your local poison control center handy. Have syrup of ipecac on hand to induce vomiting.

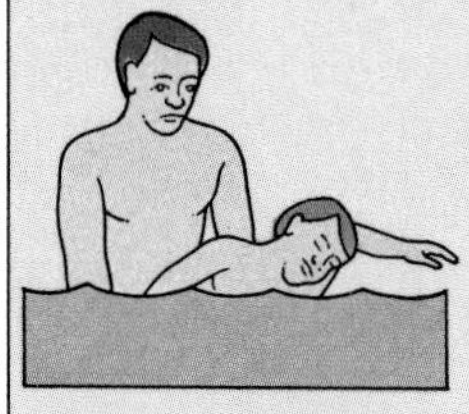

Preventing drowning
Young children can drown in very shallow water and should never be left alone in or near a tub or swimming pool. A toddler can even drown in a bucket of water or in the toilet bowl. Teach your child to swim and to observe water safety precautions as early as possible.

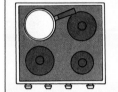

Preventing burns
Scalding can be prevented by turning pot handles inward when cooking. Keep electrical cables short and out of your children's reach. Use safety covers on all unused electrical outlets. Cover open fires with a screen. Keep matches out of reach.

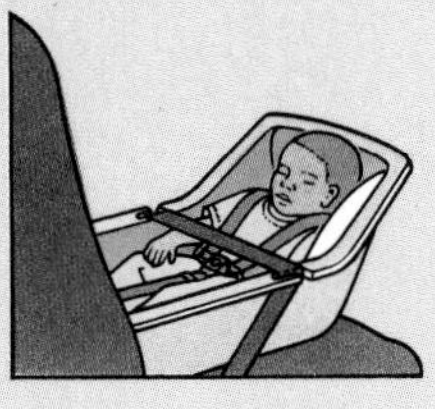

Traveling safely
Children younger than 10 should travel in the back seat of vehicles inside car seats. Put childproof locks on doors so that children cannot open them. Keep windows closed or opened only partially so that your children cannot put their arms or head outside the car.

Number of deaths in children aged 1 to 18 (1987)

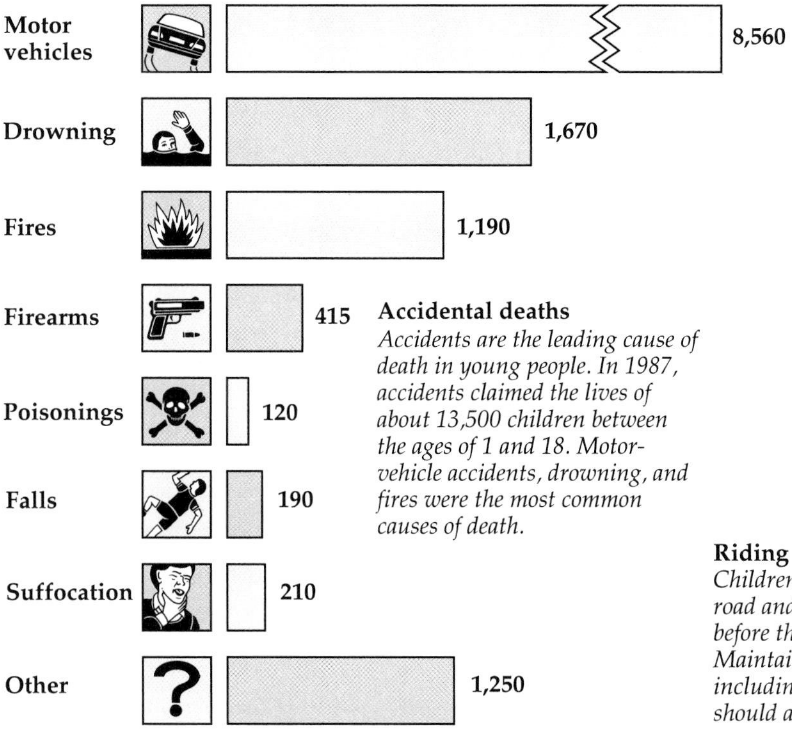

Accidental deaths
Accidents are the leading cause of death in young people. In 1987, accidents claimed the lives of about 13,500 children between the ages of 1 and 18. Motor-vehicle accidents, drowning, and fires were the most common causes of death.

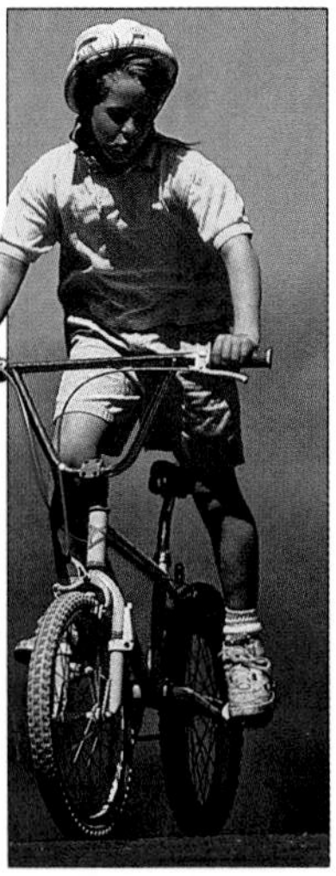

Riding a bike
Children should know the rules of the road and should be at least 8 years old before they ride a bike on the street. Maintain your child's bicycle, including lights and brakes. Children should always wear bicycle helmets.

TELEVISION IN THE HOME

Television is an important influence on children in the US. With your guidance, television can become a positive and valuable educational resource.

◆ Limit the amount of time your children watch television.
◆ Make sure that at least some of the programs they watch have educational value.
◆ Plan viewing times and allow your children to watch only specific programs that you have chosen in advance.
◆ Watch television with your children and discuss the program content with them.
◆ Monitor the programs that your children watch for violence and subject matter inappropriate for their age.
◆ Explain to your children why a particular program is not suitable for them to watch.

EDUCATION

A child's education begins at birth. Children learn how to speak and act by observing and imitating the example set by those around them. To encourage good language and problem-solving skills, you need to instruct your children from an early age and try to answer their questions clearly and honestly.

Helping your child learn

A child's performance at school reflects inherited intelligence and the amount of stimulation received at home. Learning should be fun rather than a chore. Parents can increase their child's motivation to learn by asking them about their progress at school and by offering help and advice. Children become easily distracted from schoolwork and benefit from having their own quiet place to study at home. Help your children to establish good study habits by setting aside a certain amount of time for homework each night.

Encourage after-school activities that the child enjoys, such as playing a musical instrument. Such activities boost confidence, help the child to relax, and provide a way to keep physically fit.

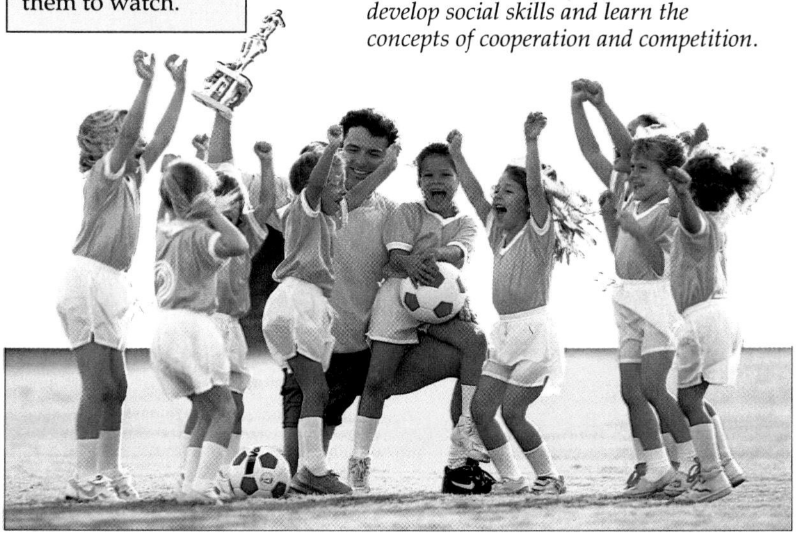

Learning through play
Play encourages the development of physical skills, such as hand-eye coordination. Through play with other children and adults, your children can develop social skills and learn the concepts of cooperation and competition.

ASK YOUR DOCTOR PLAY AND LEARNING

Q My 3-year-old likes to play on her own even when she is with other children. Is this unusual?

A Children of this age often play alongside rather than with other children. It takes time for toddlers to learn how to share, take turns, and interact with other children, especially if they have no siblings. Children develop social skills through experience. In time, your child will learn how to communicate and play with other children.

Q I want to buy toys for my grandson that are safe and educational. What should I look for?

A Make sure toys are appropriate for the child's age and abilities. Look for the manufacturer's age-approved labeling. Toys should be sturdy and should not have small parts that can be swallowed or inhaled. Do not buy loud toys that could damage the child's hearing. Books or brightly colored toys such as blocks help children learn about colors, sizes, and shapes.

Q My 5-year-old daughter cannot read at all yet. Is this kind of delay unusual?

A Children develop the memory and visual skills needed for reading at different rates and ages. Healthy children who start reading at a later age than average usually catch up with their peers if they're motivated. Children learn to read sooner if they are read to from an early age, are given plenty of encouragement, and see other family members reading. If you are worried because your daughter cannot yet read, discuss it with her teachers.

CARING FOR A SICK CHILD

When your child is sick, you must decide the best way to care for him or her. You can usually identify and treat common illnesses, such as a cold or stomach upset, at home. For more serious illnesses, such as measles, you may need help and advice from your doctor. Children under 2 years can become sick very quickly. It is best to seek your doctor's advice in the event of an unexplained illness.

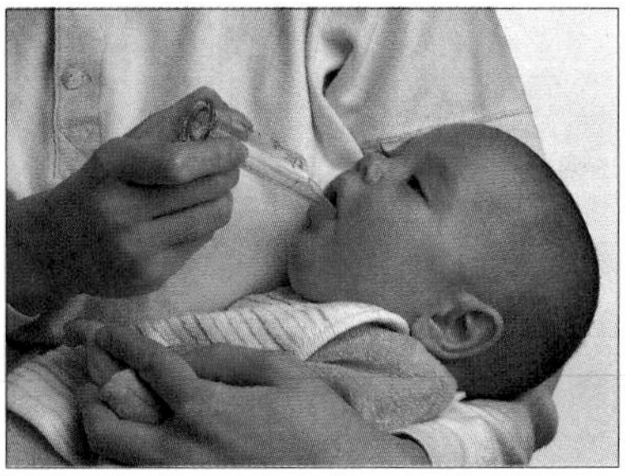

Giving medicines
Minor illnesses go away whether or not you give medicines. If your doctor has prescribed a medicine, follow the instructions exactly. The doses of medicines for children are much smaller than those for adults. Medicines given in too large a dose may be poisonous.

CHECKING FOR SYMPTOMS OF ILLNESS

Children who are irritable, clinging, pale, or listless or who eat less than usual are almost certainly sick. An unresponsive or inconsolable child is often very sick. Check the signs and symptoms below. If you notice any of these in your child, call your doctor.

WARNING

Call your doctor immediately if your baby has the following symptoms.
- ◆ No urine passed in 12 hours.
- ◆ A red or purple rash.
- ◆ Inconsolable crying for more than 1 hour.
- ◆ Persistent fever higher than 102°F.
- ◆ Lethargy that makes it difficult to arouse or feed your child.

Call a doctor when a child of any age has one or more of the following symptoms.
- ◆ Drowsiness and reluctance to eat, speak, or drink.
- ◆ Acute pain that does not improve quickly.
- ◆ Persistent wheezing or difficulty breathing.
- ◆ Repeated vomiting or diarrhea.
- ◆ Persistent fever of 104°F.
- ◆ Convulsions after a fall.

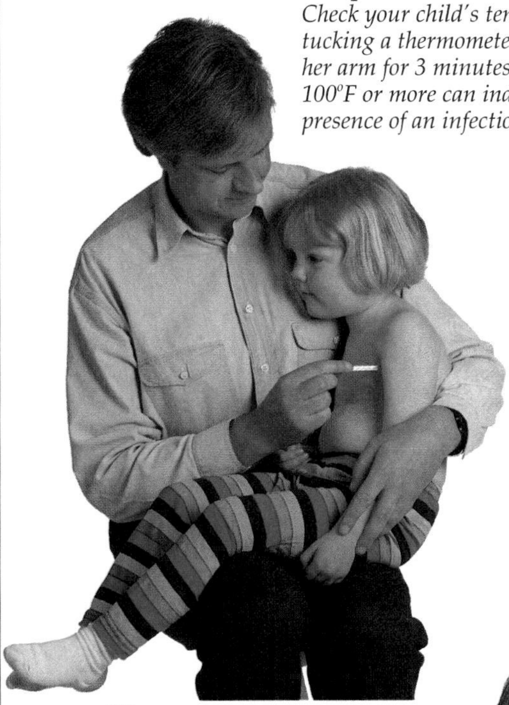

Temperature
Check your child's temperature by tucking a thermometer under his or her arm for 3 minutes. A fever of 100°F or more can indicate the presence of an infection.

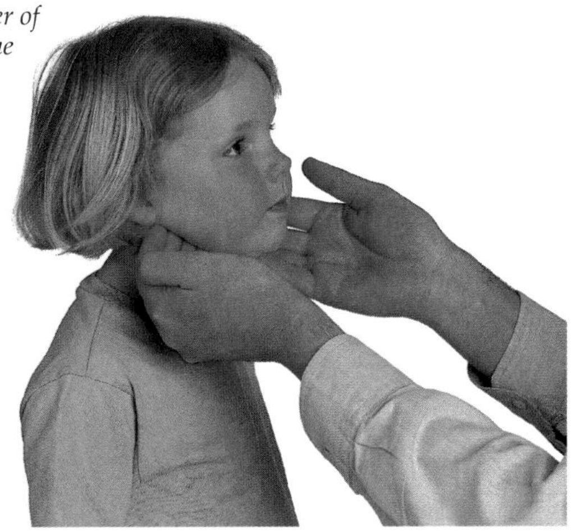

Swollen glands
Feel gently under your child's jawbone and on either side of the front and back of his or her neck. Swelling and tenderness in these areas are common signs of illness.

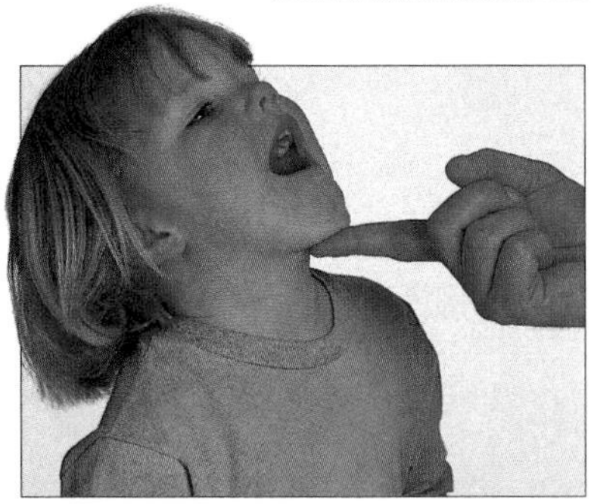

Throat infection
Examine your child's throat in good light. Redness or creamy spots in the throat and swollen tonsils indicate the presence of an infection.

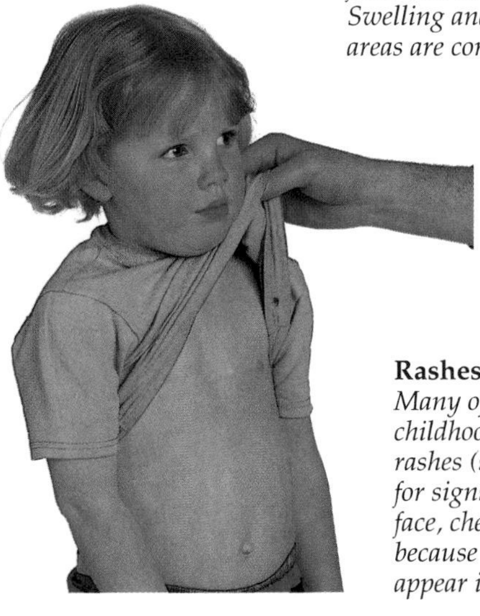

Rashes
Many of the common childhood infections produce rashes (see page 102). Check for signs of a rash on the face, chest, or abdomen, because rashes often first appear in these areas.

TREATING A FEVER

A fever signals that your child's body is fighting off an infection. Fevers usually last for a few days; during this time, children feel tired and sleep intermittently. Keep feverish children cool and comfortable. Give a feverish child plenty of fluids to prevent dehydration, especially if he or she is vomiting or has diarrhea.

WARNING

Never give aspirin to an infant, child, or teenager. Doctors have found a link between aspirin and Reye's syndrome, a rare disorder characterized by brain and liver damage.

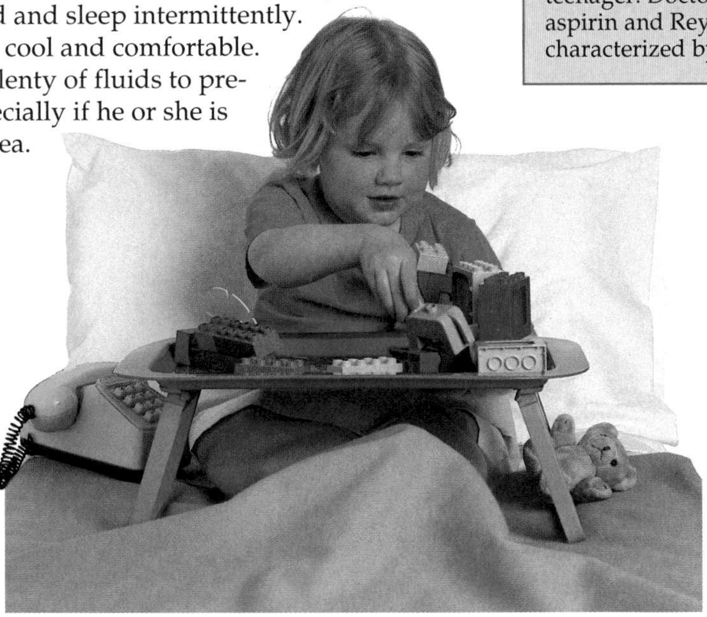

Favorite foods
To encourage sick children to eat, give them their favorite foods in small quantities.

Fluids
Encourage feverish children to drink fluids by offering them their favorite soft drinks, juices, or popsicles.

Entertainment
Recuperating children need to be entertained. During this period, they usually prefer quiet, simple games that are well within their capabilities.

Reducing a fever
Sponging down a feverish child with cool water (never alcohol) helps to lower body temperature and increase comfort. Medications such as acetaminophen also help to reduce a fever, but be sure to follow the recommended dose. Do not wrap the child in blankets.

The doctor's examination
To diagnose an illness, your doctor may listen to sounds in your child's chest with a stethoscope; examine his or her ears, nose, and throat; feel his or her abdomen; take his or her temperature; and check for swollen glands or lymph nodes. The doctor will ask you what your child's symptoms are and how long they have been present. If the doctor suspects a particular illness, he or she may recommend further tests.

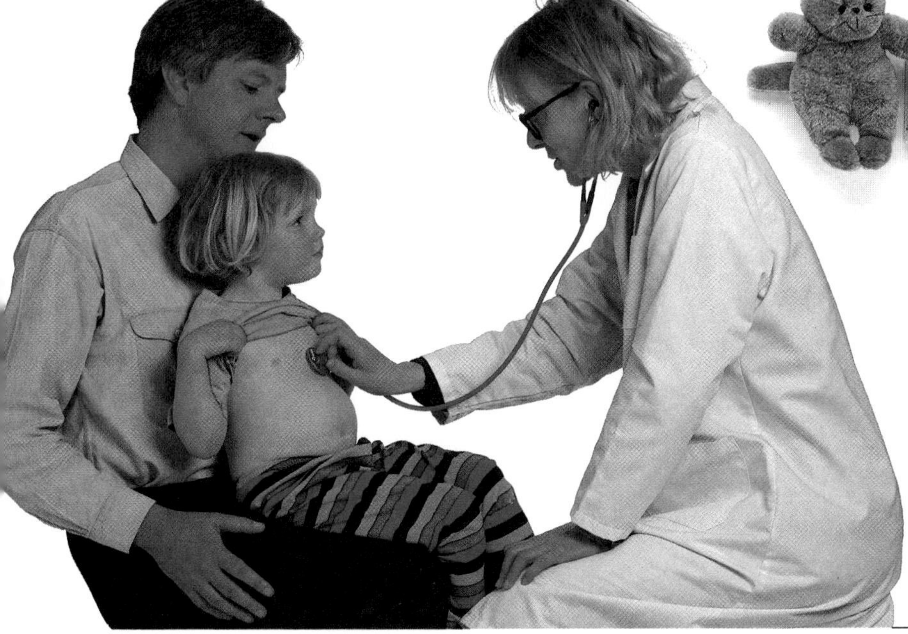

A HOSPITAL STAY

A stay in the hospital is frightening for a young child who has never been away from home. Explain why the child needs to go into the hospital and tell the child what is going to happen there. Ask if you and your child can take a get-acquainted tour before your child checks in.

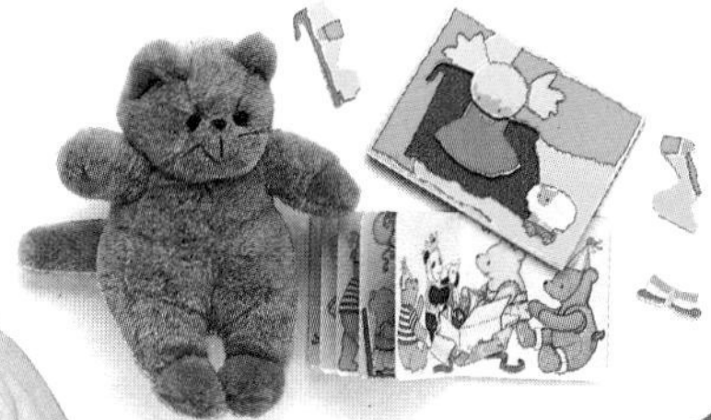

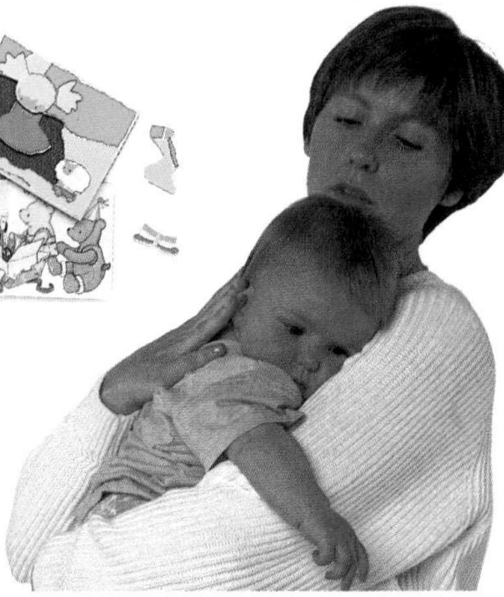

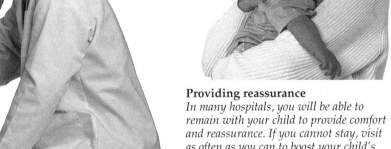

Providing reassurance
In many hospitals, you will be able to remain with your child to provide comfort and reassurance. If you cannot stay, visit as often as you can to boost your child's morale and to reduce his or her feelings of fear or loneliness. Favorite toys are a great source of comfort to an anxious child.

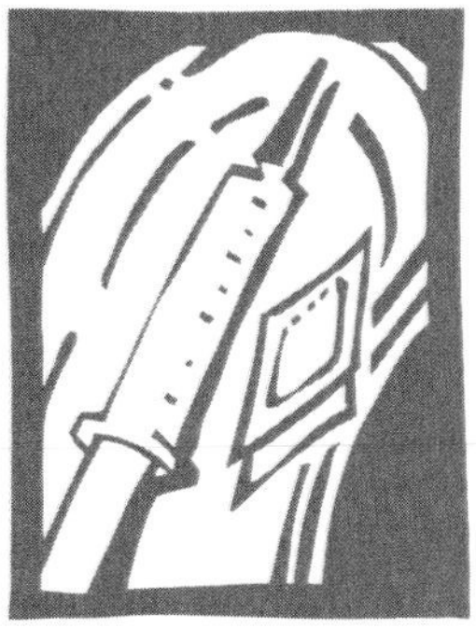

CHECKUPS AND IMMUNIZATIONS

YOUR PEDIATRICIAN WILL tell you how often to bring your child in for periodic checkups. Regular checkups enable the doctor to detect medical problems at an early stage when treatment may be more effective. Immunizations provide protection against a number of life-threatening and disabling diseases, such as whooping cough and poliomyelitis, that once struck thousands of children.

Children should see the doctor regularly throughout the year so that the doctor can monitor their height, weight, and health status. Because children can become seriously ill very quickly, call your doctor whenever your child's symptoms seem troubling or severe.

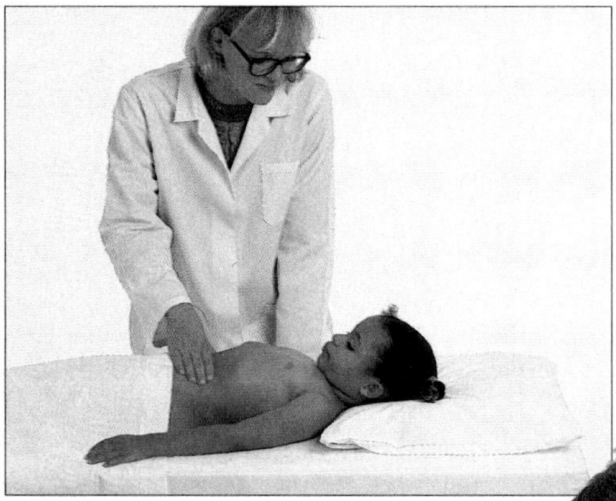

Examining abdominal organs
By gently pressing on your child's abdomen, the doctor can detect any swelling or abnormal growth in such abdominal organs as the liver or pancreas.

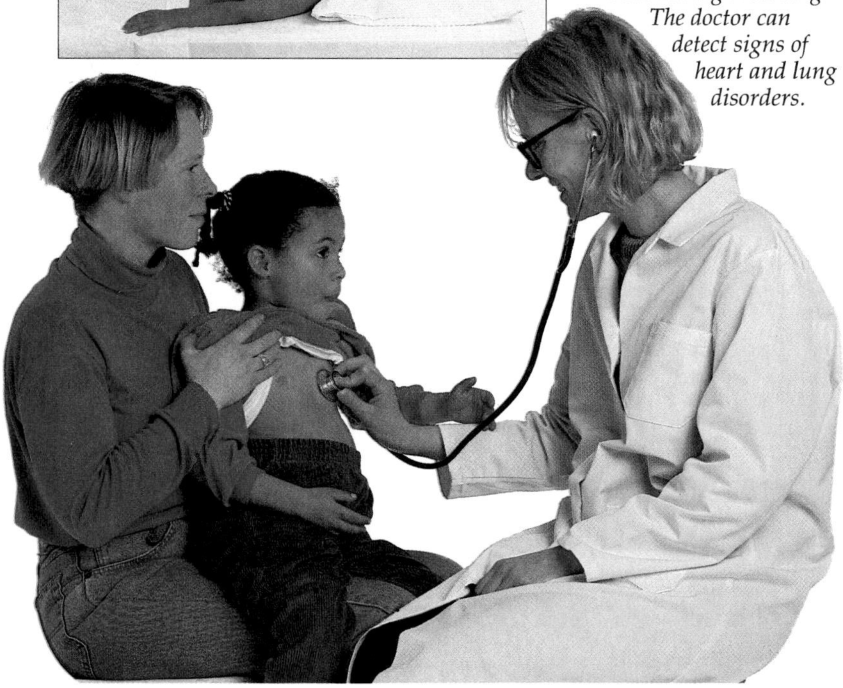

Checking heart and lung sounds
By placing a stethoscope on different areas of your child's chest, the doctor can listen to his or her heartbeat and the sounds made during breathing. The doctor can detect signs of heart and lung disorders.

YOUR CHILD'S DOCTOR

A doctor can best treat your child's problems when he or she is familiar with your child's medical history. Seeing the doctor regularly gives you a chance to discuss any concerns you may have about your child's health, behavior, or development. Your doctor can give you plenty of information about every aspect of child care, from diet and home safety to immunization. He or she will also make sure that your child is protected against disease by giving him or her the appropriate immunizations (see page 70).

Regular medical checkups are especially important during the first few years of your child's life, when growth and development are rapid. By performing a number of routine physical tests, the doctor can detect signs of illness or developmental delay at an early stage. The table on page 69 outlines the recommended ages for most routine checkups.

Monitoring growth

Your pediatrician regularly measures increases in your child's height and weight and plots the measurements on standard growth charts (see page 45). If your child's rate of growth changes, the doctor may order medical tests. Failure to grow is the only indication of some disorders. A slow growth rate can stem from some uncommon, treatable disorders, such as a hormone deficiency.

RECOMMENDED MEDICAL TESTS AND CHECKUPS FOR CHILDREN UNDER AGE 18

TEST	PURPOSE	FREQUENCY
Growth and development 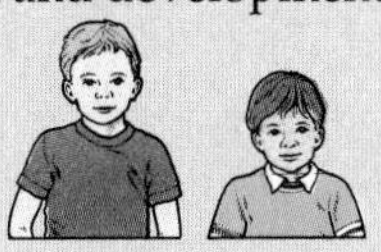	To detect signs of illness and any unusual delays in growth or development.	The doctor performs developmental and growth checks at birth, 2 to 4 weeks, 2, 4, 6, 9, 12, 15, and 18 months, 2, 2 1/2, and 3 years, and then yearly.
Hearing 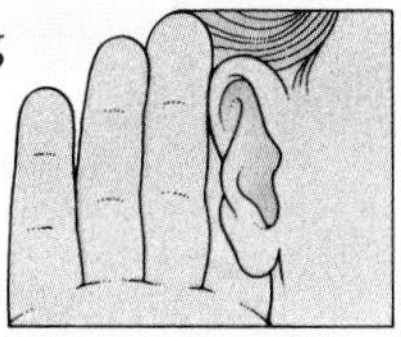	To detect any abnormality or infection in the ear that could impair hearing.	The doctor examines your child's ears at each routine physical examination. A hearing evaluation screening is performed when the child is 4 to 5 years old. Obvious delays in speech or hearing problems require a hearing evaluation.
Eyesight 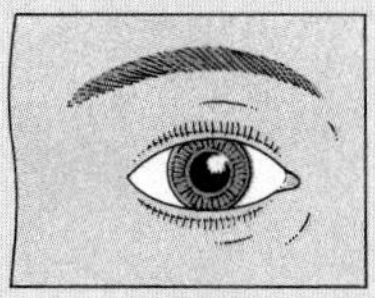	To detect any vision problems or irregularities in the eye muscles and to check for some medical conditions.	The doctor performs eye examinations at birth and at each routine visit. Eye movement, alignment, and sharpness of vision are checked at 4 to 6 months and then yearly. Yearly examination by an eye specialist is recommended if your child has eye problems. If not, eye tests are done every 3 years.
Dental 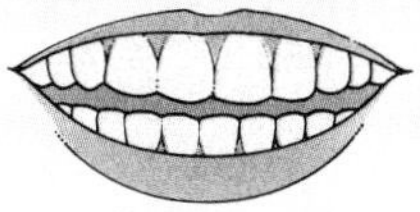	To detect signs of tooth decay, infection, and misalignment of teeth.	Starting at age 3, children should visit the dentist for a checkup every 6 months.

Monitoring development

A young child's physical growth normally coincides with improvements in hand-eye coordination, speech, problem-solving, and social skills (see DEVELOPMENTAL MILESTONES IN INFANCY AND CHILDHOOD on pages 22 and 48). By questioning you and your child, and by observing your child playing or performing simple tasks, the doctor can evaluate his or her current stage of mental and physical development. It is not useful to think in terms of your child passing or failing developmental tests. They are designed to assess your child's progress and to determine whether your child has acquired the skills that most of his or her peers have. If your child has not mastered a certain skill, such as walking or talking, by a particular time, your doctor will test for the skill again later. A child who has not developed a particular skill well beyond the usual age could be experiencing a delay in development.

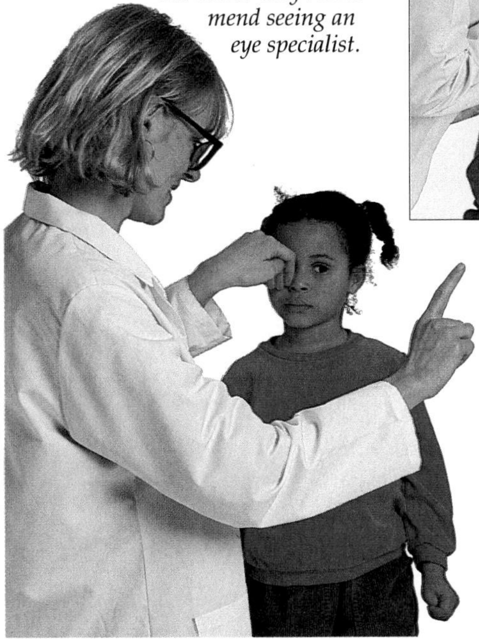

Examining the eyes
During a vision test, the doctor may cover each of the child's eyes in turn to find out whether the uncovered eye can focus on and follow a moving object. If the child has difficulty with a visual test, the doctor may recommend seeing an eye specialist.

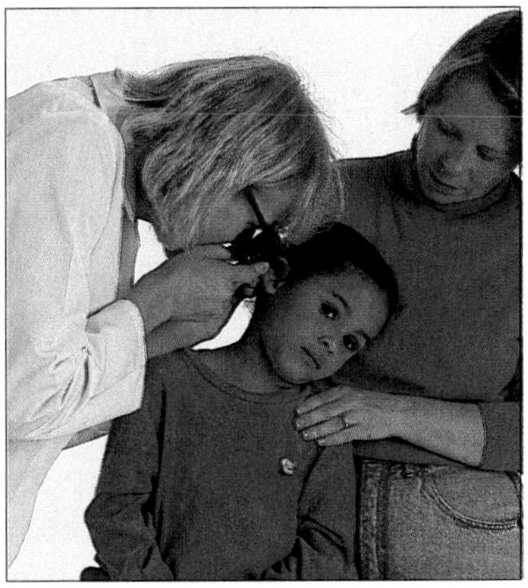

Examining the ears
Ear infections are common during childhood. Using a viewing instrument called an otoscope, the doctor checks to make sure that the ear canal is not blocked or that the eardrum is not infected. An accumulation of wax in the ear canal or fluid behind the eardrum can impair hearing.

LIFE-SAVING VACCINATIONS

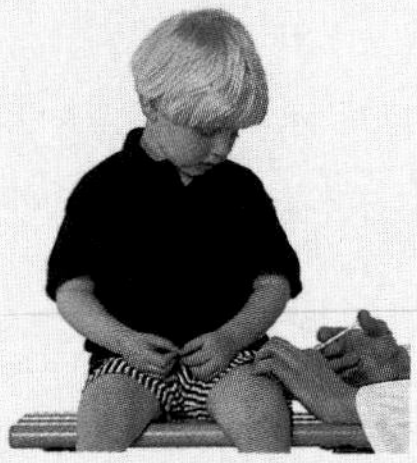

Vaccinations can protect against:

◆ Diphtheria – a disease characterized by high fever, severe sore throat, and heart and breathing problems.

◆ Poliomyelitis – a disease that can cause paralysis.

◆ Infection with *Haemophilus influenzae* type b (Hib) – a bacterium that can cause meningitis, inflammation of the membranes surrounding the brain.

◆ Tetanus – a bacterial infection that can cause muscle spasms and death.

◆ Whooping cough (pertussis) – a disease that causes a cough that disrupts breathing and can last several weeks.

◆ Measles – infection by a virus that can spread to the lungs or brain.

◆ Mumps – infection by a virus that causes swelling of the salivary glands; it can infect the testicles after puberty, causing sterility.

◆ Rubella (German measles) – infection by a virus that can cause birth defects in pregnant women.

◆ Hepatitis B – infection by a virus that causes inflammation of the liver.

IMMUNIZATIONS

Today, immunization can prevent several serious infectious diseases, such as measles, diphtheria, poliomyelitis, and whooping cough, that once killed and disabled thousands of children each year. Children are especially susceptible to infection because their immune systems have not been exposed to common diseases and so have not developed natural resistance to them. Without such resistance, or immunity, exposure to the organisms that cause infectious diseases can lead to life-threatening illness and permanent disabilities, such as paralysis, brain damage, and heart problems.

Immunization increases a child's resistance to infectious disease by artificially stimulating his or her immune system to produce substances called antibodies that attack the disease-causing organisms. Your child may need more than one immunization to provide long-lasting resistance. The initial immunization starts the body's production of antibodies against the disease, and later immunizations, sometimes called boosters, reinforce the existing protection.

Travel vaccinations
Travel in a foreign country may require immunization against diseases common in the destination country. To find out whether your family needs immunization, call your doctor 3 months before you leave.

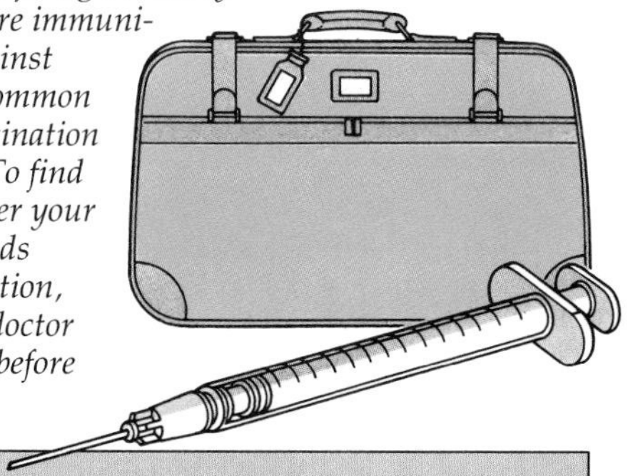

RECOMMENDED IMMUNIZATION SCHEDULE FOR CHILDREN UP TO AGE 18		
AGE	**DISEASE**	**ROUTE**
2 months	Diphtheria, whooping cough, and tetanus *Haemophilus influenzae* type b (Hib) infection (a cause of meningitis) Hepatitis B Poliomyelitis	Combined injection Separate injection Separate injection Oral
4 months	Diphtheria, whooping cough, and tetanus *Haemophilus influenzae* type b (Hib) infection Hepatitis B Poliomyelitis	Combined injection Separate injection Separate injection Oral
6 months	Diphtheria, whooping cough, and tetanus *Haemophilus influenzae* type b (Hib) infection Hepatitis B	Combined injection Separate injection Separate injection
15 months	Measles, mumps, and rubella (German measles) *Haemophilus influenzae* type b (Hib) infection	Combined injection Separate injection
18 months	Diphtheria, whooping cough, and tetanus Poliomyelitis	Combined injection Oral
4 to 6 years	Diphtheria, whooping cough, and tetanus Poliomyelitis	Combined injection Oral
11 to 12 years	Measles, mumps, and rubella	Combined injection
14 to 16 years	Diphtheria and tetanus	Combined injection

TUBERCULOSIS SKIN TEST

Tuberculosis is a chronic (long-term) disease that affects the lungs, causing pain, coughing, and shortness of breath. Tuberculosis tends to occur in economically depressed areas of cities and in nonindustrialized countries but it can occur anywhere. People whose immune systems are compromised, such as people undergoing chemotherapy, are more susceptible than the general population. In the US, doctors recommend that children have a periodic tuberculosis skin test. Doctors treat children who have a positive skin test with medication.

Immunization programs

Immunizations can provide the maximum protection against a disease only when children receive them at specific ages. For this reason, you need to follow a recommended immunization program (see table on page 70). You should keep a record of your child's immunizations so you know when he or she is due for the next one. If your child starts the immunization program late, or misses some vaccinations, your doctor can adjust the schedule to bring him or her up to date.

Possible aftereffects

Some immunizations may make your child feel sick for a short time. For example, after the measles-mumps-rubella vaccine, your child may develop a rash within a week to 10 days. Joint aches may begin 7 to 10 days after your child receives the rubella vaccine. After any injected vaccination, a small lump may develop at the injection site. The lump should subside in about a week or two. Remember that the life-saving benefits of immunization far outweigh the possible risks of minor side effects.

PREPARING YOUR CHILD FOR A SHOT

All shots hurt a little. Babies often react by crying for a few minutes, but they quickly forget the experience, especially if you comfort them right away with a feeding. Explain to an older child what to expect from a shot and why he or she is getting it. If your child is apprehensive, try to divert his or her attention from the needle by holding or comforting him or her. A reward can often make the experience less upsetting.

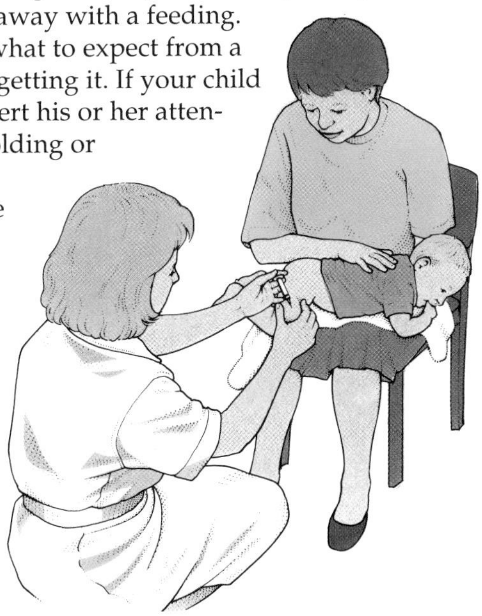

Getting a shot
To provide comfort and reassurance, hold your child gently but firmly during an injection. Babies usually receive injections in the thigh; older children may receive them in the upper arm.

ASK YOUR DOCTOR IMMUNIZATIONS

Q I have heard that the vaccine for whooping cough can cause brain damage. Is this true?

A Recent research done on possible adverse effects of the diphtheria, pertussis (whooping cough), and tetanus (DPT) vaccine found that no clear evidence exists linking the vaccine and the occurrence of brain damage. The vaccine infrequently causes febrile seizures (see page 118). The benefits of vaccination outweigh this very small risk.

Q My child is terrified of shots. Why can't all vaccines be given to children by mouth?

A Because the digestive tract would destroy most vaccines. To ensure that they are effectively absorbed into the bloodstream, most vaccines are injected into a muscle or into fat underneath the skin.

Q My daughter received all of her vaccinations against whooping cough but she still got the disease. Why did this happen?

A Vaccinations reduce but don't eliminate the likelihood of developing a given disease. Children who have been vaccinated against whooping cough occasionally contract the disease, but they are usually less severely affected than children who have not been vaccinated.

Q Is there a vaccine that protects against chickenpox?

A A vaccine for chickenpox is available only for children with weakened immune systems. Use of the vaccine in healthy children is still being tested.

CHAPTER FOUR

DISORDERS OF INFANCY AND CHILDHOOD

A sick child is always a source of concern for parents. The anxiety may spring from your inability to identify the problem and your questions about how serious the illness might be. Always remember that you might be able to influence your sick child's condition for the better simply by learning more about it. Knowledgeable parents exude confidence, and the child feels safer and less upset by the symptoms.

All children get sick at some time but, thanks to widespread immunization and new treatments, few illnesses pose the threat to a child's life that they once did. As a parent, you must be on the lookout for early warning signs of illness. Sometimes the earliest indication of illness in a child is a sudden change in his or her behavior, such as refusing to eat or being quieter – or crankier – than usual. Such subtle changes are usually perceived only by a person who knows the child very well.

Most childhood illnesses are minor. In such cases, your child needs nothing more from you than sympathy and reassurance. As a parent, you must decide when to let your child's illness run its course, when to consult your doctor, or, in serious cases, when to take your child to the nearest hospital emergency department. As a basic guideline, you should always seek medical advice if you are uncertain about what to do.

In general, babies, toddlers, and older children do not get the same illnesses as adults, but children are especially susceptible to certain infections, such as measles, chickenpox, and whooping cough. By learning in advance about these infections, you will know what to expect should they ever occur in your child. This chapter describes the most common disorders of infancy and childhood and explains how doctors diagnose and treat them. Many of these disorders, such as heat rash, are not serious and respond quickly to simple treatment. Serious disorders are far less common in children than are minor conditions, such as a sore throat. But serious childhood disorders often have characteristic symptoms, so doctors can diagnose them more easily.

Some young children have health problems that are present from birth (congenital), such as cerebral palsy, but doctors may not be able to discover these problems immediately. The extent to which a child is disabled by a congenital disorder depends on its severity, but doctors routinely screen for most birth defects. Prompt treatment improves the outlook for an affected child. This chapter also describes childhood behavioral problems, such as temper tantrums, and offers advice on ways to handle them.

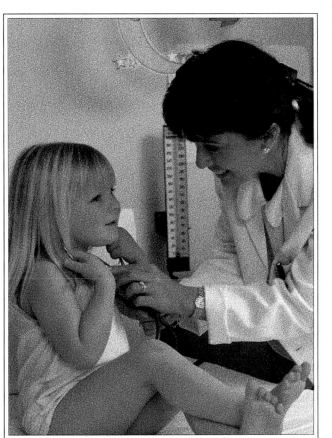

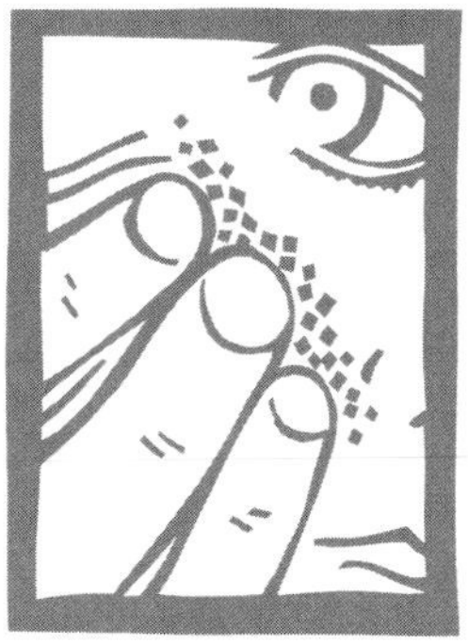

SKIN PROBLEMS

SUNLIGHT, HARSH DETERGENTS, and cold, dry air can all damage a person's skin. But your child's sensitive skin is especially vulnerable to injury and infection. Most skin problems that affect children are minor and respond rapidly to treatment. Serious skin conditions rarely occur in infants and young children.

HEAT RASH

Heat rash, or prickly heat, is a rash that consists of numerous tiny red pimples. The rash usually occurs in areas where sweat gathers, such as around the neck. Alleviate heat rash by ensuring that your child avoids excess heat, wears loose clothing, and takes cool baths or showers regularly.

Because your child's skin is so soft and new, changes in his or her skin become readily apparent. Doctors can identify and treat most childhood skin problems at an early stage. A change in the skin may arise from irritation or damage by agents as diverse as insect bites, rough or tight clothing, infectious organisms, soaps, allergens, or sunlight.

CHILDHOOD RASHES

Doctors define a rash as a group of spots or blisters or an area of red, inflamed skin that may be accompanied by itching or fever. A rash may be localized (affecting only a small area of skin) or generalized (covering the entire body). Rashes and itching characterize some common childhood infections, such as chickenpox and measles. But many rashes signal a disorder affecting the skin itself.

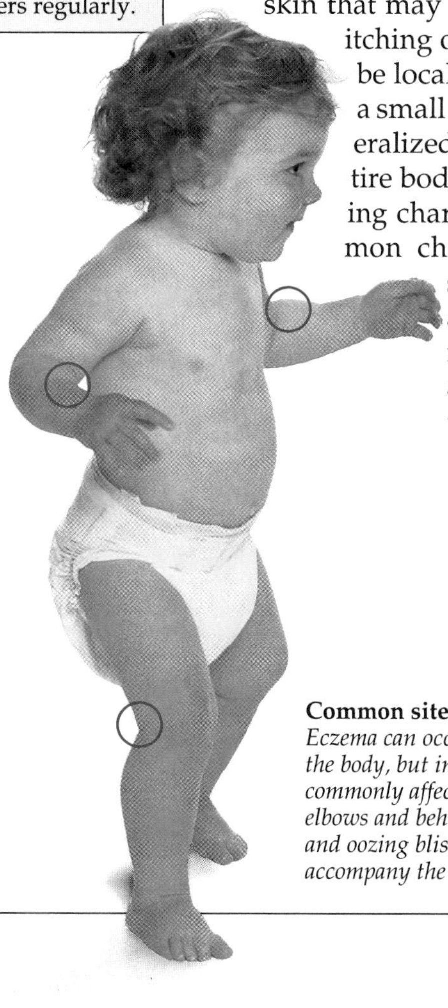

Affected areas

Common sites of eczema
Eczema can occur anywhere on the body, but in children it most commonly affects the areas inside the elbows and behind the knees. Scaling and oozing blisters sometimes accompany the rash.

Contact dermatitis
Certain substances can cause a burning, itchy, red rash if they come into contact with the child's skin. This reaction may be a direct toxic effect of the substance or may be an allergic response by the skin. Common causes of contact dermatitis include detergents and certain plants, such as poison ivy (below). Calamine lotion and inflammation-fighting creams may help relieve symptoms.

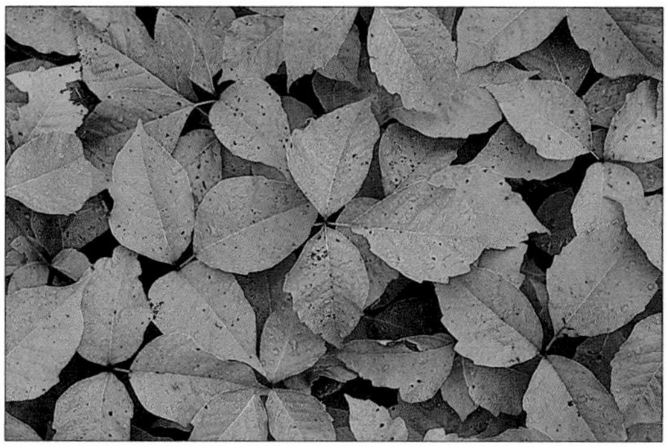

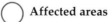

Eczema

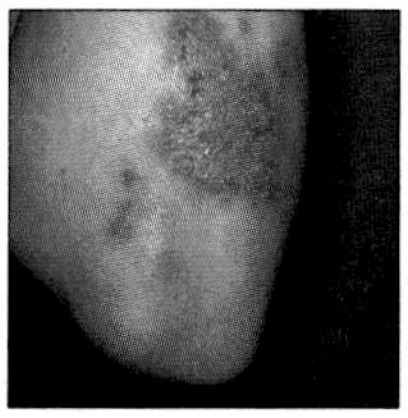

Usually caused by an allergy, eczema produces a red, itchy, and scaling rash. A child can't help scratching the rash, and scratching often disturbs sleep and causes irritability. Children with eczema are likely to have very dry skin and are also prone to other allergic conditions, such as asthma and hay fever. The condition tends to run in families. Eczema usually clears up on its own as the child grows older, although the disorder may come and go for several years before finally disappearing. Most children outgrow the condition by the time they reach puberty.

If your child has eczema, try to keep his or her skin well moisturized – use plenty of moisturizing creams and add oil or moisturizers to bath water. Even

Chilblains
Chilblains are painful, purple marks or swellings caused by excess cold. They may include areas of broken skin and occur mainly on the fingers, toes, and nose. Prevent chilblains by making sure that your child wears warm, dry footwear and gloves in cold weather. If your child develops chilblains, they will disappear on their own within a few weeks.

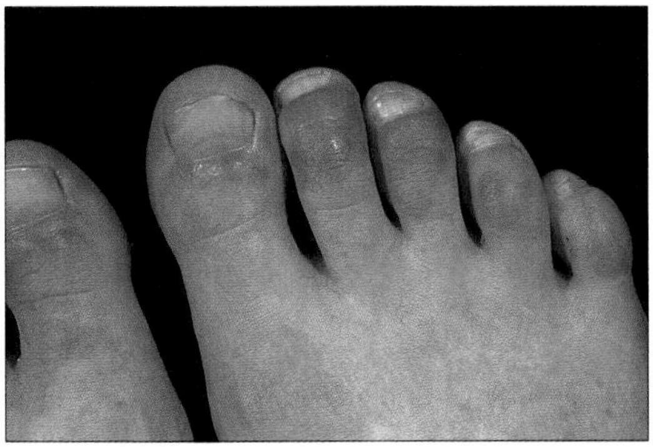

mild soaps can strip the skin of its natural oils. Use moisturizing soaps, or those with a high fat content, when bathing your child. Excessive heat aggravates itching, so avoid using too many blankets and bathe your child in lukewarm water. Do not dress your child in wool clothing that could irritate the skin.

Antihistamine drugs may relieve the irritation produced by eczema, help prevent scratching, and enable your child to sleep at night. If the eczema is severe, your doctor may prescribe a cream or ointment containing an inflammation-fighting corticosteroid drug.

Seborrheic dermatitis

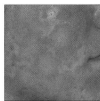

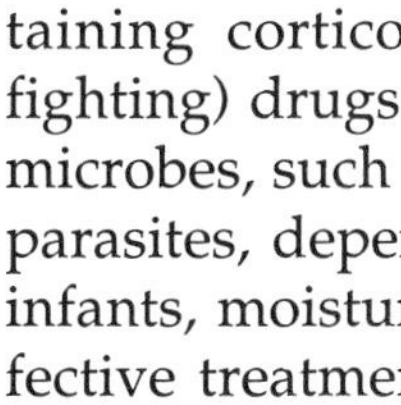

Seborrheic dermatitis is a red, scaly, itchy rash that develops on the face (especially the nose and eyebrows), scalp, chest, and back. The exact cause of the rash is unknown. Doctors treat the condition with ointments containing corticosteroid (inflammation-fighting) drugs or medications that kill microbes, such as viruses, bacteria, and parasites, depending on the cause. For infants, moisturizers or baby oil are effective treatments. Avoid using irritating substances, such as detergents, that can worsen the condition.

Psoriasis

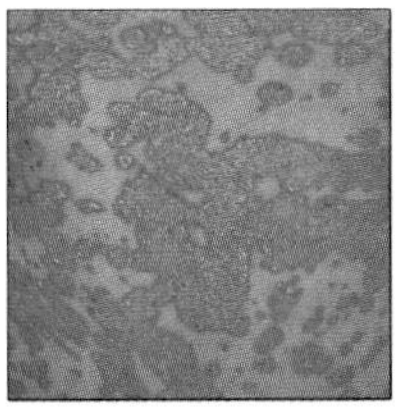

Psoriasis is characterized by round, red, thickened areas of skin covered by silvery, scaly patches. The condition does not produce itching. Psoriasis typically develops on the child's elbows, knees, or scalp, although it often starts as a scaly rash over the entire body. Doctors quite commonly see psoriasis in infants and children. In infants, psoriasis often looks like a persistent diaper rash that resists common treatments. The disorder tends to run in families. Treatment usually includes applications of coal tar ointment and shampoo. Other methods of treatment include the use of corticosteroid drugs or a form of ultraviolet light therapy.

Hives

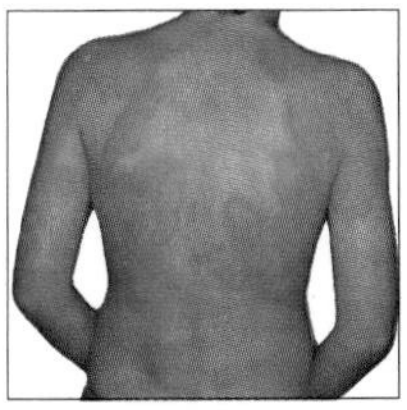

Hives (also called urticaria) is a common itchy, raised rash consisting of red blotches with white centers. The rash develops during a period of minutes or hours. Hives is usually caused by an allergic reaction triggered by, for example, eating a particular food. Often, doctors cannot find the precise cause. Try eliminating certain factors from your child's environment to identify the trigger. Calamine lotion and antihistamine drugs relieve the itching caused by hives.

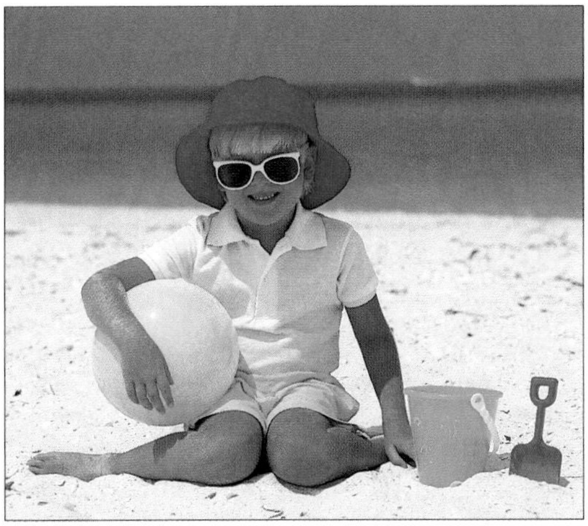

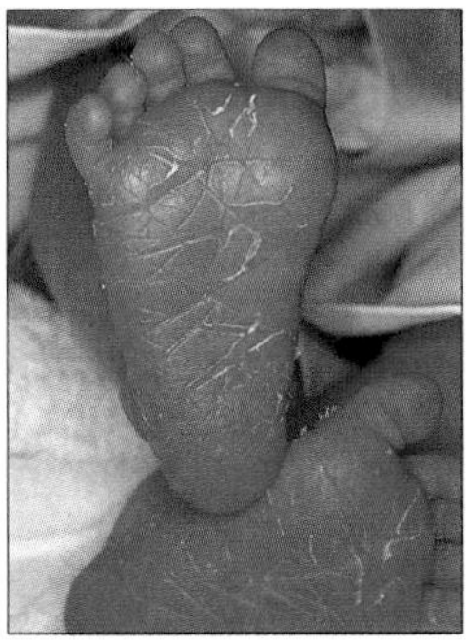

Dry, chapped skin
Cold weather and low humidity cause the skin to produce less oil. Dry skin feels rough and itchy and tends to become cracked and sore. The lips, hands, and face are especially prone to chapping. Alleviate dryness with frequent use of moisturizing creams or petroleum jelly.

DANDRUFF

Dandruff, a condition in which scaly flakes of dead skin accumulate on the scalp, is a very common problem in children. Dandruff is a mild form of seborrheic dermatitis. You can effectively treat dandruff by regularly washing your child's hair with one of the many available antidandruff shampoos.

Sunburn
A child's skin becomes sunburned easily. Protect your child's skin with light clothing, a hat, and a sunscreen, especially between 10 AM and 2 PM. Treat mild sunburn by soaking burned areas in lukewarm water.

INFECTIONS AND INFESTATIONS OF THE SKIN

Most childhood skin infections are not serious and doctors can diagnose and treat them easily. Many different infections can affect the skin, including those caused by bacteria, viruses, and fungi. The skin and hair can be invaded by both microorganisms and larger parasites, such as mites, ticks, and lice. Doctors can easily treat infestations of these organisms by applying antiparasitic preparations to the affected area.

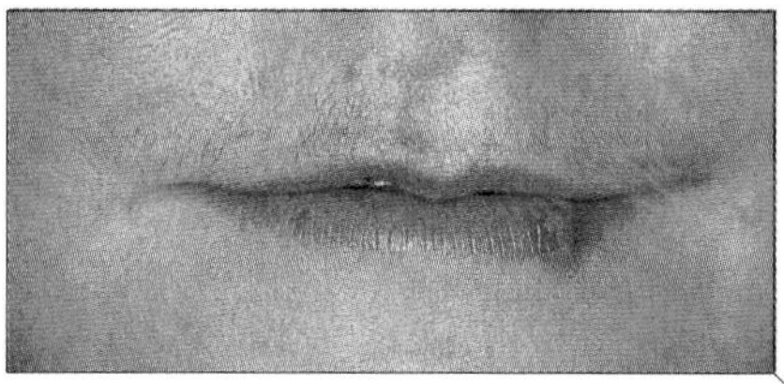

Cold sores
Infection with the herpes simplex virus causes cold sores. They begin as small, irritating blisters on the lips and around the mouth. Within a day or two, the blisters burst and form a sore. A crust forms over the sore, which heals in about a week. Cold sores tend to recur during periods of illness or after exposure to direct sunlight or cold wind.

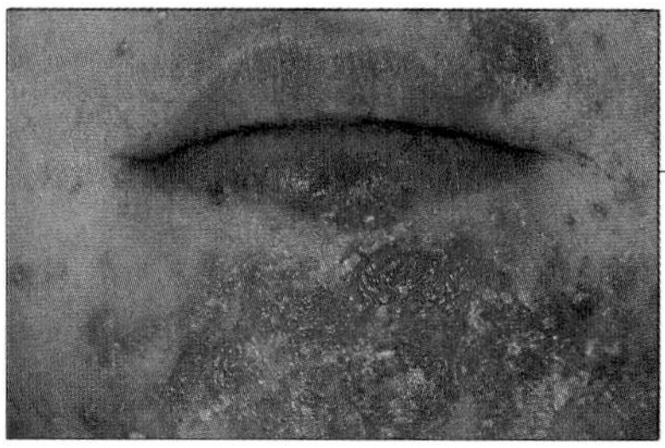

Impetigo
Impetigo is an infection caused by bacteria that usually occurs around the nose, mouth, and chin. It begins as small, red spots that break down, forming a weeping area covered by a brown crust. Impetigo is highly contagious. A child with impetigo should not interact with other children until the infection has healed. Doctors treat impetigo with antibiotics.

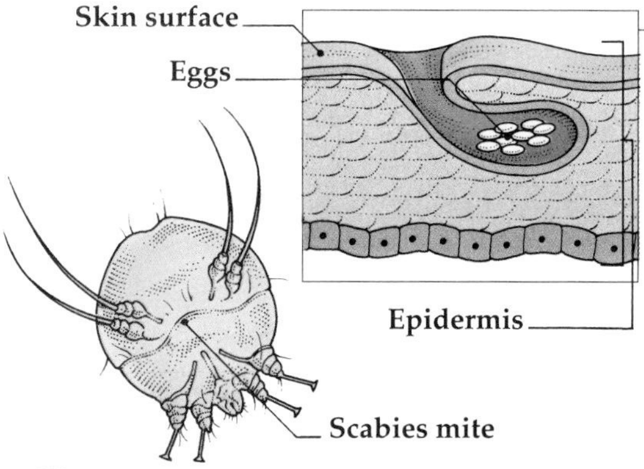

Scabies
Scabies is a highly contagious condition caused by tiny mites that burrow into the skin to lay eggs. The mites produce a red, very itchy rash. Sites affected are the areas between the fingers and the wrists, elbows, feet, underarms, and genital area. Physical contact spreads scabies. Doctors treat scabies by applying insecticide lotion over the child's entire body, except the head. The whole family must be treated at the same time.

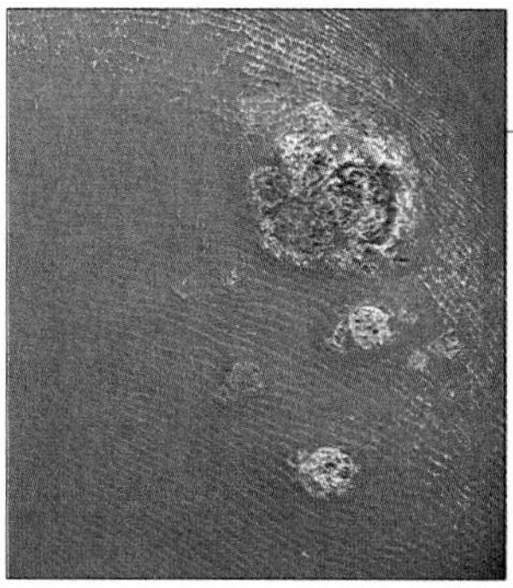

Warts
The growths known as warts are caused by a virus infection of the skin. Many children get warts on their hands or feet at some time. Warts on the soles of the feet are called plantar warts, and you may need to take your child to a dermatologist (a doctor who specializes in skin disorders) to have one removed. Other warts usually clear up on their own after a few months. Applications of a mild acid are often effective. Your doctor may also remove warts by cryotherapy (freezing).

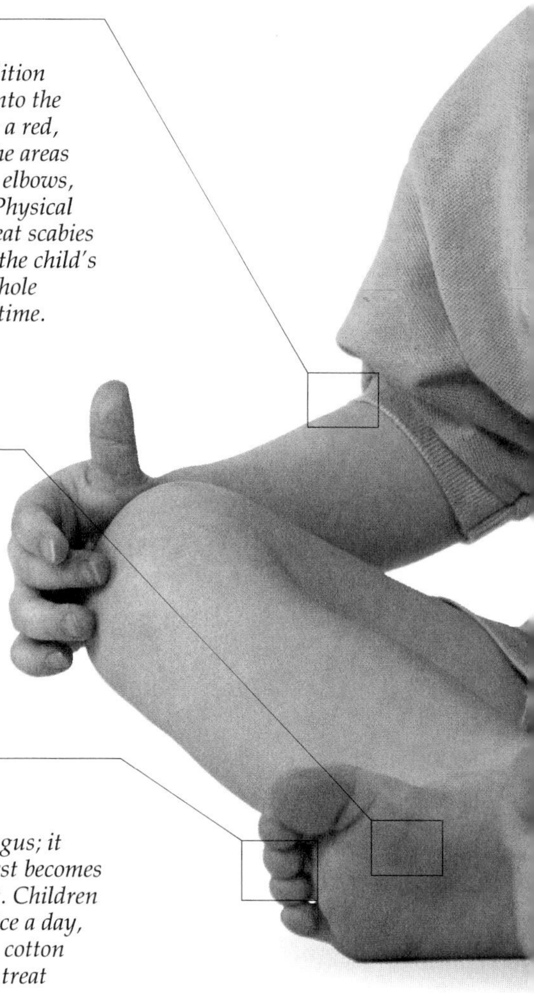

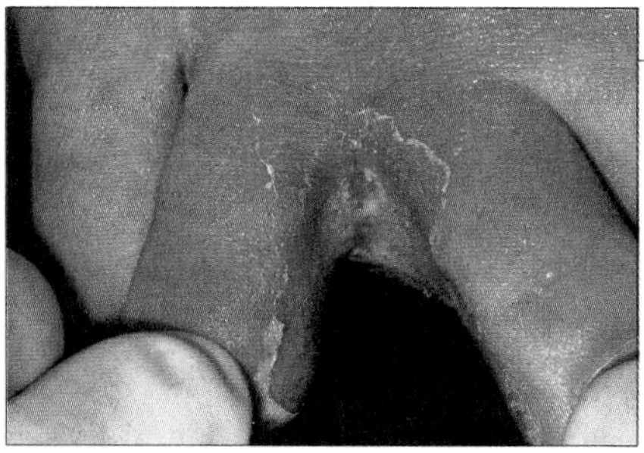

Athlete's foot
Athlete's foot is an infection caused by a fungus; it affects the skin between the toes. The skin first becomes red, scaly, and itchy, then cracked and moist. Children with athlete's foot should wash their feet twice a day, and dry them thoroughly. They should wear cotton socks and try to keep their feet cool. Doctors treat athlete's foot with an antifungal cream.

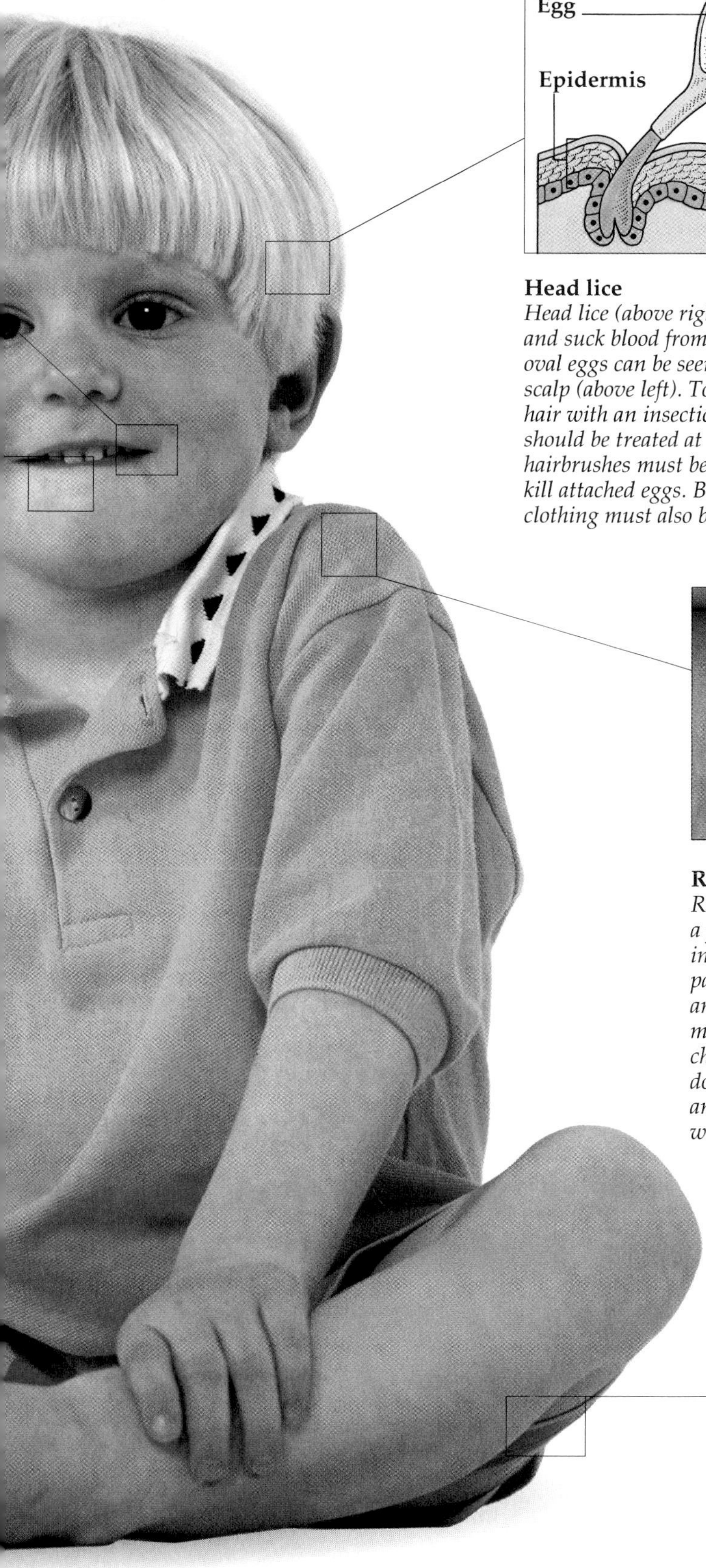

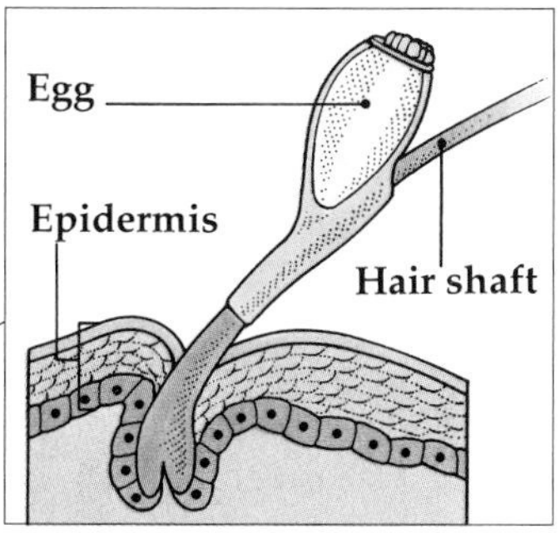

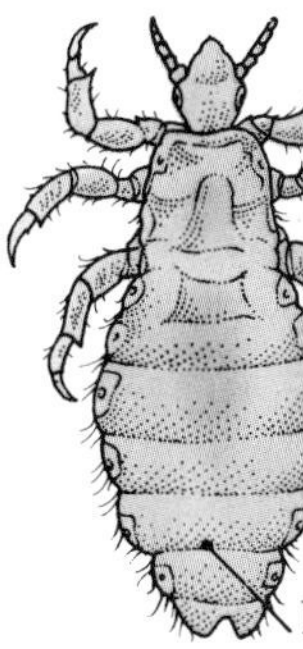

Head lice
Head lice (above right) are tiny insects that live on and suck blood from the scalp. Their small, white, oval eggs can be seen attached to hairs close to the scalp (above left). To treat head lice, wash the child's hair with an insecticidal shampoo. The entire family should be treated at the same time. Combs and hairbrushes must be cleaned in very hot water to kill attached eggs. Bed linens, hats, and hoods on clothing must also be cleaned.

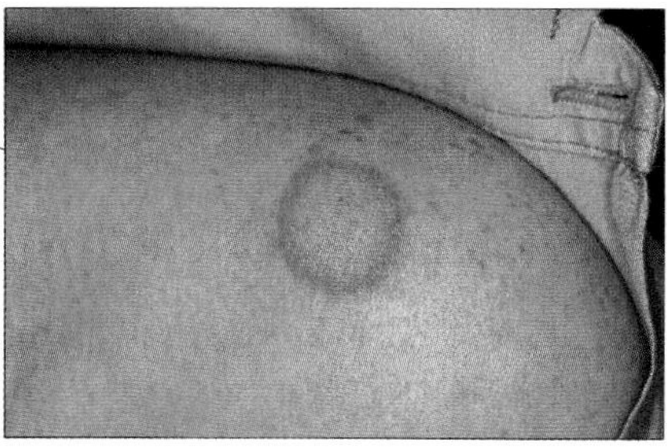

Ringworm
Ringworm is a common infection caused by a fungus that affects the skin or scalp. The infection produces itchy, red, ring-shaped patches with tiny blisters around the edges and a pale center. On the scalp, ringworm may cause bald patches. In many cases, children catch the infection from cats or dogs. Doctors treat ringworm with an antifungal ointment or, in severe cases, with a course of medication taken by mouth.

TICKS

Ticks attach themselves to human or animal skin and feed on blood. In the US, certain ticks can transmit Lyme disease and Rocky Mountain spotted fever. If your child walks in a tick-infested area, make sure that he or she wears long pants tucked into socks, a long-sleeved shirt, and boots. Apply a tick repellent to clothing. Check your child's skin for ticks when he or she returns home. If a tick becomes attached to the skin, remove it by grasping it by its head with tweezers and pulling slowly. Do not try to use your fingers because the tick's head may break off and remain in your child's skin. Swab the bitten area with rubbing alcohol. If the tick's head remains embedded, or if you see a large reddened area, call your doctor.

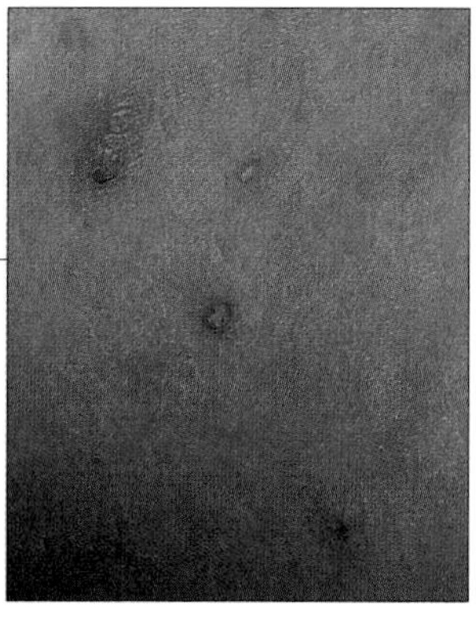

Molluscum contagiosum
Molluscum contagiosum is a harmless skin infection caused by a virus and characterized by small, round, pearllike spots. Each spot has a cloudy-white depressed center. The condition most often occurs on covered areas of skin. The spots eventually disappear on their own, but doctors can treat the condition using a medication that kills the virus and causes the spots to blister.

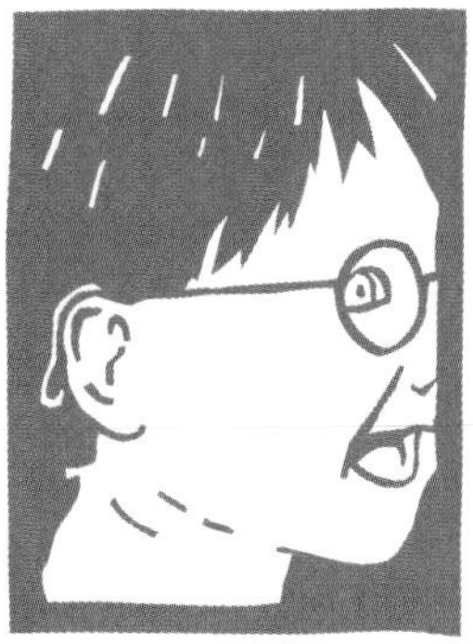

EYE AND EAR PROBLEMS

CHILDREN WHO HAVE a vision or hearing problem are often completely unaware that there is anything wrong with their eyes or ears. Affected children may not draw your attention to the possibility of a problem, so you must carefully watch your child for any signs of difficulty with these two vital senses.

A disorder that affects a child's eyes is potentially more serious in the first 6 years of life, when the nerve connections between the child's eye and brain are still developing. This explains why poor vision needs to be diagnosed and corrected as soon as possible. The same is true for a child's hearing. Early deprivation of sound can delay a child's speech and mental development dramatically because the child gains so much important information through hearing.

AMBLYOPIA

If a child has a defective eye, an abnormal optical image may fall on one or both retinas. A distorted pattern of nerve impulses travels to the brain, and the links between the outside world, the eyes, and the brain are not made.

Amblyopia, a permanent condition of defective vision, can result from any disorder that affects vision in one or both

HOW DOES YOUR CHILD SEE?

Vision is the perception in the brain of images that have registered on the retinas of the eyes a split-second earlier. The brain can interpret these images only if the eyes can form clear, sharp images. If you suspect that your child has a vision problem, take your child to the doctor. It is unlikely that the child will "grow out of" a vision problem.

Image formation
Perfect vision depends on the formation of normal images on the retina, the sensory membrane located at the back of each eye. The parts of the eye that work together to focus light rays on the retina are the cornea and the lens. Although the images on the retina have exactly the same shapes as the objects being viewed, they are upside down (see below).

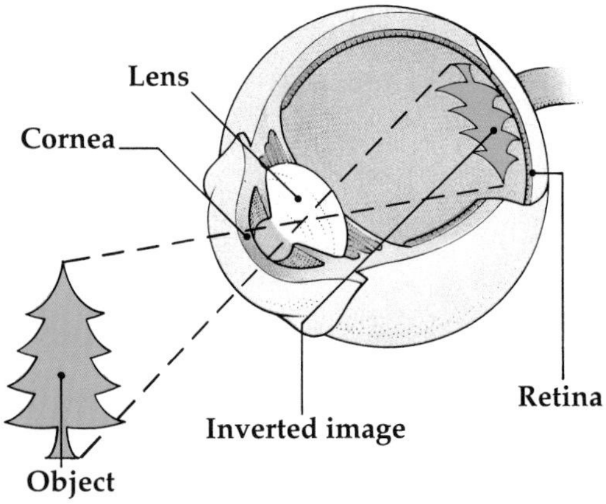

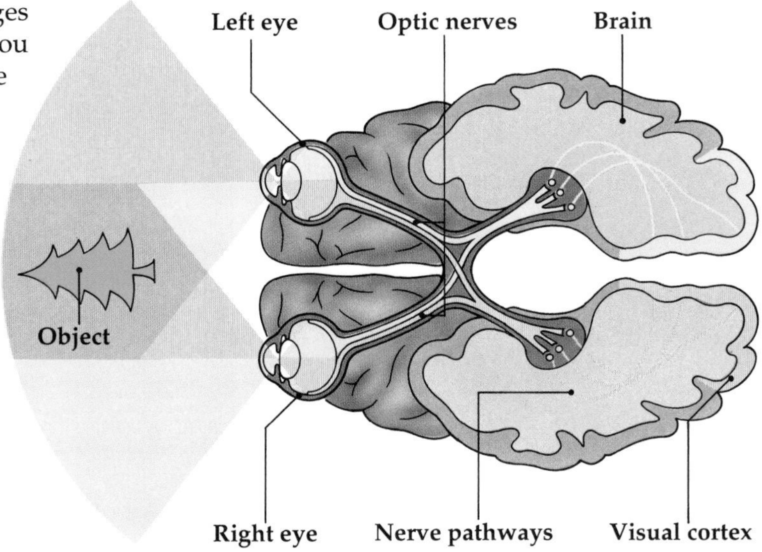

Image interpretation
The retina codes images in the form of electrical signals, which then travel along nerve pathways to the visual cortex of the brain. The visual cortex interprets the coded signals and turns the images right side up. The right side of the visual cortex perceives objects in the left field of vision and the left side perceives objects in the right field of vision. The brain compares the images from both eyes and then gives you a single three-dimensional view.

eyes. Such conditions include strabismus (crossed eyes), severe focusing errors, cataracts, a tumor on the retina, and drooping eyelids (see DEFECTIVE VISION IN CHILDHOOD on page 80). Early eye problem detection is critical. After a child reaches the age of 7, it is very difficult for doctors to correct a visual defect caused by an early, untreated eye disorder.

A failure of normal visual development in one or both eyes during childhood rarely leads to blindness. The child has some sight but cannot see detail very well. The child usually does not know that his or her eyesight is defective unless injury or disease disturbs vision in the unaffected eye, forcing the child to rely on the amblyoptic eye.

EYE TESTS

It can be difficult to evaluate a young child's visual ability accurately. Ophthalmologists (doctors who specialize in the care of the eyes) use the eye tests described below to assess a child's ability to see.

Refraction test
Doctors use refraction tests to write a prescription for eyeglasses. The doctor places eye drops into both eyes that cause the child's eyes to become temporarily unfocused. The doctor then illuminates the interior of each eye with a narrow beam of light. By placing different lenses in front of the child's eye and observing the effect of the light reflected off each lens, the doctor can calculate how much correction each eye needs.

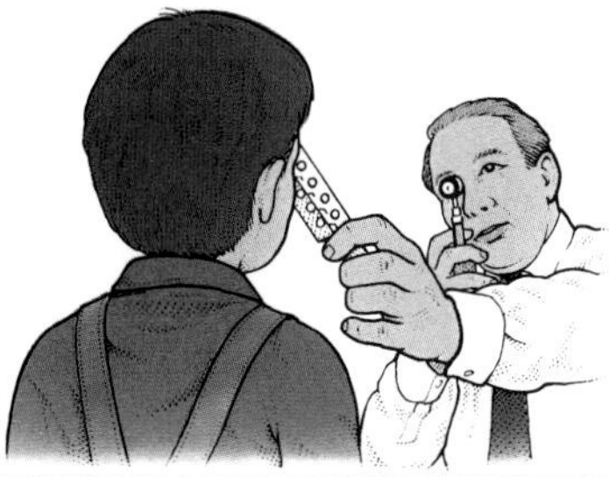

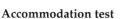

Using a retinoscope
The ophthalmologist uses an instrument called a retinoscope to perform a refraction test. The retinoscope projects a narrow beam of light, which reflects off the retina in the child's eye. The doctor observes how different lenses affect the light reflected from the eye and calculates the eyeglass prescription.

Accommodation test
When the eye is at rest, it focuses on distant objects. An accommodation test assesses the ability of the eye to change focus. The doctor performs the test after correcting the ability to focus on distant objects with eyeglasses.

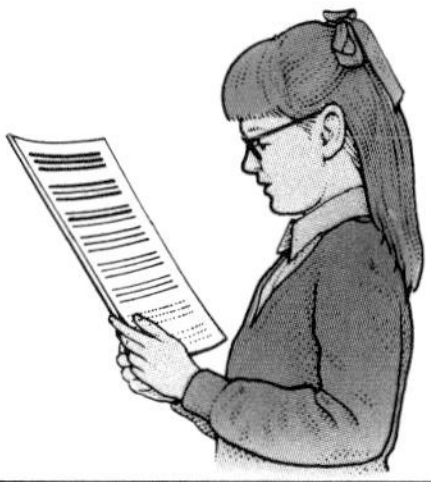

Focusing ability
To test the ability of the eye to change focus, the tester will ask an older child to read lines of type of various sizes. A younger child will be asked to match shapes held up at various distances.

Visual acuity test
Sharpness of vision (visual acuity) is tested by asking a child to read letters from a standard chart, first with one eye and then with the other (see right). For children who are too young to read, doctors use cards showing the letter E in different sizes and positions. The doctor asks the child to indicate the direction in which the arms of the letter are pointing.

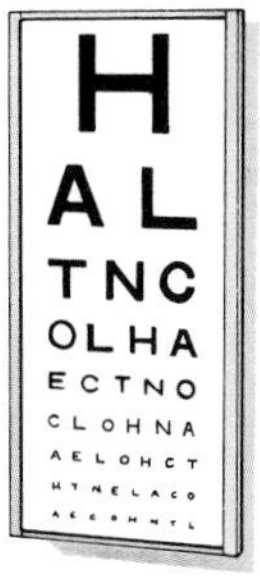

Snellen's chart
Doctors measure sharpness of vision with the Snellen's test chart. The tester places the child 20 feet away from the chart and asks him or her to read lines of letters, which decrease in size. Vision is rated 20/20 when the child can read the bottom line of letters from a distance of 20 feet.

Visual field tests
Visual field tests assess whether the retina and the optic nerves function properly and provide a full field of vision. If the child is old enough to talk and count, the test is easy to perform. Someone holds the child's head still and covers each eye in turn. Lights shine briefly on a screen in front of the child, who must indicate the number and positions of the lights.

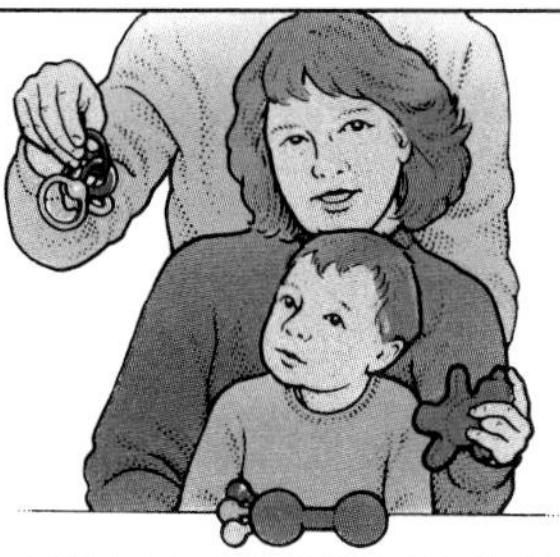

A full field of vision
To test a young child's visual field, the tester holds up a toy in front of him or her, while another toy is introduced from the side. The tester notes when the child becomes aware of the second toy.

DEFECTIVE VISION IN CHILDHOOD

Nearly all the eye conditions that affect adults can also affect children. But because of the importance of normal early visual development, many of these conditions have more serious long-term effects if they occur during early childhood. Babies do not always have coordinated control of their eyes in the first couple of months of life, but if you notice that your baby's eyes are crossed, you should have him or her examined by an ophthalmologist promptly.

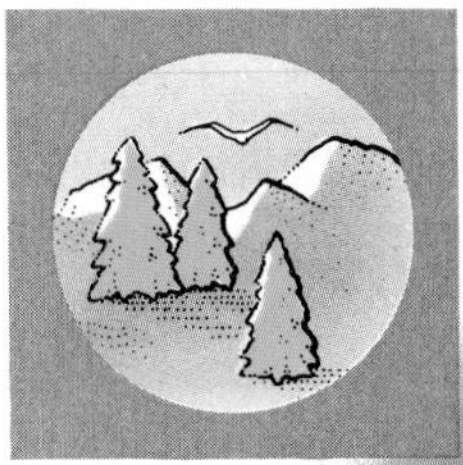

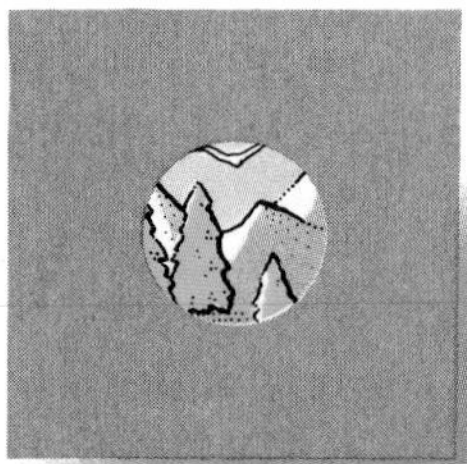

Glaucoma
Glaucoma that is present from birth needs immediate treatment. Fluid builds up inside the eyeball. The cornea (the transparent dome at the front of the eye) increases in size, and the eye waters and becomes sensitive to light. At first, only a partial loss of vision occurs (above left), which progresses (above right) to blindness without treatment.

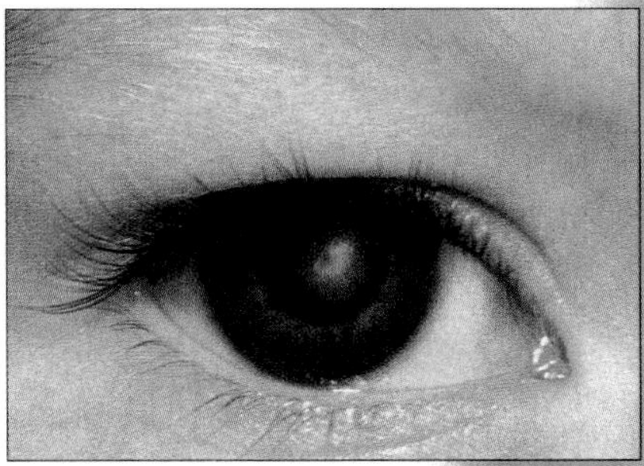

Cataract
Normally, the lens in the eye is transparent. Sometimes changes occur in the fibers of the lens, causing it to become opaque. Doctors call this condition a cataract. A cataract can be present from birth, can result from injury to the eye, can be caused by an infection the mother had during pregnancy, or, less commonly, can result from diabetes or other disorders. A cataract rarely causes complete blindness.

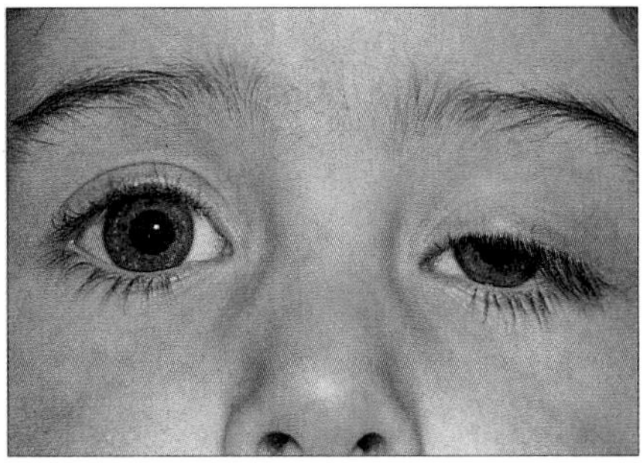

Drooping eyelid
If a baby's eyelid droops so far that it covers more than one half of the pupil of the eye at birth, it may interfere with his or her normal visual development. Surgery may be needed to shorten the muscle that lifts the eyelid. If your child develops a drooping eyelid suddenly during childhood, you should ask your doctor to check it immediately because it may signal a serious disorder, such as a brain tumor.

TYPES OF "CROSSED EYES" (STRABISMUS)

Strabismus refers to any condition in which the two eyes do not point in the same direction when looking at an object. Walleye, cross-eye, and vertical strabismus are three varieties. Surgery may be needed to correct any type of strabismus. Sometimes a patch is placed over the unaffected eye to force the child to use the affected eye and to prevent it from developing a permanent defect. Ophthalmologists may use corrective eyeglasses to treat strabismus.

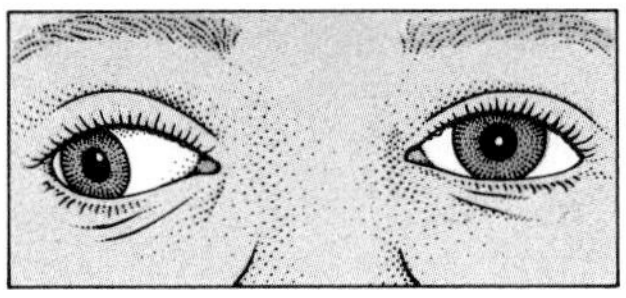

Walleye
One eye points outward in relation to the other eye. In rare cases, walleye can be caused by nearsightedness.

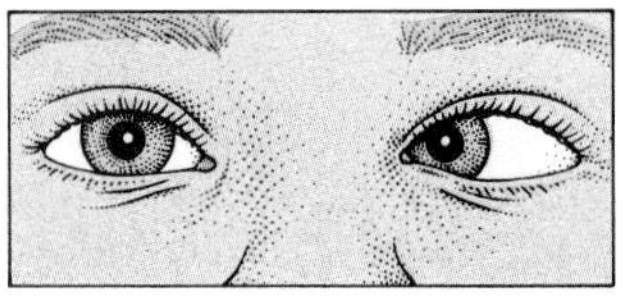

Cross-eye
One eye points inward in relation to the other eye. Cross-eye often results from farsightedness.

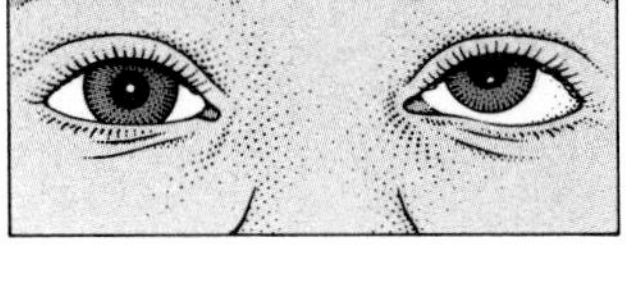

Vertical strabismus
One eye points upward or downward in relation to the other eye.

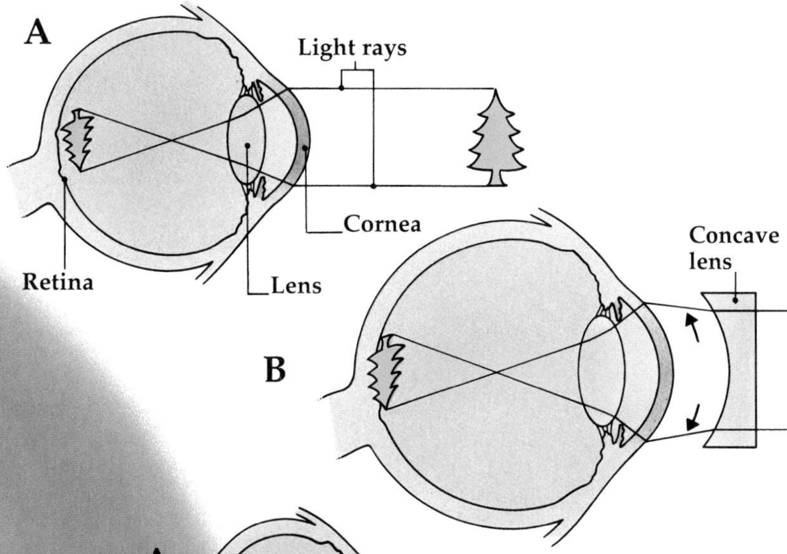

Nearsightedness
Distant objects look blurred to a person with nearsightedness (myopia) because the cornea (the transparent dome at the front of the eye) and lens focus the image at a point that falls short of the retina (A). An ophthalmologist prescribes a concave eyeglass lens so that the image becomes focused directly on the retina (B).

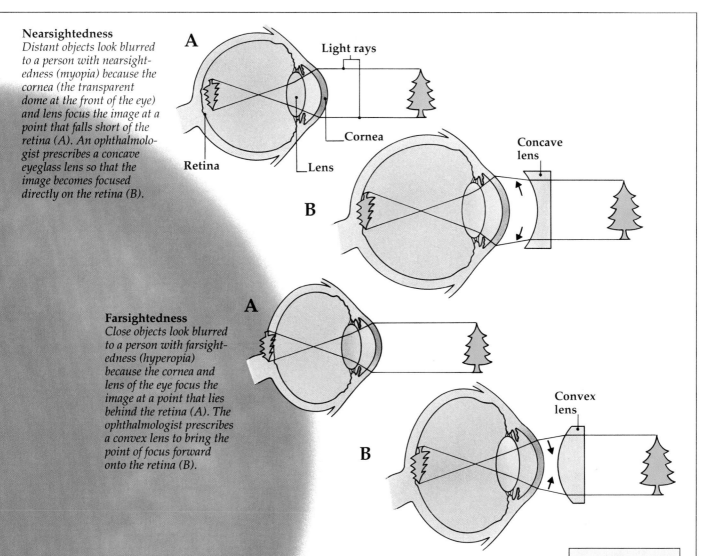

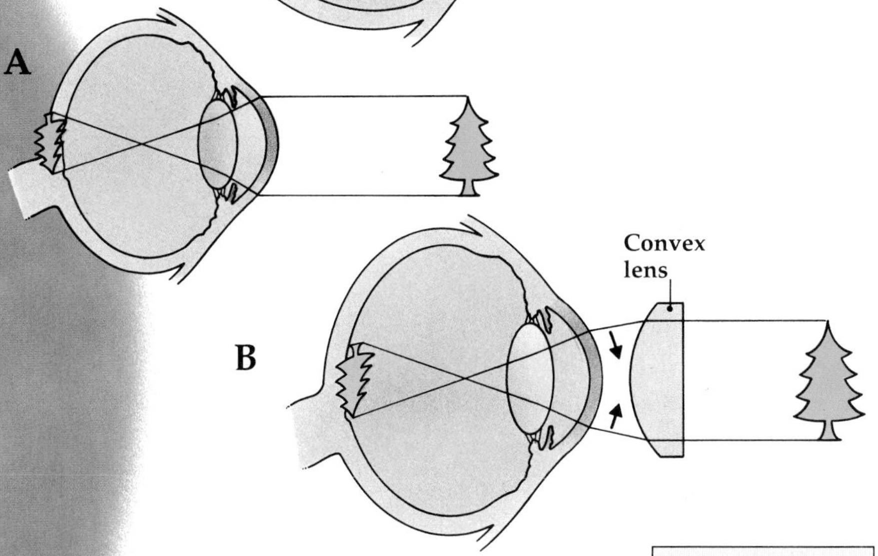

Farsightedness
Close objects look blurred to a person with farsightedness (hyperopia) because the cornea and lens of the eye focus the image at a point that lies behind the retina (A). The ophthalmologist prescribes a convex lens to bring the point of focus forward onto the retina (B).

Color-blindness
Color-blindness (color vision deficiency) more often affects boys than girls. In the most common types, there is a decreased sensitivity to red or green or difficulty distinguishing between shades of red and green. No medical cure exists. The photograph below shows how the apples at right might look to a child with simple decreased sensitivity to red.

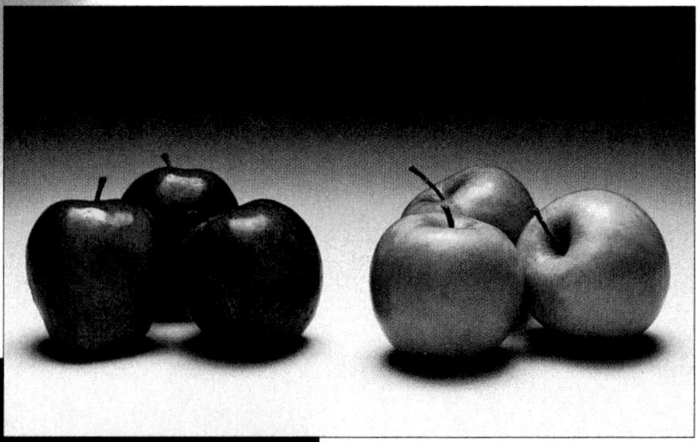

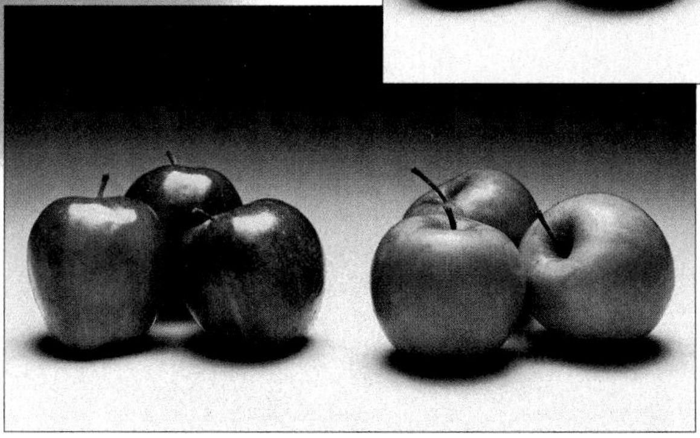

UVEITIS

Uveitis is an inflammation of the iris and the focusing muscle that surrounds its root. In childhood, uveitis is a common complication of juvenile rheumatoid arthritis (a disease that affects the joints and other parts of the body). An affected child has blurred vision, redness around the cornea, and pain. Doctors treat the condition with inflammation-fighting drugs.

MINOR EYE PROBLEMS

Several common eye problems, such as styes, can occur during infancy and childhood. Although these problems are uncomfortable and can be persistent, they will not affect a child's vision.

Clearing a blocked duct
To clear a blockage in a tear duct, press gently with a clean fingertip on the skin next to and just below the inner corner of the eye. Massage regularly for several days or weeks.

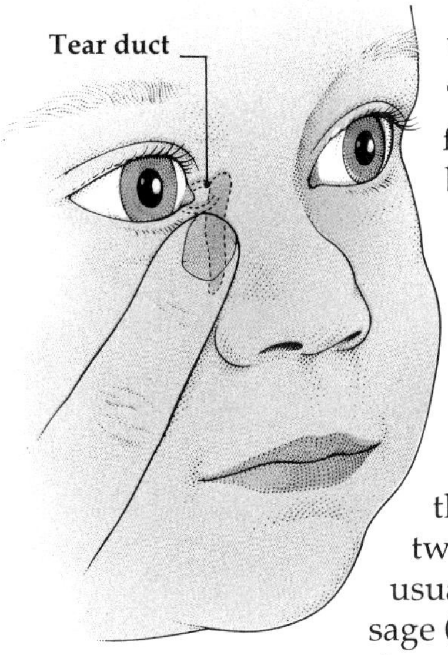

Watering eyes

The tear ducts normally carry extra fluid from the eyes into the nose, but if a duct has remained blocked from birth, a baby's eyes may water persistently. Infection can affect the upper part of the tear duct because bacteria that are not being drained with tears can accumulate. The infection can cause a swelling below the inner corner of the eye and a collection of pus between the eyelids. Clogged tear ducts usually open on their own or with massage (see left) by 6 or 8 months of age. If the problem persists, call your doctor. He or she may need to pass a thin metal probe down the tear duct to clear the obstruction if the ducts do not open by 8 months of age. During this operation, the baby must be under anesthesia.

Styes

A stye is an infection of the follicle of an eyelash (the small pit in which the root of the eyelash is embedded). Apply a warm, wet cloth and antibiotic ointment to help heal the infection. Try not to let your child touch an infected eye.

Stye formation
A stye forms when bacteria invade the follicle of an eyelash and multiply, producing poisons that cause redness, swelling, and pain. The white blood cells of the body's immune system attack the bacteria and kill the infected cells, causing the formation of a yellow nodule filled with pus.

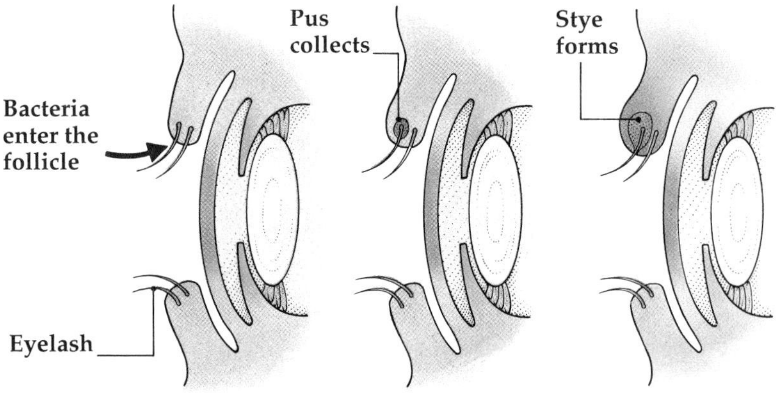

Applying eye drops
Have your child lie across your lap or on a bed. Put your arm around the top of the child's head so your hand reaches the face. Gently hold each of the child's eyelids apart with your finger and thumb. After the child blinks, put the drops into the corner of the eye. Keep the child still for a few minutes so the drops can spread across the eyeball.

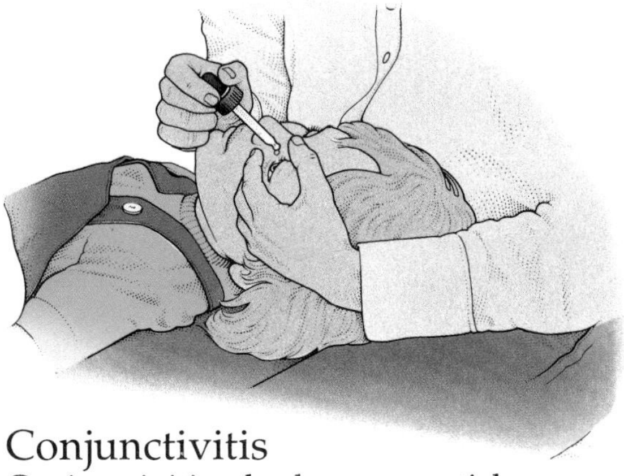

Conjunctivitis

Conjunctivitis, also known as sticky eye or pinkeye, refers to inflammation of the conjunctiva (the transparent membrane that covers the white of the eye and the insides of the eyelids). It is usually caused by infection. The conjunctiva is prone to infection because bacteria and viruses can collect and multiply behind the lower lid, where it is warm, moist, and dark. Your child's eye will water and the eyelid will become sore and inflamed. During sleep, when the child's eyes are closed for some time, his or her eyelashes may stick together with pus. To open the child's eyes, swab them gently with cotton balls soaked in warm water. Your doctor can clear up the condition with an antibiotic ointment or eye drops.

Blepharitis

Blepharitis is the medical term for inflammation of the edge of the eyelid. The eyelid becomes red and swollen, the skin at the root of the eyelashes becomes greasy, and flakes of skin stick to the eyelashes. Blepharitis often accompanies dandruff or seborrheic dermatitis (a scaly, itchy skin rash). Gently swab the child's eyelids with warm water. Your doctor can prescribe a soothing ointment to control the inflammation.

CASE HISTORY
FALLING BEHIND AT SCHOOL

MICHAEL ENJOYED FIRST AND SECOND GRADE and seemed to be doing well. But his third grade teacher said that Michael was starting to fall behind. At about the same time, Michael's father noticed that he had become unwilling to play basketball with his friends, although he spent hours watching TV. Michael's father became worried and made a doctor's appointment for Michael.

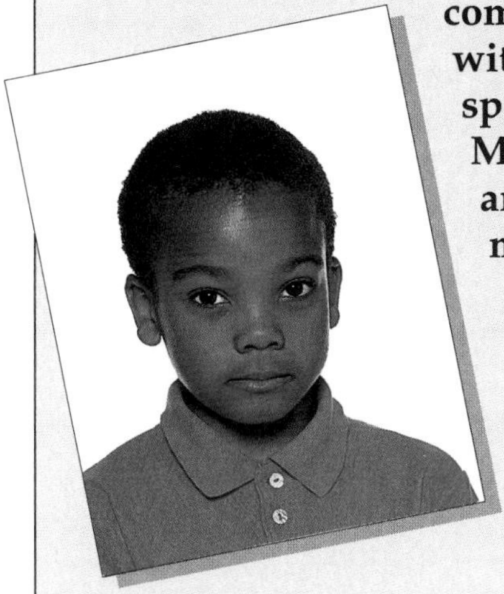

PERSONAL DETAILS
Name Michael Jefferson
Age 8
Occupation Student
Family Michael's parents and two older sisters are healthy.

MEDICAL BACKGROUND
Michael has always been very healthy and has rarely needed any kind of medical care.

THE CONSULTATION
The doctor asks Michael's parents about his growth and development, appetite, energy level, sleep pattern, and after-school activities. Then he gives Michael a comprehensive physical examination. The doctor tells Michael's parents that he cannot find anything wrong with their son. Then the doctor asks Michael to read the letters on an eye chart. When Michael says he can only read the top two lines, the doctor suggests that his parents make an appointment with an eye specialist (ophthalmologist) immediately.

FURTHER INVESTIGATION
The ophthalmologist carefully examines Michael's eyes. He puts eye drops into Michael's eyes to widen his pupils and temporarily block his ability to focus. The ophthalmologist then projects light into Michael's eyes from a retinoscope and holds up different lenses in a frame in front of Michael's eyes. The doctor asks Michael to look at red and green letters illuminated on the wall, while the doctor tries out more lenses. When he's finished, the eye specialist tells Michael's parents that their son's eyes are perfectly healthy, but that Michael has MYOPIA (nearsightedness) and needs a pair of glasses to correct his vision.

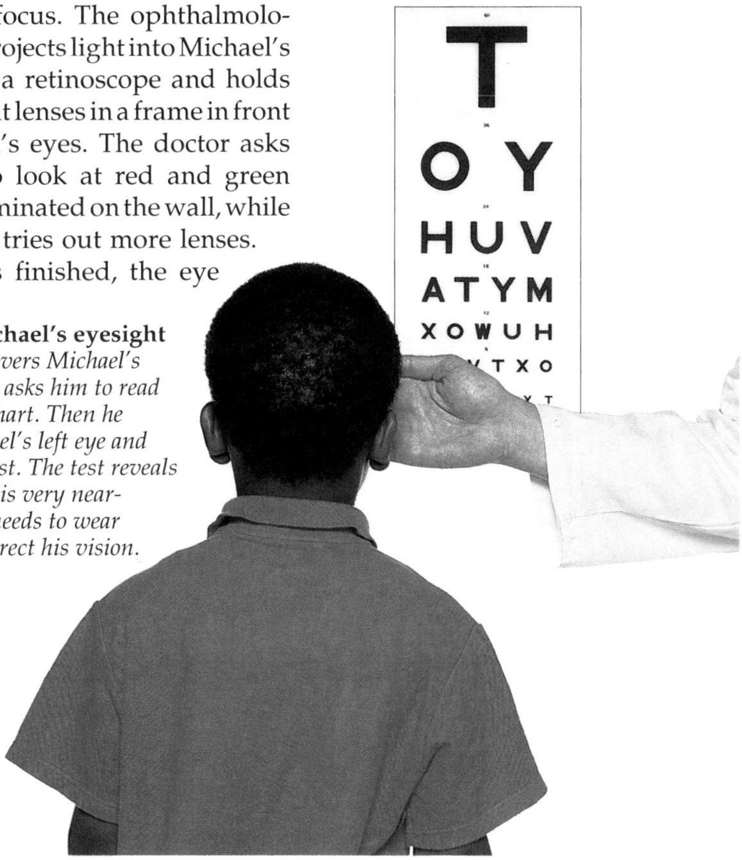

Testing Michael's eyesight
The doctor covers Michael's right eye and asks him to read letters on a chart. Then he covers Michael's left eye and repeats the test. The test reveals that Michael is very nearsighted and needs to wear glasses to correct his vision.

THE OUTCOME
The ophthalmologist measures Michael's eyes for glasses. At first, Michael resents having to wear glasses. But when he puts on the glasses for the first time, Michael realizes how much better he can see. Michael's schoolwork improves almost immediately. He regains his enthusiasm for basketball and spends less time watching TV. His parents promise him that he can have contact lenses when he gets older if he wants them, as long as the ophthalmologist confirms that he can wear them without any problems.

EAR PROBLEMS

A child who is severely deaf from birth probably will not learn to speak unless the condition is detected early and special efforts, such as speech therapy, are made to compensate for his or her inability to hear. All babies should be screened for deafness before the age of about 8 months. If you suspect that your child has a hearing defect, take your child to your doctor.

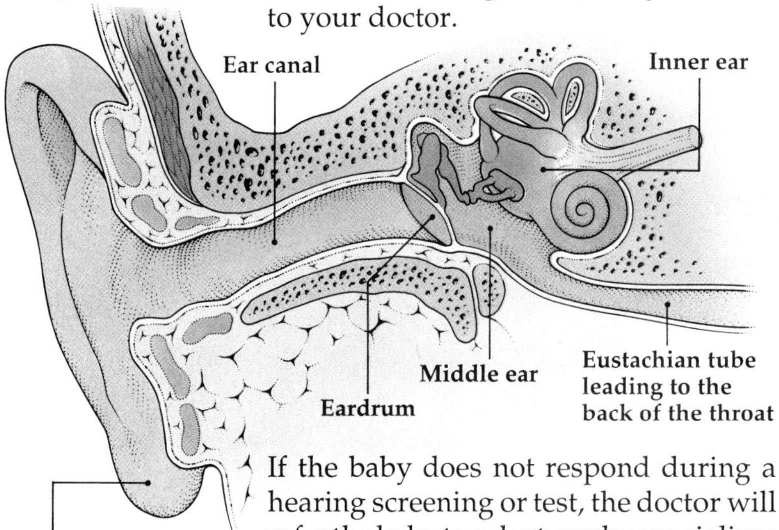

Inside the ear
The ear canal runs between the outer ear and the membrane called the eardrum. On the inner side of the eardrum lies the middle ear, which is connected to the back of the throat by the eustachian tube. The inner ear controls hearing and balance.

If the baby does not respond during a hearing screening or test, the doctor will refer the baby to a doctor who specializes in hearing problems for further investigation. A hearing aid fitted at the earliest possible opportunity can make a big difference in a child's ability to speak and in his or her learning potential.

EAR INFECTIONS

Children are much more likely to have middle ear infections than are adults because of the shape and position of their eustachian tubes (tubes that connect each middle ear to the back of the throat). Call your doctor promptly if you suspect that your child has an ear infection. Early treatment of ear infections can prevent rupture of the eardrum or long-term infection. Hearing defects and speech problems can result from long-term ear infections and fluid accumulation.

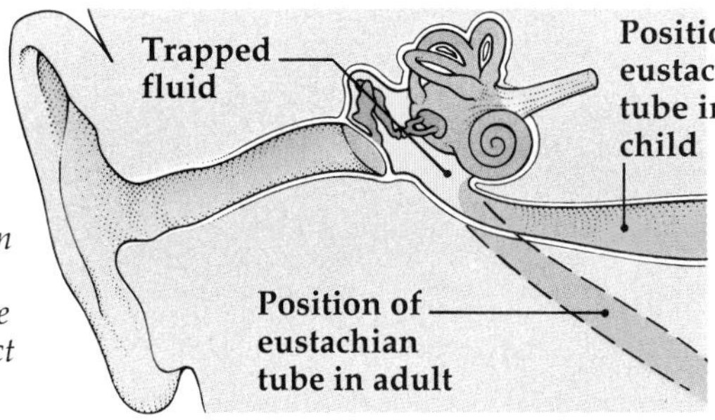

Ear infections
Middle ear infections occur often in children, because a child's eustachian tubes are shorter, wider, and more horizontal than an adult's. Fluid in the middle ear may not drain down the throat because of swelling in the eustachian tube from infection. Swollen adenoids (clusters of tissue at the back of the nose) may also obstruct drainage.

Outer ear infections

When a child has an outer ear infection, the ear canal and ear flap become swollen, painful, and itchy. Children who swim regularly are more prone to the

CHECK YOUR CHILD'S HEARING

Check your child's hearing regularly, especially if he or she has recently been sick. Call your doctor if the answer to any of the questions below is "no."

◆ At 5 to 6 weeks, if you speak to your baby when you are outside the range of vision, does your baby react and turn his or her head toward you?
◆ At 6 to 12 months, does your baby respond to the sound of paper being crumpled and his or her name? Does your baby make verbal sounds?
◆ By 18 months, can your child speak his or her first words?
◆ At 2 years, can your child hear you when you call from another room?
◆ At 3 years, does your child speak clearly, except for "s" and "th"?

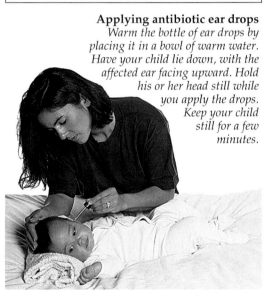

Applying antibiotic ear drops
Warm the bottle of ear drops by placing it in a bowl of warm water. Have your child lie down, with the affected ear facing upward. Hold his or her head still while you apply the drops. Keep your child still for a few minutes.

disorder because of irritants in water that can enter the ear. Your doctor may treat the condition with antibiotic ear drops. Do not allow water to enter the child's ear until the infection clears up.

Middle ear infection

Otitis media is the medical term for inflammation of the chamber between the eardrum and the inner ear. The most common cause is infection. The condition causes fever and pain. Your doctor can confirm the diagnosis by examining the child's eardrum with a viewing instrument. Antibiotics usually relieve the pain and fever within 48 hours. Hearing loss caused by accumulation of fluid in the middle ear may last 1 to 2 weeks.

Middle ear effusion

Middle ear effusion is the accumulation of sticky fluid or mucus in the middle ear. The fluid may build up following a cold or an attack of otitis media (see above). Other causes include hay fever or enlarged adenoids (clusters of tissue at the back of the nose) that block the openings of the eustachian tubes. Traveling in an airplane while having a cold can also cause middle ear effusion when cabin pressure changes. For reasons that are unclear, smoking by the parents may also contribute to middle ear effusion in children. Fluid in the middle ear interferes with the transmission of sound from the eardrum to the inner ear and can cause partial or total hearing loss. Doctors recognize the condition during a checkup or when testing for hearing loss.

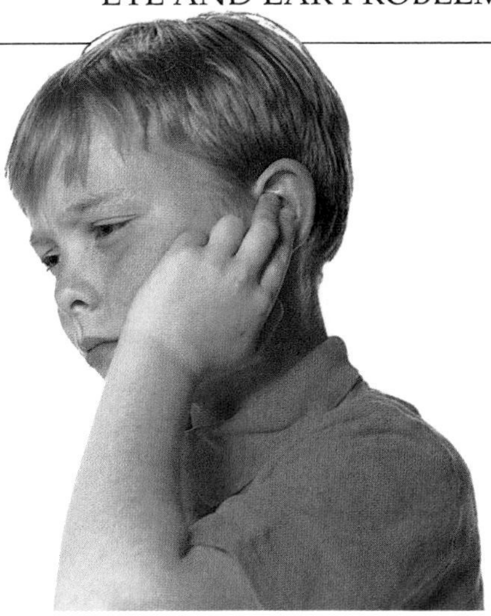

Symptoms of infection
You may not immediately recognize the symptoms of a middle ear infection in a small child. The child may have no pain in the ear or may only have mild discomfort. Your child may cry, be irritable, stop eating, or sleep poorly. He or she may have a fever and may keep pulling at the affected ear.

Treating middle ear blockage

Fluid in the middle ear often dries up without treatment, but your doctor will probably observe your child for a short time to make sure this happens. Antibiotics can help if infection by bacteria is present. Hearing loss from a blocked middle ear may require surgery.

REMOVING EAR WAX

If you think that there is too much wax in your child's ear, do not try to remove it or flush it out yourself. Your doctor will give you ear drops designed to dissolve the accumulated wax in your child's ear. If the wax does not dissolve, take your child back to your doctor, who can remove the wax in his or her office.

OBJECTS IN THE EAR

Children often put small objects, such as peas, beads, or bits of paper, into their ears. Such foreign objects may cause pain or temporary hearing loss. Deep penetration of the ear by a foreign object, or attempts to remove an object at home, can damage the eardrum. If your child puts something in his or her ear, do not attempt to wash the object out. It could swell and make removal more difficult. Foreign objects in the ear should always be removed by your child's doctor.

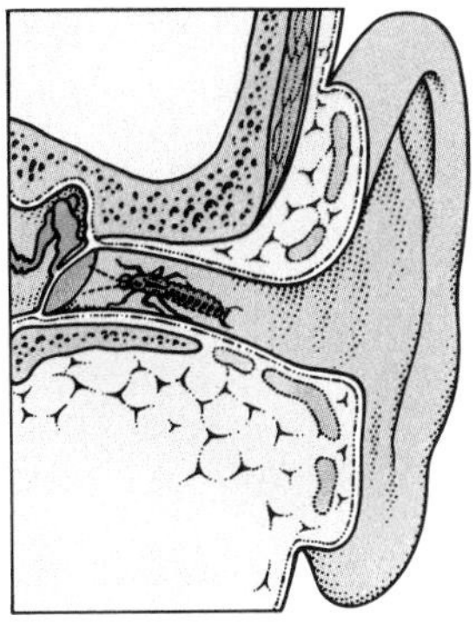

Insects in the ear
Insects can fly or crawl into the ear and become trapped. A child can become frightened by loud buzzing or tickling from the trapped insect. To kill the insect before it is removed at the doctor's office, put several drops of warm oil, such as baby oil or olive oil, into your child's ear.

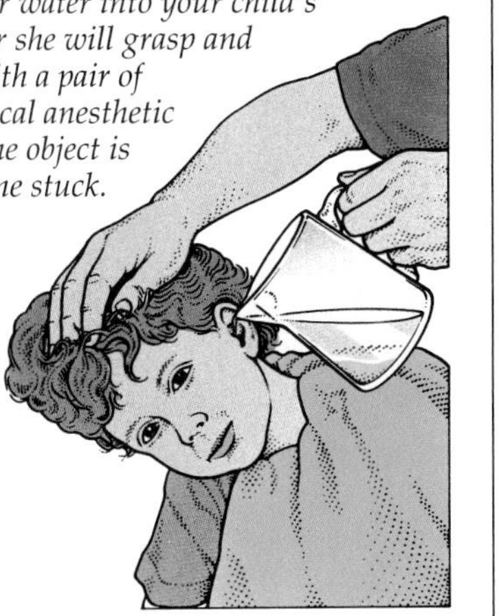

At the doctor's office
The doctor will examine your child's ear with a viewing instrument before removing the object. If the object can be floated out, the doctor may pour lukewarm oil or water into your child's ear. Otherwise, he or she will grasp and remove the object with a pair of slender forceps. A local anesthetic may be required if the object is swollen or has become stuck.

DIGESTIVE SYSTEM DISORDERS

THE DIGESTIVE SYSTEM is the series of organs that process the food you eat and expel waste products from food. The digestive system breaks down food so the body can absorb and use it. Children often have mild digestive system infections that cause diarrhea or vomiting. More serious digestive tract disorders, such as appendicitis, occur much less frequently.

Some disorders of the digestive system produce easily identifiable symptoms, such as diarrhea, vomiting, fever, and pain. Others only cause generalized abdominal pain. Such pain usually goes away without treatment.

ABDOMINAL PAIN

Abdominal pain is a symptom of many common childhood illnesses, including some that do not directly begin in the digestive system. For example, children with measles often complain about having abdominal pain. Recurring pain in the abdomen can signal anxiety, insecurity, or stress. Sometimes older children use a stomach ache as an excuse to avoid school or an activity they dislike. If your child has abdominal pain but is eating, sleeping, and playing normally, he or she is probably not seriously ill. But severe, prolonged, or recurrent abdominal pain may be a sign of an underlying disease, such as appendicitis, so you should call your doctor promptly if severe abdominal pain lasts more than 3 hours.

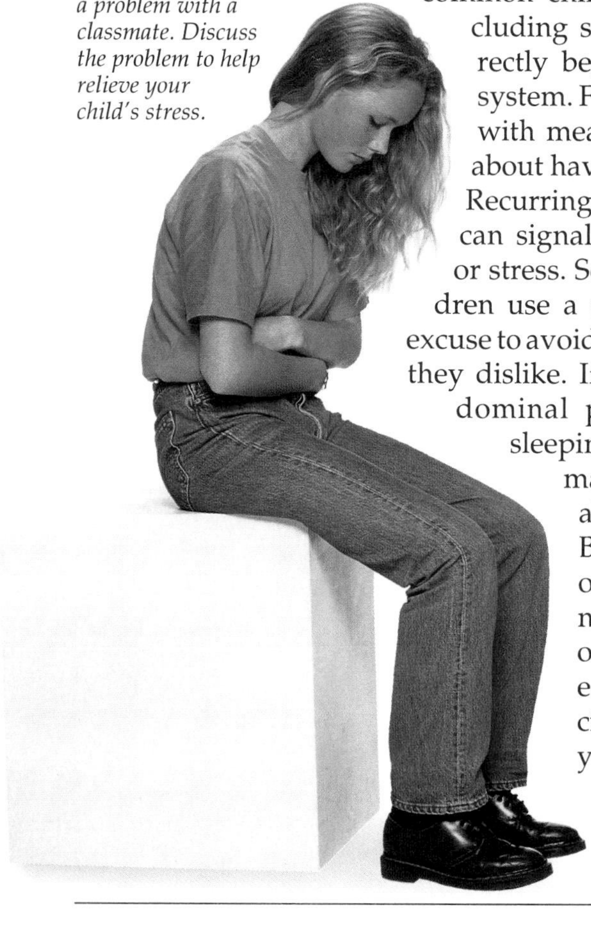

Recurrent abdominal pain
School-age children often have recurrent abdominal pain of unknown cause. Such pain is usually caused by stress. Sources of anxiety can include schoolwork or a problem with a classmate. Discuss the problem to help relieve your child's stress.

Severe abdominal pain
Children with severe abdominal pain often draw their knees up to their chest to make themselves more comfortable. Call your doctor if the pain lasts for more than 3 hours, causes your child to cry or scream, or is accompanied by blood-stained feces, vomiting, or a high fever (above 102°F).

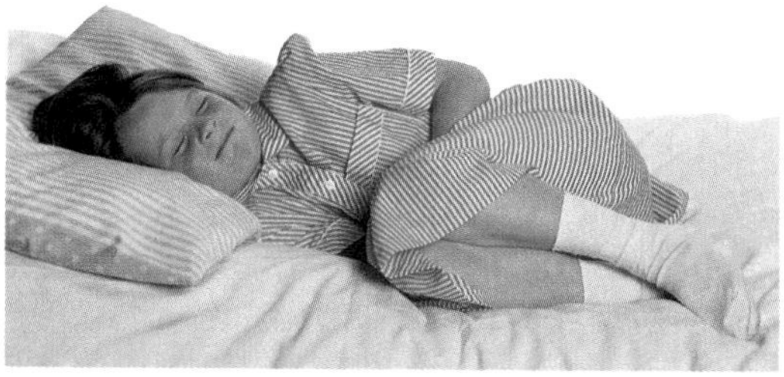

APPENDICITIS

Appendicitis is the most common abdominal emergency in children, although it is very rare in children younger than 2 years. Sudden, severe inflammation of the appendix, a narrow tube that branches off the large intestine, is usually caused by obstruction and infection. Children with appendicitis have a stomach ache for several hours and then severe pain in the lower right part of the abdomen. A child with appendicitis may vomit, refuse to eat, have a high fever, and become constipated. The pain gets worse when the child moves, and he or she usually prefers to lie still in a curled-up position. Surgeons must remove the inflamed and infected appendix before it ruptures and spreads infection throughout the child's abdomen.

GASTROESOPHAGEAL REFLUX

Gastroesophageal reflux occurs when a very young baby brings up a small part of his or her feeding from the stomach. It is caused by the immature coordination of the muscle contractions that move food and liquids down the esophagus (the tube that connects the throat and the stomach) and keep them in the stomach. Babies with mild and infrequent spitting up usually grow out of the condition by the time they are 12 months of age. Severe and frequent gastroesophageal reflux can lead to weight loss, poor growth, painful ulcers in the esophagus, and inhalation of the stomach contents that can cause a lung infection.

MALABSORPTION

Some children have digestive system disorders that impede the body's ability to break down and absorb nutrients from food. Doctors call this impaired absorption of nutrients malabsorption.

CAUSES OF GASTROESOPHAGEAL REFLUX

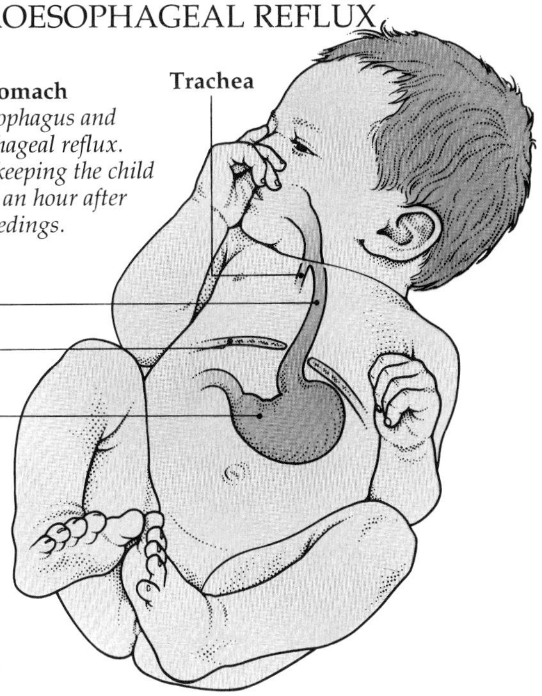

Weakened junction between esophagus and stomach
A weakened junction of the esophagus and stomach can cause gastroesophageal reflux. Symptoms can be relieved by keeping the child in an upright position for half an hour after feeding or by giving thicker feedings.

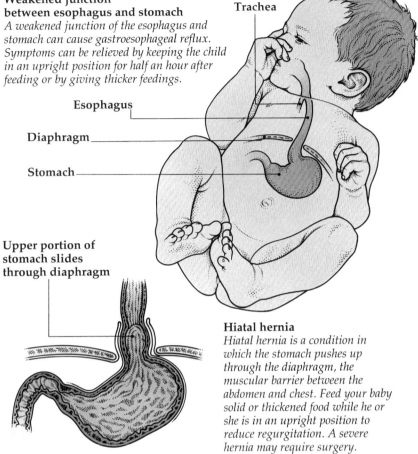

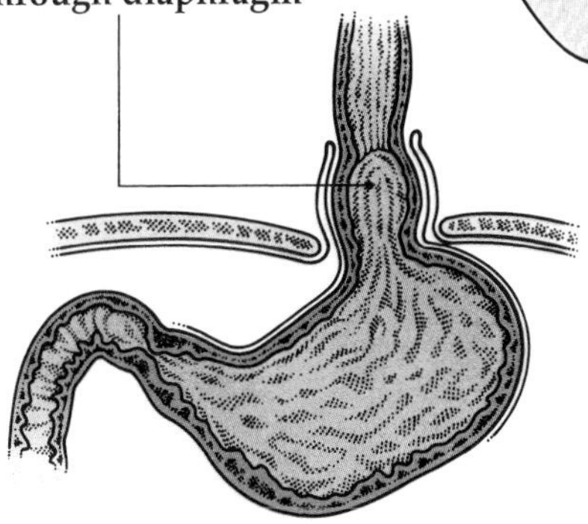

Hiatal hernia
Hiatal hernia is a condition in which the stomach pushes up through the diaphragm, the muscular barrier between the abdomen and chest. Feed your baby solid or thickened food while he or she is in an upright position to reduce regurgitation. A severe hernia may require surgery.

Celiac sprue

Celiac sprue is a rare condition characterized by sensitivity of the intestine to substances called glutens that are present in cereals, such as wheat, rye, barley, and oats. When a parent introduces foods containing these cereals into the diet of a baby with celiac sprue, the gluten damages the lining of the baby's small intestine and interferes with further absorption of food, leading to weight loss.

Children with celiac sprue often have a characteristic appearance: fair skin, light-colored hair, and long eyelashes. Affected children have a poor appetite, seem to be miserable, and appear pale because of anemia. Children with celiac sprue whose condition is not recognized and treated develop pot bellies and fail to grow normally. Their development may be slowed. Treatment with a gluten-free diet causes rapid improvement. Children with celiac sprue must adhere to dietary restrictions for life. Occasionally, an infant's sensitivity to gluten decreases as he or she gets older.

Lactose intolerance

Children who cannot digest a sugar called lactose that is present in milk and other dairy products are said to be lactose intolerant. In the small intestine, bacteria ferment the undigested lactose, causing symptoms such as abdominal cramps, excess gas, and diarrhea. The condition may arise from a hereditary deficiency of the enzyme lactase, a temporary complication of an infection in the stomach or intestines, celiac sprue, or cystic fibrosis.

A lactose-free diet improves the child's symptoms dramatically. Lactase supplements are now available in stores.

UMBILICAL HERNIA

An umbilical hernia occurs when a small loop of bowel protrudes through a tiny defect in the center of the baby's navel. The bulge may increase in size when the baby cries. Most umbilical hernias disappear without treatment by the time the baby is 2 years old (or as late as 5 years).

COMMON MOUTH PROBLEMS

In the first stage of the digestive process, your teeth break down food in your mouth. Your tongue, cheeks, and lips all have muscles designed to manipulate your food. Mouth problems that cause pain, such as infections or dental cavities, can cause a decreased appetite in children. Good oral hygiene and regular visits to the dentist can reduce the likelihood of your child developing mouth problems.

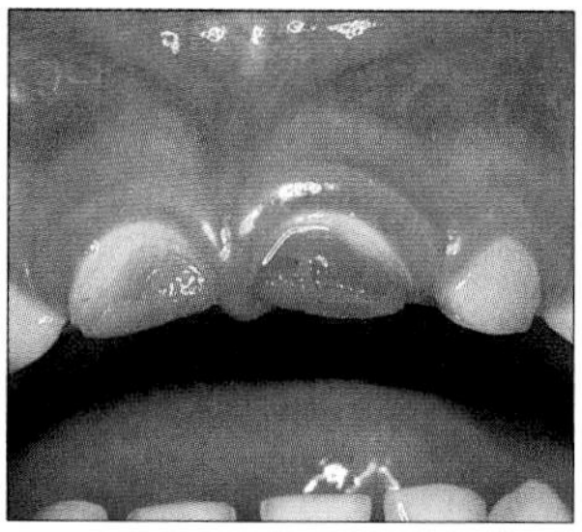

Tooth decay
Toothache brought on by eating sweet, hot, or cold foods is caused by tooth decay. Decay often appears as a blackened area on a tooth. But the advanced decay produced when a child frequently sleeps with a bottle of milk or juice in his or her mouth for several hours often appears brown and leathery (see left).

Mouth ulcers
Mouth ulcers are small, painful patches of open sores with pale yellowish centers and reddened edges that occur singly or in clusters inside the mouth and on the tongue. Infection by a virus often causes mouth ulcers, and they are common in children aged 10 or younger. If the ulcers fail to heal on their own in a week, consult your doctor.

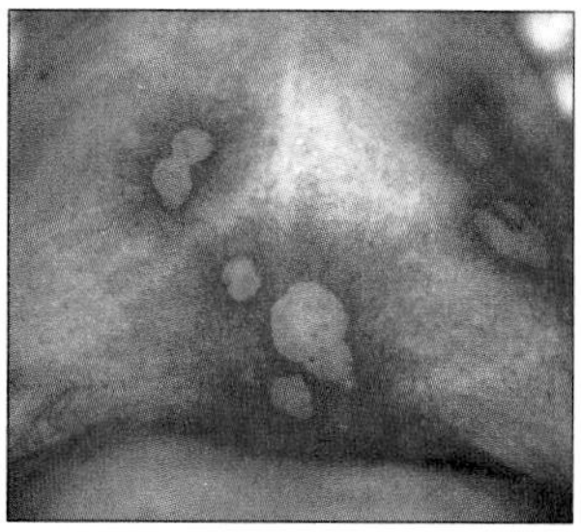

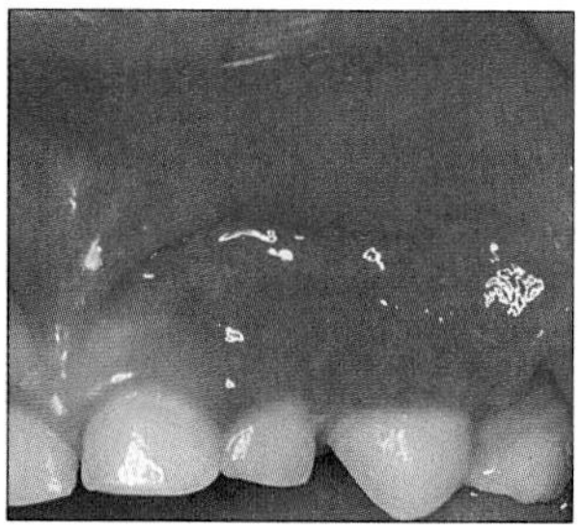

Gingivitis
Gingivitis (inflammation of the gums) is a stage of gum disease that you can reverse with good oral hygiene. Gums often become tender and swollen, and toothbrushing often causes the gums of people with gingivitis to bleed. Untreated gingivitis can erode the tissue that supports the teeth, leading to tooth loss.

Rehydration solutions
Rehydration solutions are better than water for a dehydrated child. They not only replace lost body fluids but also provide minerals that have been lost through vomiting. You can buy a commercial rehydration solution at a drug store or make one at home. Add half a teaspoon of salt, 2 teaspoons of sugar, and a quarter of a teaspoon of baking soda to 1 pint of water.

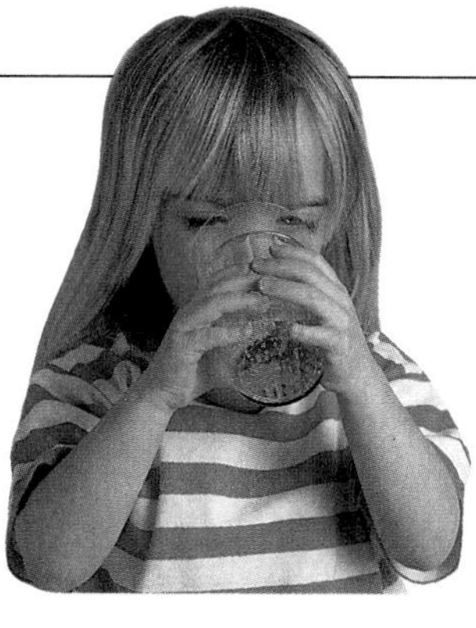

VOMITING

Doctors do not consider the bringing up of small amounts of swallowed food to be vomiting. The term vomiting refers to a more complete emptying of the stomach or to a strenuous and repeated regurgitation of any food or liquid the child consumes. The vomit may initially contain food but prolonged vomiting eventually brings up only stomach juices.

A common cause of vomiting is infection. Malabsorption of nutrients from food, motion sickness, psychological problems, and certain serious medical disorders can also cause vomiting. For example, a thickening of the muscle at the outlet of the stomach, known as congenital (present at birth) hypertrophic pyloric stenosis, may produce an obstruction that causes projectile vomiting. When a child experiences projectile vomiting, his or her stomach contents may be ejected several feet. Doctors must perform surgery to correct congenital hypertrophic pyloric stenosis.

Call your doctor immediately if your child's vomiting is projectile or bloody or if it lasts longer than 6 hours.

Preventing dehydration

Persistent vomiting and diarrhea can cause the water content of the child's body to become dangerously low. Fluid loss is accompanied by the loss of many essential body chemicals, such as potassium and magnesium.

Symptoms of dehydration include dark-colored concentrated urine, a dry mouth, a lack of tears, sunken eyes, and lethargy. If your child has been vomiting, stop giving fluids and solids for 2 hours, to forestall further vomiting. After that, give your child rehydration solutions (see left) frequently in small amounts. Do not give solids for 12 to 24 hours.

Extreme dehydration is a medical emergency. Doctors will hospitalize the child and give him or her fluids intravenously (into a vein).

ABNORMAL FECES

A child who passes watery feces several times a day has diarrhea. Causes of diarrhea include eating food that is too rich or contains too much fiber, infections of the digestive tract, malabsorption (defective absorption of nutrients from food), and food intolerance. Parents should remember that normal bowel movements vary according to a child's age – breast-fed babies pass "seedy," loose, bright-yellow, odorless feces four or more times a day, while toddlers can have three or four soft bowel movements a day. Call your doctor if your child's diarrhea lasts for more than 6 hours or contains blood or mucus, if your child is also vomiting, or if he or she is dehydrated (see the GASTROENTERITIS box below).

Food poisoning
Sudden bouts of vomiting, diarrhea, and abdominal pain may occur after eating food contaminated with bacteria, such as Salmonella. *Foods that carry a high risk of contamination include eggs and egg-based dishes, shellfish, poultry, and cooked meats that have either been eaten cold or have not been reheated thoroughly before eating.*

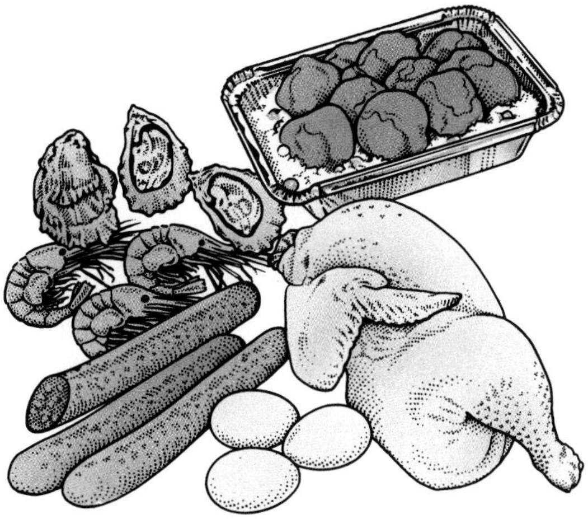

HIRSCHSPRUNG'S DISEASE

Severe constipation and slowed growth in infancy can be signs of Hirschsprung's disease, caused by the absence of nerve tissue in the rectum, colon (large intestine), or small intestine. Muscles in the affected section of intestine cannot contract, causing feces to accumulate above the affected area. Doctors must remove the accumulation surgically.

GASTROENTERITIS – INFECTION OF THE INTESTINE

Gastroenteritis is an infection of the intestine, by bacteria or viruses, that causes vomiting, abdominal pain, and diarrhea. Affected children lose their appetite and usually have a fever. Gastroenteritis is infectious, meaning that it can spread from one person to another. So it is important to wash your hands after caring for or feeding an affected child to prevent the organism responsible for the infection from contaminating food and work surfaces.

Signs of dehydration
Children who are vomiting and have diarrhea can quickly become dehydrated. Call your doctor if your child shows these signs of dehydration.

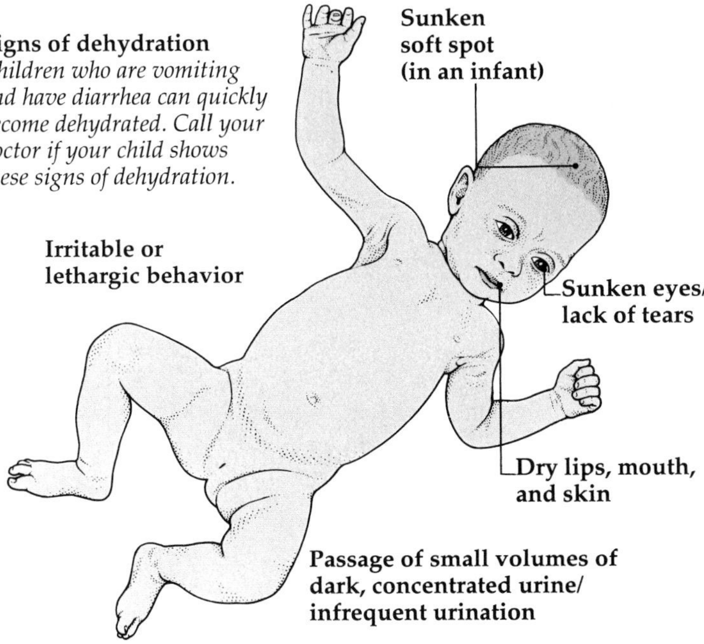

Constipation

A child whose feces are hard and who has less than one bowel movement every 3 to 4 days is constipated. Some causes of constipation, which is common in children, are dehydration, inadequate intake of fluids and fiber in the diet, or emotional stress. Passing hard feces can split the lining of the child's anus, creating a fissure that causes pain and bleeding when the child defecates. To avoid the pain, a child with an anal fissure often ignores the urge to defecate and becomes even more severely constipated.

To treat constipation, doctors advise eating more fiber and drinking more fluids. In hot weather, your child needs more fluids to make up for increased perspiration. Never hurry your child when he or she is having a bowel movement and do not leave him or her sitting for too long on an uncomfortable potty chair or in a cold bathroom. Such tension or discomfort can inhibit your child's ability to have a bowel movement. Call your doctor if constipation does not improve with increased dietary fiber and fluids. Do not give your child laxatives unless your doctor orders them.

CASE HISTORY
RESTLESS NIGHTS

BEN HAD ALWAYS been a cheerful boy who enjoyed playing with other children at nursery school. But during the past few weeks, his mother became concerned because he was not sleeping well. She noticed that he became restless and irritable every night and that he had a habit of scratching hard around the anal area. She decided to discuss the problem with the family doctor.

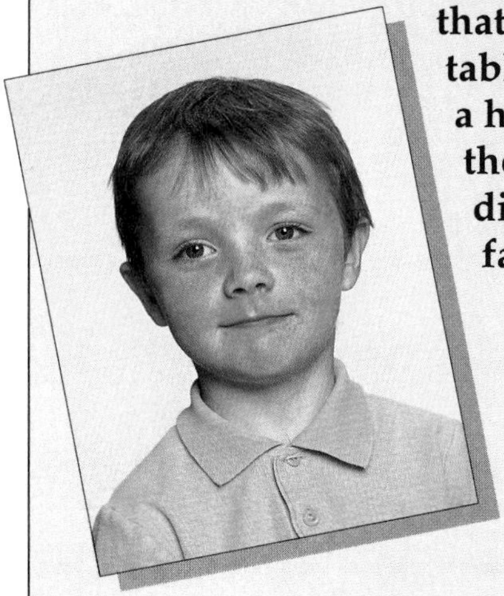

PERSONAL DETAILS
Name Ben Donahue
Age 4 years
Occupation Preschool student
Family Ben's parents are both healthy. His sister, aged 8, has no medical problems.

MEDICAL BACKGROUND
Ben has never had any serious health problems, and he has had all the recommended immunizations.

THE CONSULTATION
The doctor questions Ben and his mother about the problem and asks how he is doing in school. The doctor gives Ben a physical examination and finds that he seems healthy. But the doctor notices that the area around Ben's anus is reddened and severely scratched.

THE DIAGNOSIS
The doctor tells Ben's mother that he probably has PINWORMS. These tiny parasitic worms live inside the intestines, but the adult females come out through the anus at night to lay eggs on the surrounding skin. This activity causes anal itching and disturbed sleep. Ben's mother is concerned by this information, but the doctor reassures her that pinworms are common – they occur in one fifth of all children – and do not cause serious problems. The doctor asks Ben's mother to perform a test (see below) at home to confirm the diagnosis.

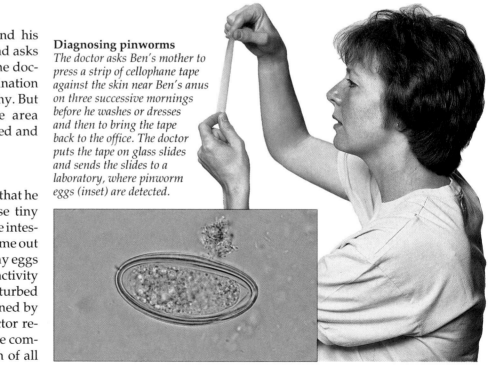

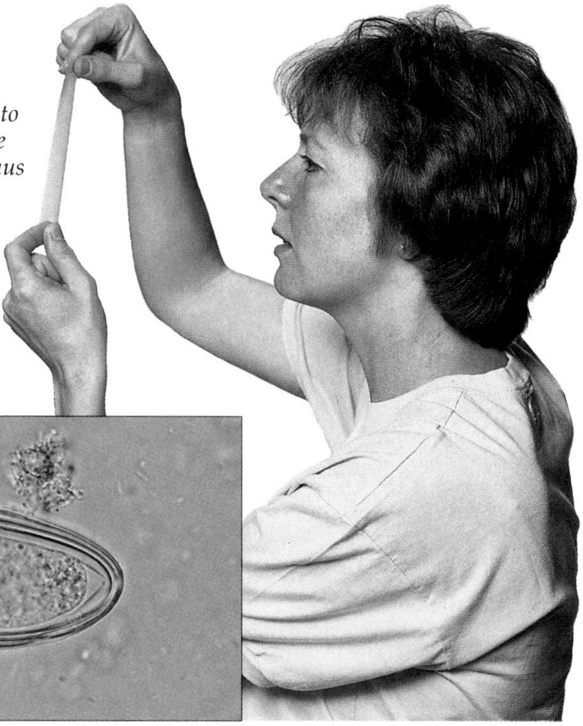

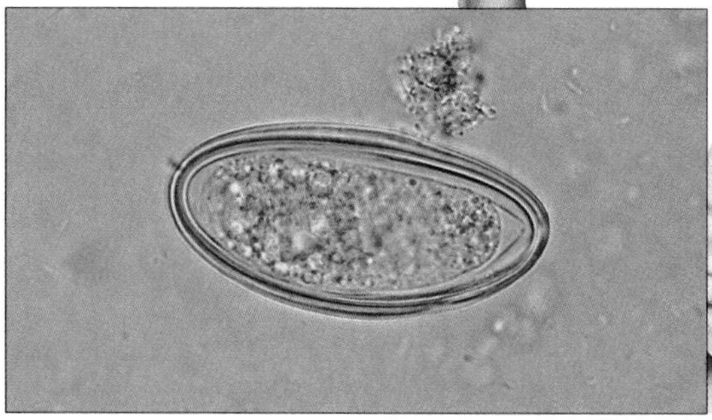

Diagnosing pinworms
The doctor asks Ben's mother to press a strip of cellophane tape against the skin near Ben's anus on three successive mornings before he washes or dresses and then to bring the tape back to the office. The doctor puts the tape on glass slides and sends the slides to a laboratory, where pinworm eggs (inset) are detected.

THE TREATMENT
The doctor describes how infestation can begin when someone accidentally swallows eggs from contaminated clothing or from fingernails contaminated during scratching. She adds that it is not unusual for young school children to have repeated infestations. The doctor explains that a pinworm infestation can pass from one member of the family to another. She treats Ben's whole family with a drug designed to kill and expel intestinal worms.

The doctor recommends that the family's bedclothes be washed daily and that Ben's underclothes and pajamas be changed daily during treatment. She also explains that keeping the family's fingernails short and clean helps cut down the chances of reinfestation.

THE OUTCOME
Ben's symptoms clear up quickly after treatment. He is able to sleep through the night once again.

BLOOD IN FECES

Always call your doctor if you see blood in your child's feces. Keep a sample of the feces to help your doctor reach a diagnosis. Your doctor can usually tell the approximate location of the bleeding by the color and nature of the blood in the feces. Dark blood can come from any site along the upper digestive tract. The darkened blood may come from a site in or above the stomach, or even from a nosebleed. Bright red blood comes from the lower colon (large intestine) and rectum. Blood from the upper digestive tract and from the small intestine and colon is usually mixed in with the feces; blood from the anus or rectum usually appears on the surface of the feces.

Children who are constipated or have an anal fissure (a crack in the lining of the anus) may find defecation painful and may pass a small amount of blood with their feces or find blood staining the toilet paper. A child who has a rectal polyp (an outgrowth of the lining of the colon or rectum) has recurrent bleeding but experiences no pain during defecation.

Serious digestive tract problems can cause bleeding. A condition called intussusception (see below) causes bleeding that gives a child's feces the appearance of red currant jam. A small bleeding pocket called a diverticulum in the wall of the upper part of the digestive tract produces black or dark feces.

MECKEL'S DIVERTICULUM

When a fetus is in the mother's uterus, part of its intestine is connected to the umbilical cord at the navel. Normally, the connection shrivels at birth. But in one out of 50 babies it remains after birth, resembling a little sac and called a Meckel's diverticulum. Occasionally, a Meckel's diverticulum causes an intussusception (see below), a twisting of the intestine, or bleeding and requires surgery.

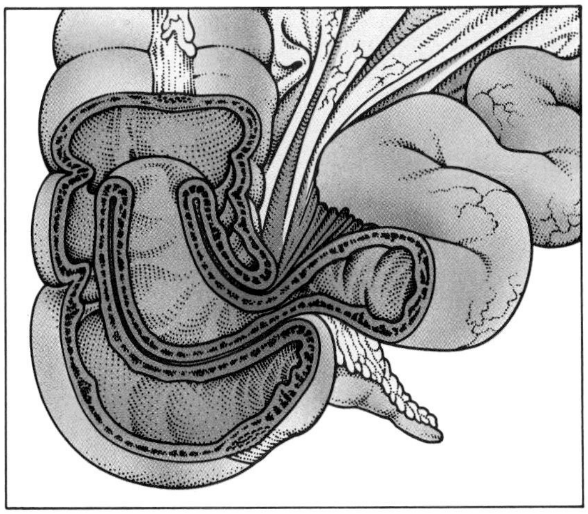

Intussusception
An intussusception occurs when part of the intestine telescopes in on itself. It is the most common cause of intestinal blockage in children under 2. Although doctors do not know what causes an intussusception, they think the condition is linked to infection or to the presence of a small pocket in the intestinal wall called Meckel's diverticulum.

ASK YOUR DOCTOR
DIGESTIVE TRACT DISORDERS

Q My 12-year-old daughter has Crohn's disease. What is it and how can it be treated?

A Crohn's disease is an inflammation that can affect any part of the digestive system, from the mouth to the anus, causing such symptoms as diarrhea, pain, fever, and weight loss. Doctors usually treat Crohn's disease with drugs and a special diet. In severe cases, treatment may include surgery to remove badly affected parts of the intestines, but Crohn's disease usually recurs.

Q My 3-year-old son swallowed a button that came off of his shirt. Is this dangerous?

A Most small, smooth objects that children accidently swallow pass safely out of their bodies in feces. But sharp objects and items such as watch batteries that contain harmful chemicals can damage a child's digestive tract. Surgeons must remove a smooth object that has failed to pass out of the digestive tract after 7 days, one that causes vomiting, or a sharp object that is causing pain.

Q My 7-year-old son has a lump in the right side of his groin that gets bigger when he stands up but disappears when he lies down. What could it be?

A Your son may have a hernia. Hernias are common in children, especially boys. They occur when the intestine protrudes through a weakened area in the abdominal wall. Your son will probably need an operation to strengthen the abdominal wall. A hernia in a newborn is surgically repaired immediately.

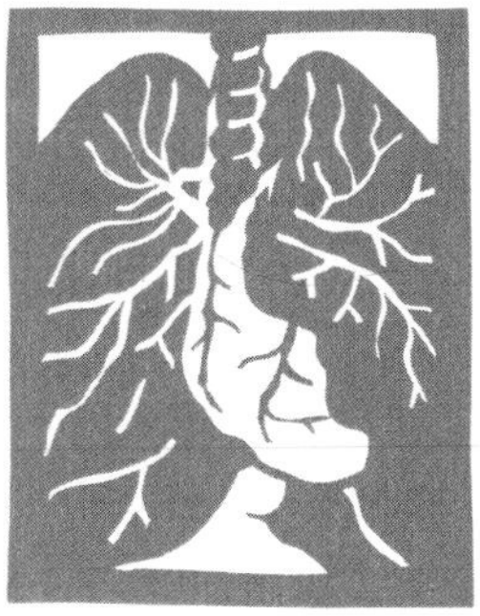

HEART AND RESPIRATORY CONDITIONS

MOST CHILDHOOD HEART problems arise from defects that are present at birth. Many such defects go unnoticed until the child gets older, but a few can be life-threatening in the first weeks of life. Inefficient pumping of the heart can lead to heart failure, causing fluid to build up in the lungs or the liver. Common causes of childhood respiratory problems are infections and asthma.

Your child's heart and lungs work together to provide all the tissues in his or her body with vital oxygen. The child's lungs and kidneys then eliminate the carbon dioxide that the body's tissues produce as a waste product. During periods of stress, such as strenuous exercise, the pumping action of your child's heart and his or her breathing rate increase to meet the body's increasing demands for oxygen. But several disorders that reduce the efficiency of the heart-lung partnership can make even the slightest activity exhausting for a child.

Normal circulation
The right side of the heart pumps blood to the lungs, where the blood absorbs oxygen and releases carbon dioxide. The oxygenated blood then travels to the left side of the heart, which pumps it to all the other tissues of the body.

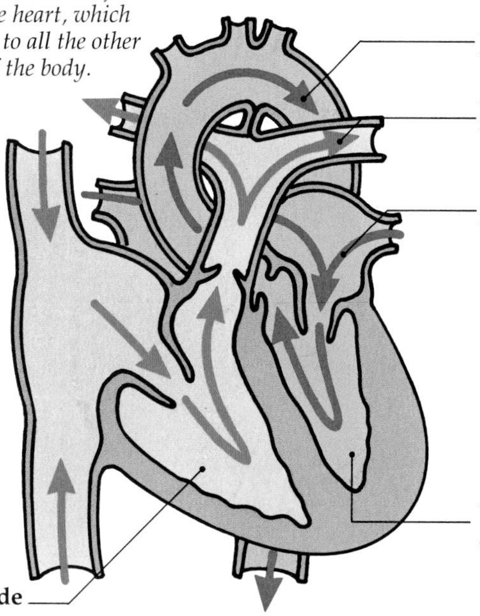

HEART PROBLEMS

About one child in 150 is born with some abnormality in the structure of the heart. Doctors call such disorders congenital (present at birth) heart defects. Major heart defects are often detected soon after birth, and affected newborns may require surgery. Minor defects can go undetected for several years. A child with a minor or even a moderate heart condition is often no more prone to infection than an unaffected child, and his or her growth may be normal or slowed. The treatment of heart defects depends on the nature of the defect.

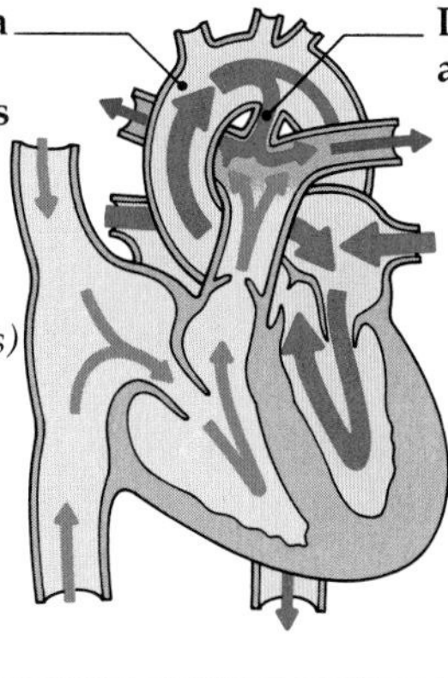

Patent ductus arteriosus
Some of the oxygenated blood pumped by the left side of the heart passes from the aorta through a duct (the ductus arteriosus) and mixes with the blood going to the lungs. This defect causes extra work for the heart, producing a murmur and breathlessness during exercise.

"Hole in the heart"
Commonly called "hole in the heart," ventricular septal defect is the most common heart disorder present at birth. This defect allows blood to flow from the left side of the heart to the right side, causing a murmur. Half of all such defects close by the time the child is 2 years old.

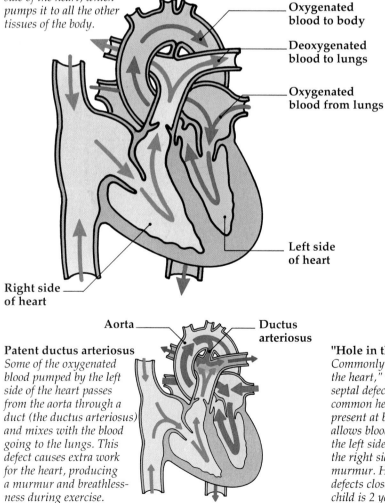

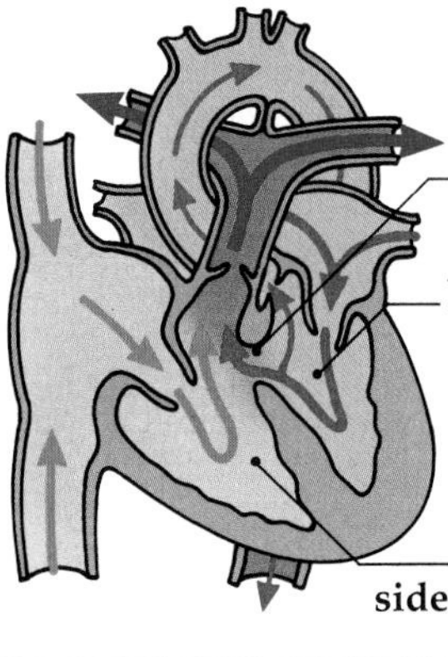

Heart murmurs

Heart murmurs are extra sounds that the heart may produce in addition to the usual sounds of the heartbeat. Murmurs do not always indicate illness. Murmurs in a child who has a structurally normal heart are said to be "innocent." About 50 percent of 2- to 5-year-old children have an innocent heart murmur, which may be present consistently or only from time to time. Doctors call a murmur caused by a structural abnormality in the heart – such as a "hole in the heart" (see page 92) or a valve that is not functioning properly – an organic murmur.

Heartbeat abnormalities

Abnormalities of the heart rhythm, especially extra heartbeats, are fairly common in healthy children and often disappear as the child grows older. Some children have a condition called paroxysmal supraventricular tachycardia, in which a heart that is otherwise normal beats rapidly for short or longer periods. An affected child may feel weak, dizzy, and short of breath. An affected infant may become quiet and less active and may not eat well. Doctors control the condition with drug therapy.

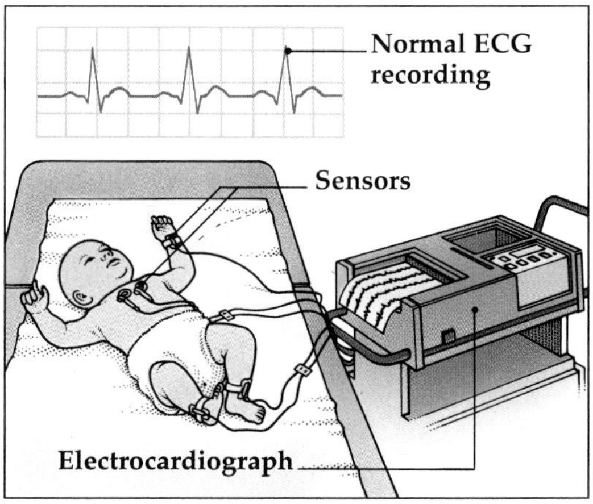

Investigating heart defects
To find out the cause of a heart murmur or heartbeat irregularities in an infant, a doctor will listen to the heart and may order tests. Such tests include electrocardiography (ECG), which records the heartbeat; a chest X-ray to measure heart size; and ultrasound scanning of the heart to measure the thickness of the walls of the heart.

Signs of abnormal breathing
A child with pneumonia often breathes rapidly. Count your child's breaths, while he or she is at rest, for a full minute. If the breathing rate is higher than normal and the skin on the neck or between or below the ribs is drawn in, the child may have a serious infection.

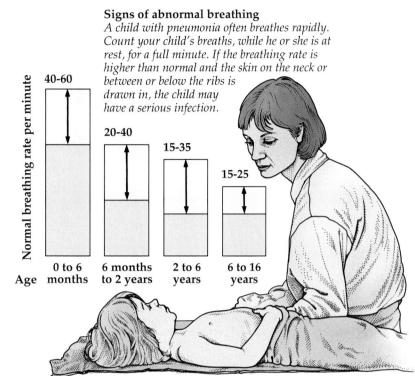

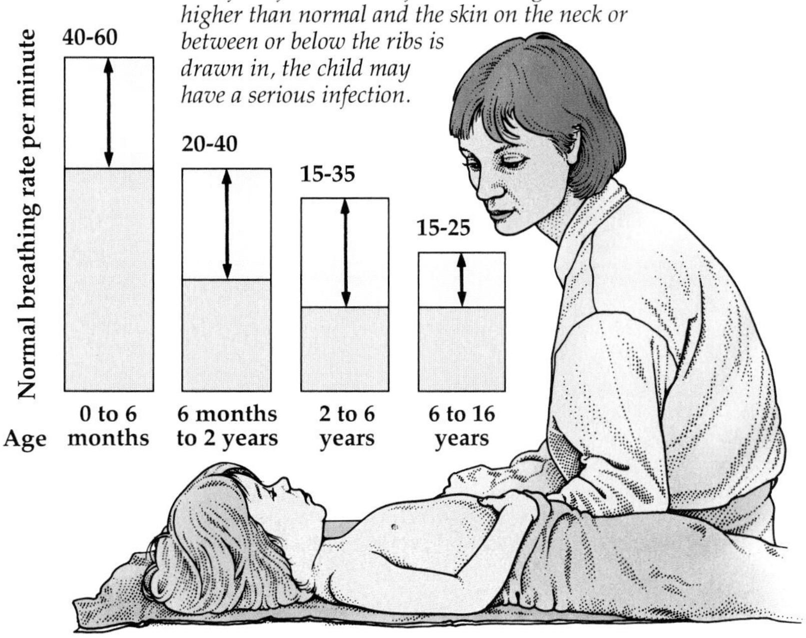

RESPIRATORY PROBLEMS

Infections by viruses or bacteria cause most childhood respiratory problems. But a number of respiratory conditions stem from inherited disorders that can affect the child's lungs.

Pneumonia

Pneumonia is an infection by a virus or bacterium that causes an accumulation of fluid inside the small air sacs of the lungs. Symptoms include a cough, rapid breathing, and a fever. Severe infection can cause the child's skin to appear blue or gray. He or she may make grunting noises when breathing, which may become painful. The child's abdomen and ribs must expand and contract more than usual so the child can breathe.

Children who have pneumonia may need to be hospitalized, but many affected children can be treated at home. In the hospital, treatment of pneumonia includes antibiotics given through a vein, drugs taken through an inhaler, and supplemental oxygen. With treatment, a child usually recovers in 2 to 3 days.

BRONCHITIS

Bronchitis is inflammation of the bronchi, the air passages of the lungs, often caused by infection by a virus or bacterium. The infection starts with a runny nose, sore throat, and muscle aches. Then, the infection spreads to the bronchi and the child begins to cough and has a slight fever. You can usually care for a child with bronchitis at home. The child should rest and take acetaminophen to reduce the fever. Drinking plenty of fluids helps to loosen the mucus in the lungs. Give cough medicine to children only on a doctor's orders. The child may also need antibiotics.

COLDS, COUGHS, AND SORE THROATS

Colds, coughs, and sore throats in children are usually caused by viral infections. Most infections occur in the first 2 years of life – an infant or toddler may have eight to 12 colds a year. Because older children gain some immunity to common viruses, they tend to have colds less frequently. Symptoms of a cold include a slight fever, a stuffy or runny nose, a sore throat, sneezing, and coughing. An infection can easily spread through the passages that link the nose, sinuses, mouth, throat, lungs, and ears.

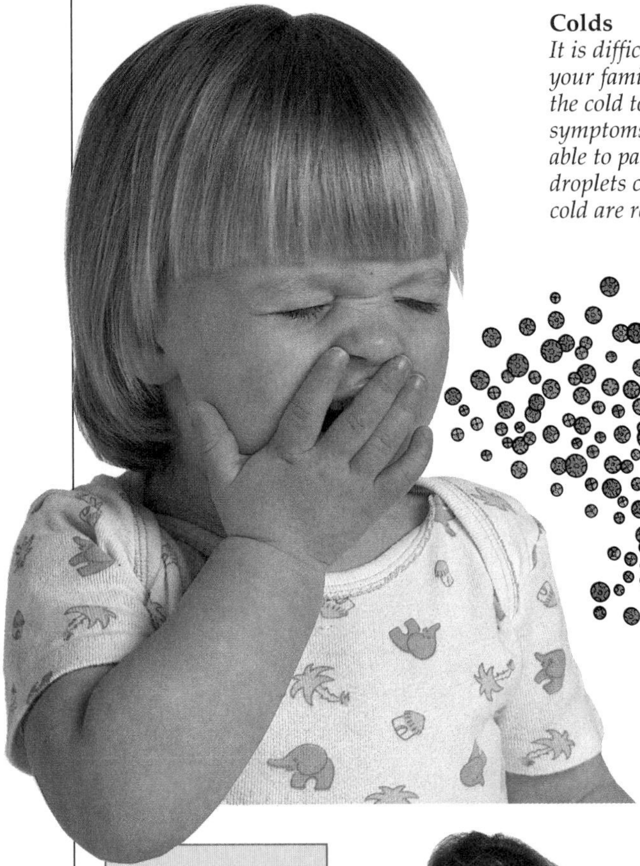

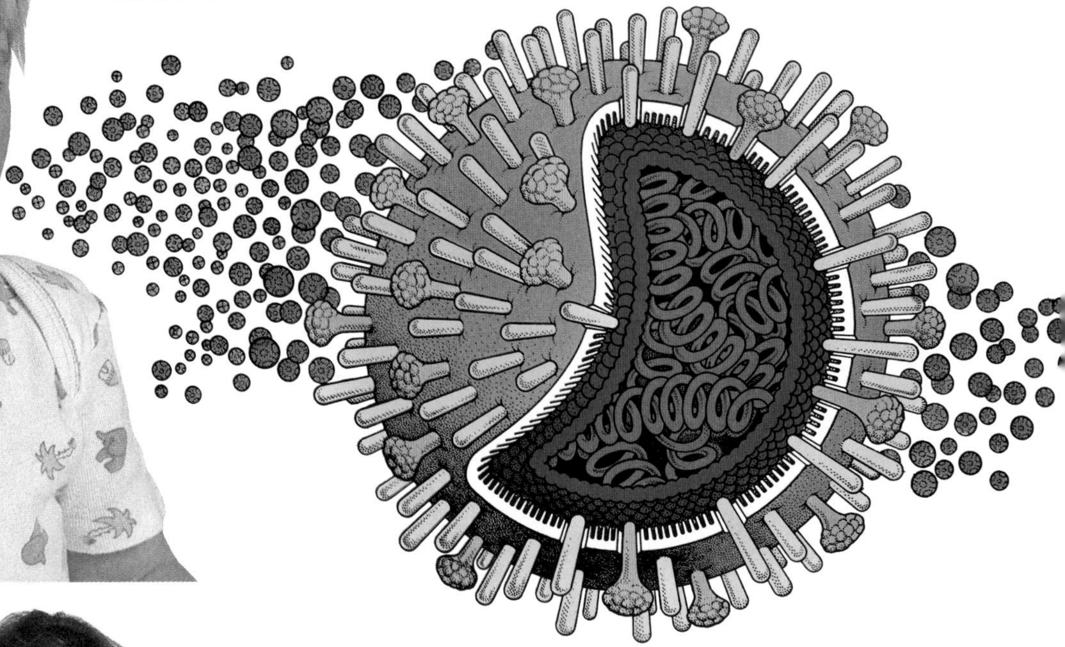

Colds
It is difficult to prevent the spread of colds within your family because an infected person can spread the cold to others a few days before and after symptoms appear. Each time a person who is able to pass on a cold sneezes, thousands of water droplets containing the virus that caused the cold are released into the air.

WARNING

Call your doctor if your child has any of these symptoms:

- A temperature higher than 102°F.
- Wheezy breathing.
- A persistent earache.
- A severe sore throat.
- A harsh cough.
- A severe headache.
- A stiff neck.
- Drowsiness.
- Irritability.
- No improvement after 3 days.

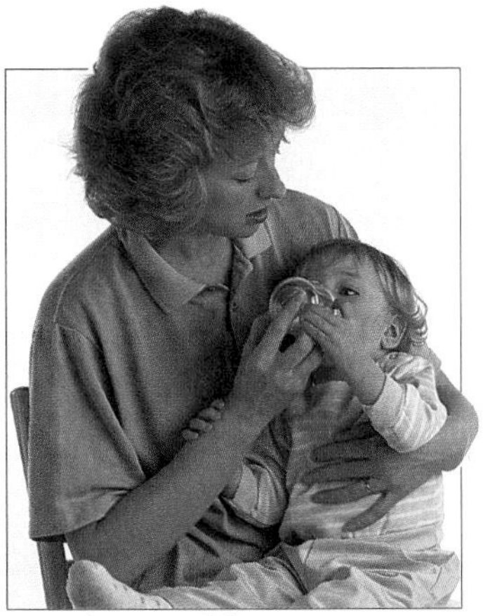

Treating a cold
To relieve symptoms, encourage your child to drink plenty of fluids and give the recommended dose of acetaminophen to reduce fever. You may use a decongestant with your doctor's approval. Cold symptoms usually go away on their own after a few days.

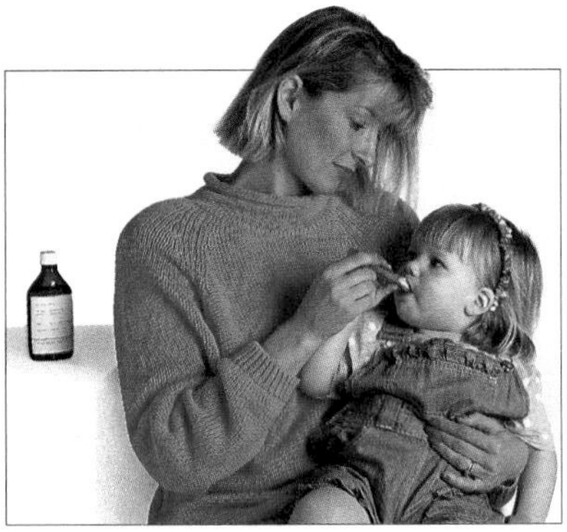

Treating a cough
Inflammation of the respiratory tract causes a buildup of mucus. The body attempts to remove the mucus through coughing. To help your child loosen mucus and bring it up, encourage your child to drink plenty of fluids. Give cough medicines only on your doctor's orders.

INFECTIONS OF THE MOUTH, NOSE, AND THROAT

Infected sinuses

Infection of the sinuses, the air spaces in the bones around the eyes and nose, is known as sinusitis. Symptoms of sinusitis are pain, fever, aching, and a nasal discharge. Persistent or recurrent sinusitis is treated with antibiotics. Recurrent infections may require surgical drainage. Sinusitis is uncommon in children under age 3 or 4.

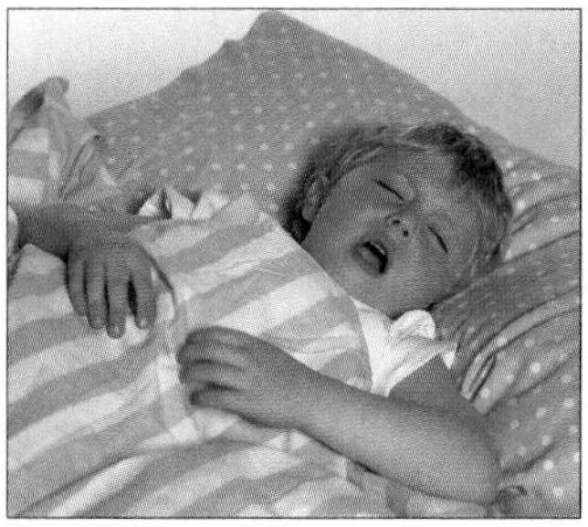

Swollen adenoids

The adenoids (clusters of tissue at the back of the nose and throat) swell when they are infected. An affected child may have a stuffy nose, forcing him or her to breathe through the mouth. Snoring is common. If your child's adenoids are frequently infected, causing loss of sleep, recurrent sinusitis, or repeated middle ear infection, your doctor may recommend that the adenoids be removed.

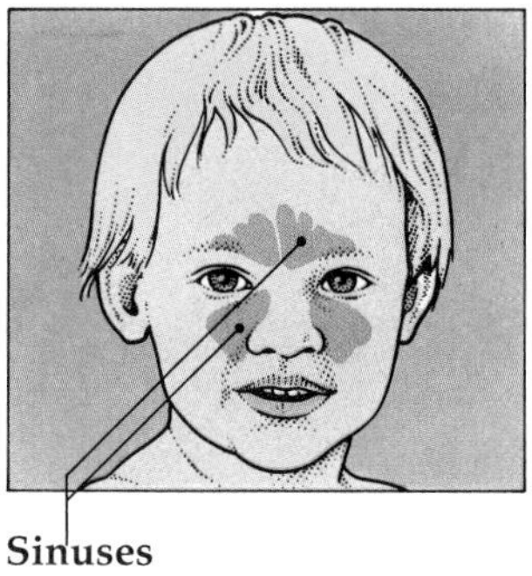

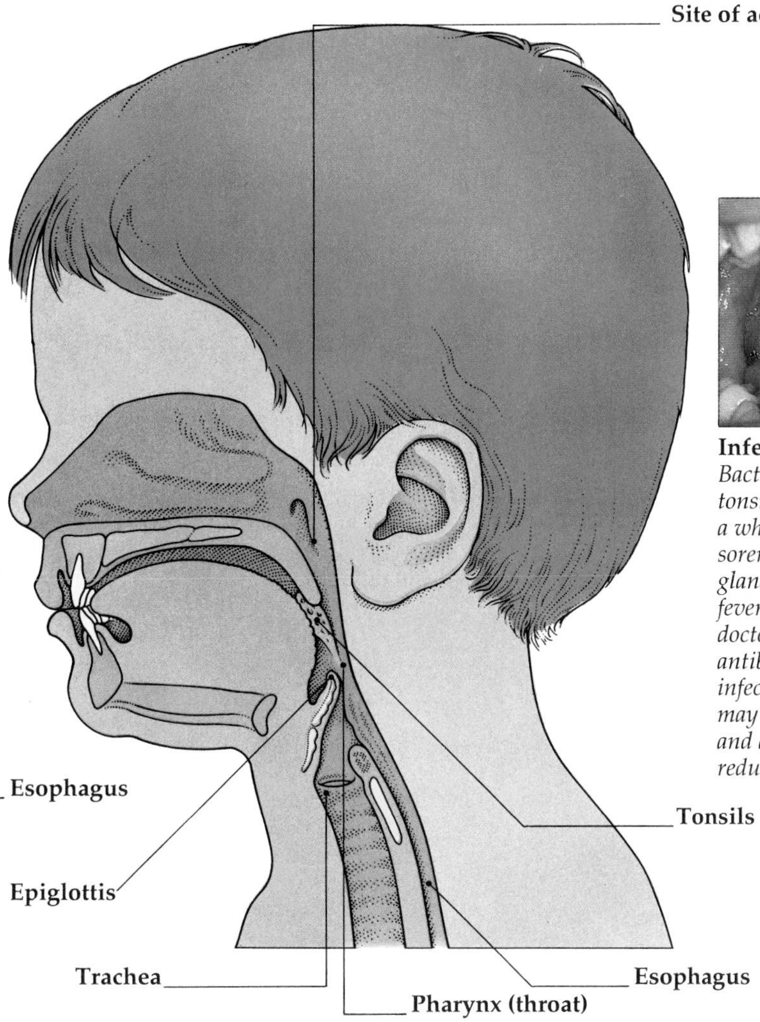

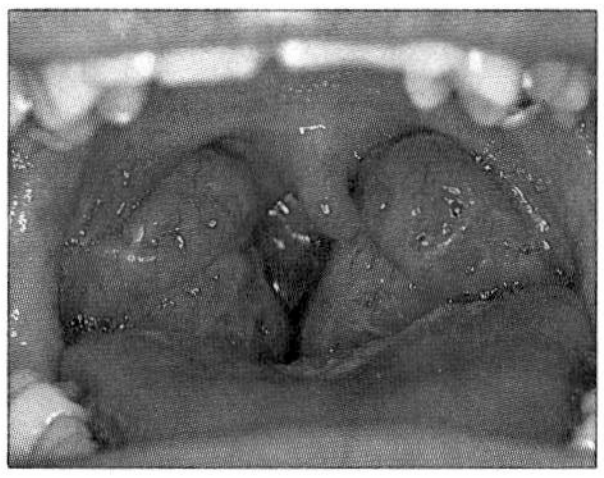

Infected tonsils

Bacterial infection of the tonsils (tonsillitis) produces a white coating and extreme soreness of the throat, swollen glands in the neck, and a fever. Take your child to your doctor, who may prescribe antibiotics to control the infection. Throat lozenges may help to relieve the pain, and acetaminophen should reduce the fever.

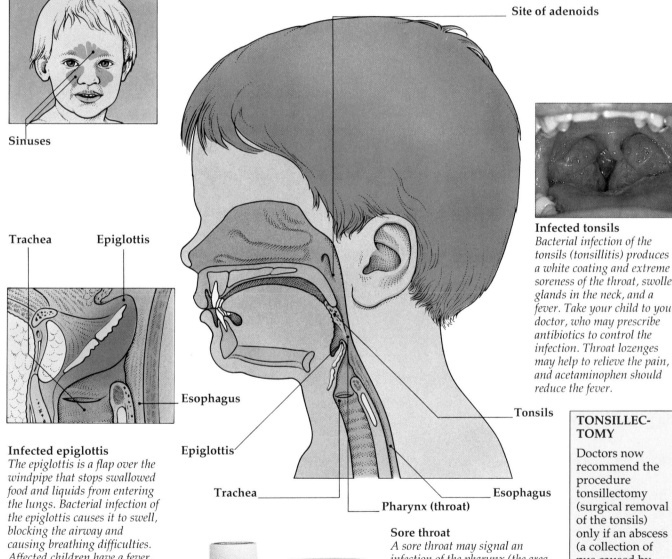

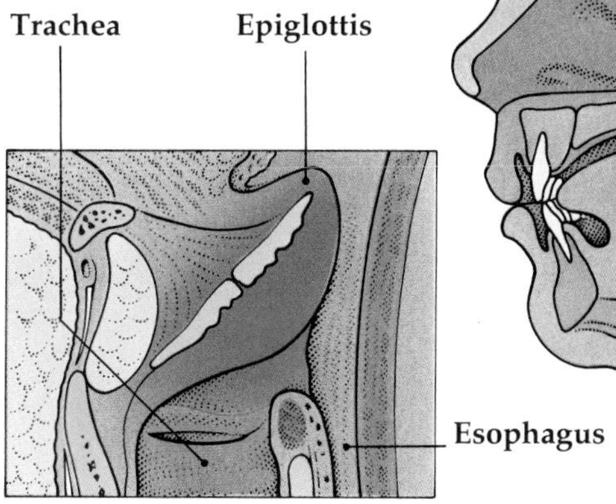

Infected epiglottis

The epiglottis is a flap over the windpipe that stops swallowed food and liquids from entering the lungs. Bacterial infection of the epiglottis causes it to swell, blocking the airway and causing breathing difficulties. Affected children have a fever, are short of breath and restless, drool, lose their voice, and produce a harsh, raspy sound when they inhale. Such children need immediate hospitalization.

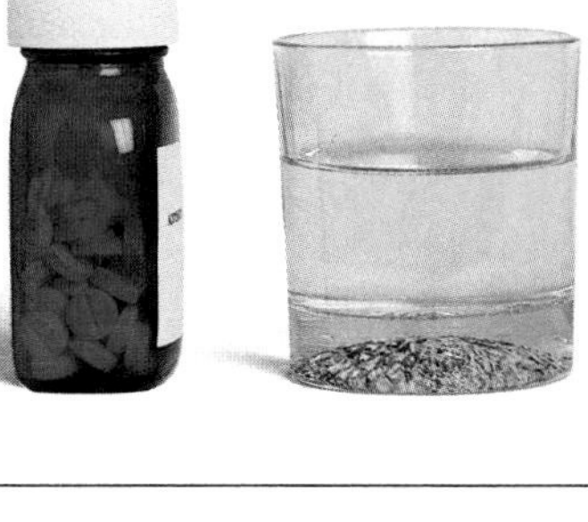

Sore throat

A sore throat may signal an infection of the pharynx (the area of the throat above the esophagus). It should be treated with acetaminophen and plenty of fluids. If the infection does not clear up in a couple of days, call your doctor, who will test to make sure that your child does not have strep throat, which is a serious infection.

TONSILLECTOMY

Doctors now recommend the procedure tonsillectomy (surgical removal of the tonsils) only if an abscess (a collection of pus caused by infection) forms around the tonsils or if the child's airway becomes obstructed and breathing is impaired.

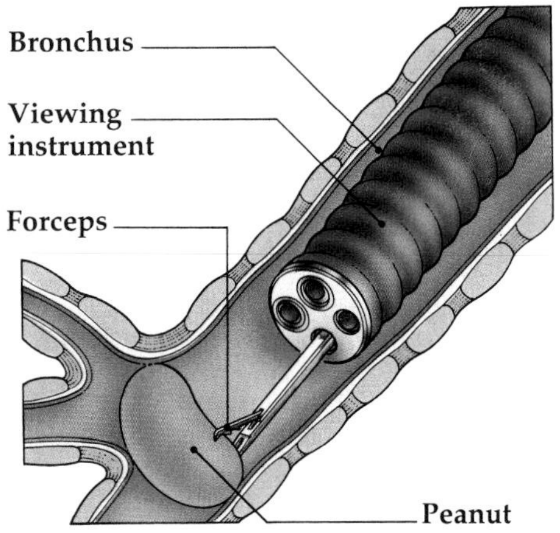

Inhaled object
Children can easily inhale a small object, such as a peanut, accidentally. Choking or coughing may follow. Contact your doctor if you think your child has inhaled an object. The doctor will obtain an X-ray to try to locate the object. He or she will then use a viewing instrument (above) to remove the object.

Whooping cough

Whooping cough, or pertussis, is a serious bacterial infection that affects a child's lungs, causing symptoms that can last for several weeks. Immunization with the pertussis vaccine (see page 70) can prevent this serious disease. Whooping cough is characterized by bouts of coughing followed by a crowing "whoop" sound as the child gasps for breath. An affected child cannot sleep well, tends to lose weight, and may vomit after bouts of coughing. The coughing spells cause mild to severe breathing difficulties. Whooping cough can be fatal or cause permanent lung or brain damage.

Cystic fibrosis

Cystic fibrosis is an inherited disease that occurs in one in 2,000 children. Affected children produce abnormally thick mucus in their pancreas (an organ that secretes digestive enzymes and insulin) that impairs the normal digestion of foods. Affected children also produce thick and profuse mucus in their bronchi, resulting in lung infections. Doctors usually diagnose cystic fibrosis soon after birth. The affected baby is slow to gain weight, has frequent chest infections, and passes loose, smelly, fatty feces. In some children, the first signs are recurrent lung infections beginning during puberty or the teenage years. Although no cure exists for cystic fibrosis, respiratory therapy and antibiotic drug treatment greatly improve the quality of life for affected children and allow most to survive well into adulthood.

ASTHMA

Asthma is characterized by attacks of wheezing, tightness in the chest, and shortness of breath. During an asthma attack, the muscle fibers surrounding the child's airways constrict, and the cells lining the airways swell and release mucus, narrowing the air passages.

Asthma affects 7 to 10 percent of children in the US. Childhood asthma is usually caused by an allergy and tends to run in families. Asthma often accompanies other allergic conditions, such as hay fever. If one parent has asthma, each child has a 50 percent chance of developing it. Asthma is a serious condition and is a leading killer of children. Call your doctor immediately if you think your child may be having an asthma attack.

CROUP

Infection of the airways by a virus, commonly called croup, starts with symptoms that resemble those of an ordinary cold, but develops into a deep, barking cough. In some children, croup can cause severe breathing difficulties, and emergency hospitalization may be needed. Croup can recur but tends to become less of a problem as the child gets older.

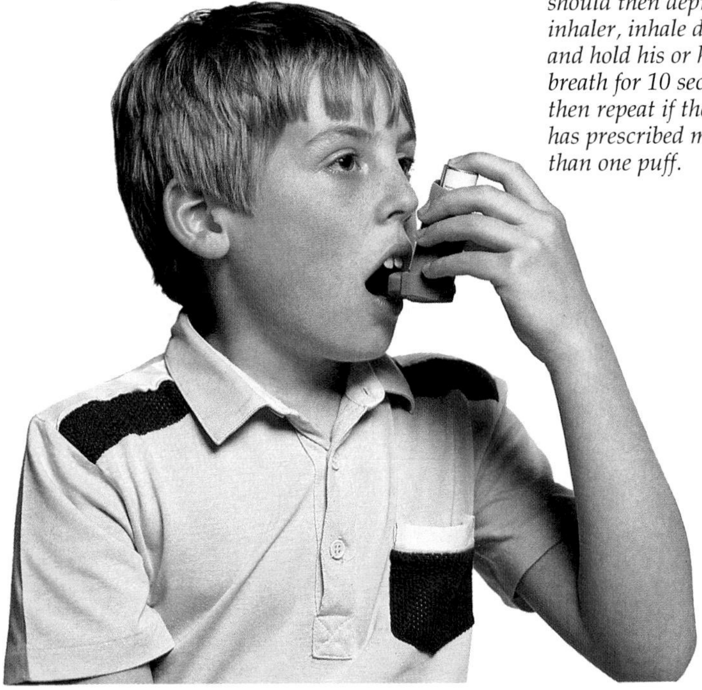

Using an inhaler
The fastest-acting antiasthma drugs are inhaled. Teach your child the correct way to use an inhaler. Shake the canister and remove the cap. After exhaling, the child should place the mouthpiece inside the lips with the mouth open wide. Your child should then depress the inhaler, inhale deeply, and hold his or her breath for 10 seconds, then repeat if the doctor has prescribed more than one puff.

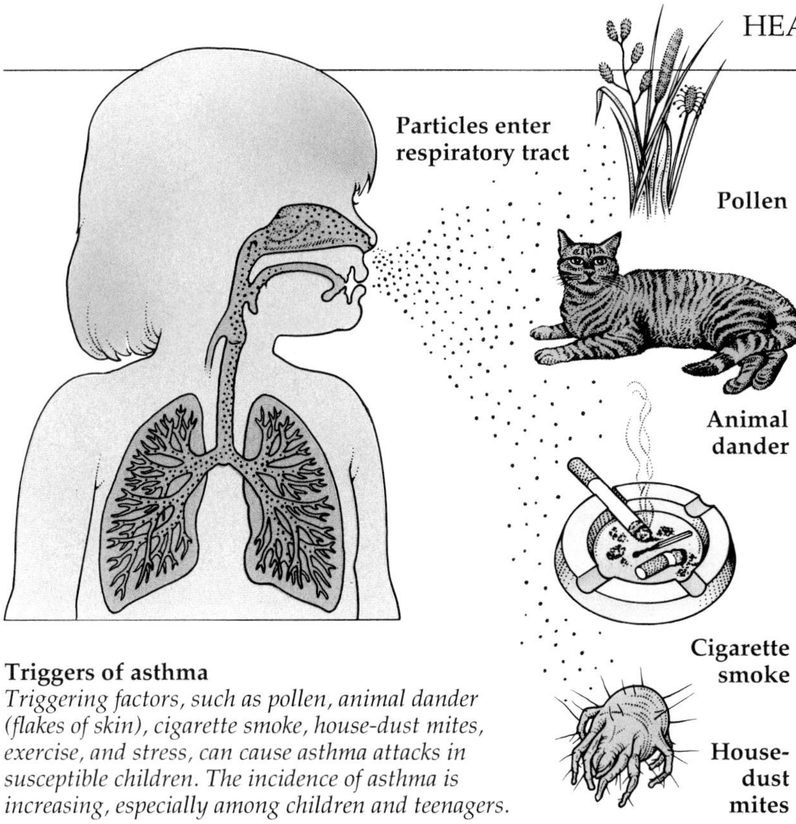

Triggers of asthma
Triggering factors, such as pollen, animal dander (flakes of skin), cigarette smoke, house-dust mites, exercise, and stress, can cause asthma attacks in susceptible children. The incidence of asthma is increasing, especially among children and teenagers.

Preventing asthma attacks

You can help your child prevent an asthma attack by limiting exposure to the factors that trigger an attack. Reduce the quantity of house-dust mites in your home by regular dusting and vacuuming. Keep rooms well ventilated. Use pillows containing artificial fibers instead of feathers. Do not have pets in your home or keep them out of your asthmatic child's bedroom. Do not allow cigarette smoking in your home.

Medications for asthma

Doctors treat asthma with inhaled drugs. When wheezing starts, an inhaler containing a drug that opens the bronchial passages can be used. The doctor may prescribe another inhaler containing a corticosteroid drug that fights the underlying inflammation in the airways. Young children may be treated with medications taken by mouth. Some treatments – sodium cromoglycate inhalers, for example – can prevent the development of an asthma attack provoked by exertion. If asthma becomes severe, hospitalization may be necessary.

HAY FEVER

In susceptible children, inhaling substances that are harmless to most people, such as particles of grass pollen, animal dander, and dust, causes an allergic reaction called hay fever or allergic rhinitis. Exposure to an irritant causes sneezing, a runny nose, and watering eyes. If your child has severe hay fever, your doctor can prescribe a medication to combat the allergic reaction and nasal sprays to alleviate the symptoms.

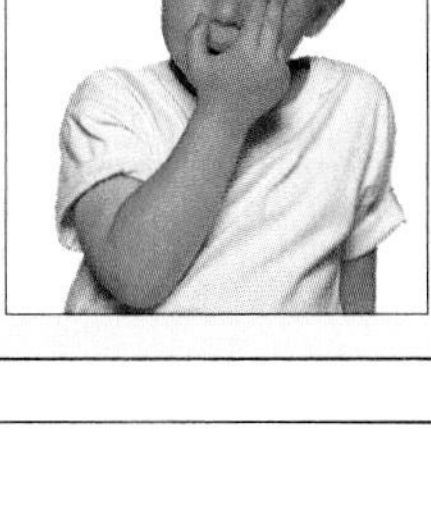

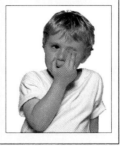

ASK YOUR DOCTOR

RESPIRATORY PROBLEMS

Q My 4-year-old son has had asthma since he was 1 year old. Is he likely to grow out of it?

A Asthma tends to become milder as a child grows older. Children who begin to wheeze before age 2 are usually symptom-free by their early teens. Those who begin wheezing after age 2 may develop more persistent asthma as they grow older, but it can be treated with inhaled drugs that widen constricted airways and fight the underlying inflammation.

Q My daughter has had repeated colds and respiratory infections. Could my husband's smoking be affecting her respiratory system?

A Yes. Research has shown that the children of parents who smoke have more respiratory infections and more severe symptoms than the children of nonsmoking parents. Passive smoking, the inhalation of smoke from someone else's cigarette, is harmful to your health too. Encourage your husband to stop smoking.

Q My friend's son was taken to the hospital with croup. Is croup always a serious infection?

A No. Croup is not especially dangerous if it is mild. But the condition causes swelling of the soft tissue of the voice box (larynx), and severe swelling can block the airway, causing a respiratory emergency. Children with severe croup must be closely observed in a hospital, where treatment with humidified oxygen and drugs can be given. If necessary, doctors pass an air tube into the windpipe to assist breathing.

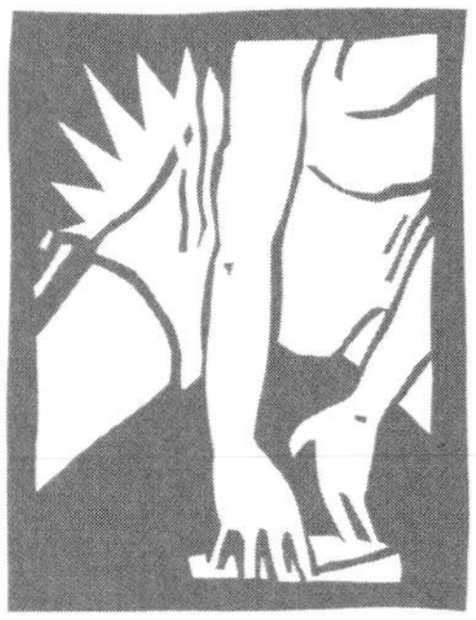

BONE AND JOINT PROBLEMS

INJURY IS THE most common cause of bone and joint problems in children. But some diseases, such as juvenile rheumatoid arthritis, can also affect a child's joints. Call your doctor if your child has persistent bone or joint pain or has an injury that restricts movement or causes a misshapen joint or bone.

GROWING PAINS

The term "growing pains" refers to the vague aches and pains that commonly occur in the limbs of children, usually when the child is at rest after exertion. Children usually feel the pains at night. Growing pains most often affect children between 3 and 8 years of age. The cause of these pains is unknown. Growing pains require no treatment and usually go away on their own. If the limb pain is severe, call your doctor.

If your child experiences temporary bone or joint pain with no other symptoms, he or she usually does not need to see a doctor. Such pain is often just the aftereffect of overexertion and disappears after a few hours of rest. But severe pain and swelling or a painful, misshapen joint probably indicate a more serious injury, such as a sprain, dislocation, or fracture. If your doctor examines and treats the affected bone or joint promptly, your child will recover rapidly and should not experience permanent impairment. If your child has a condition, such as arthritis, that is not related to injury, your doctor will monitor your child closely. Treatment, such as drug therapy, depends on the disorder.

COMMON BONE AND JOINT INJURIES

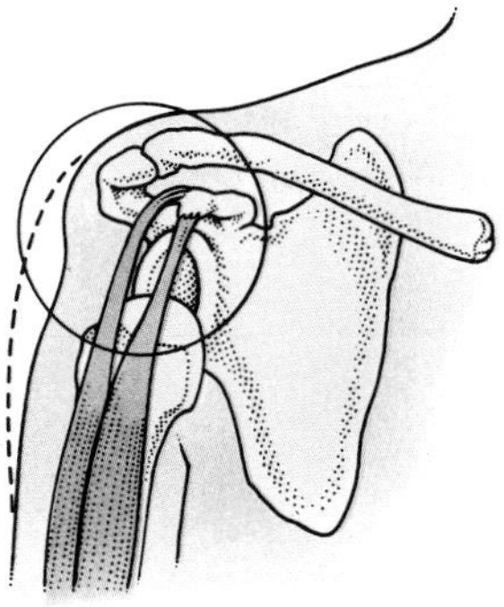

Dislocation
A dislocation is a complete displacement of the two bones in a joint so that they are no longer in their normal positions in relation to each other. Stretching or damage of the joint ligaments and damage to the capsule that encases the joint accompany dislocation. Treatment includes manipulation, to place the bones back into position, and immobilization of the joint.

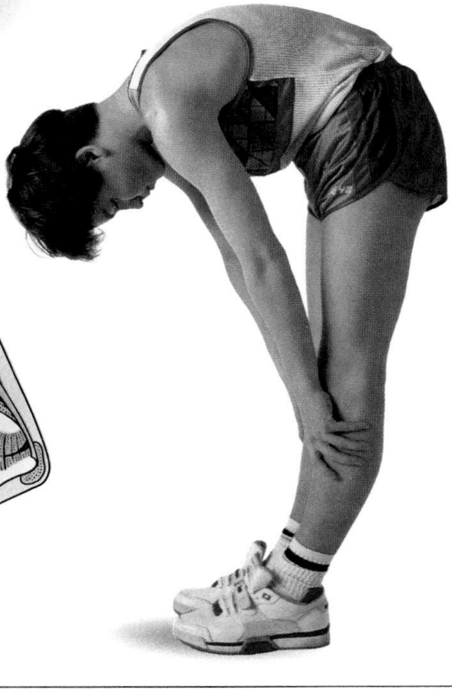

Sprain
A sprain is a tearing or overstretching of one or more of the ligaments that hold together two bones in a joint, usually from a sudden pull or twist. Sprains usually need nothing more than RICE – rest, ice, compression (a light elastic bandage), and elevation. A severe sprain may require a splint, cast, or brace.

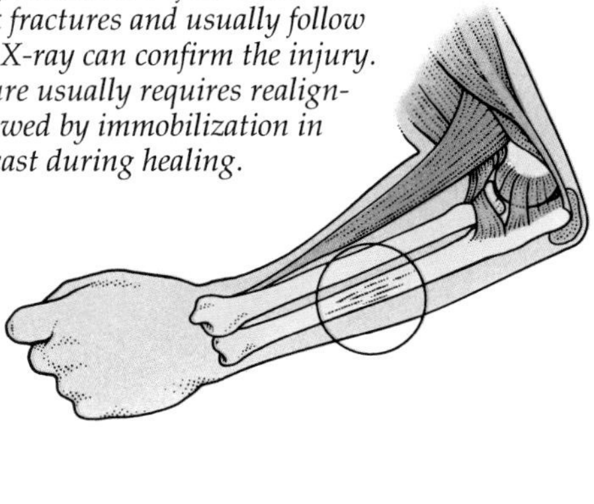

Fracture
A fracture is a partial or complete break in a bone. Partial fractures in children, in which the bone is splintered but not completely broken, are often called greenstick fractures and usually follow a fall. An X-ray can confirm the injury. The fracture usually requires realignment followed by immobilization in a plaster cast during healing.

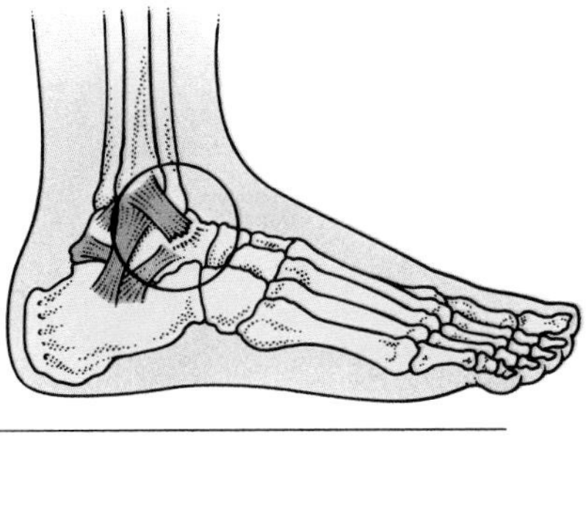

SYNOVITIS

Inflammation of the thin membrane that lines a joint (the synovium) is called synovitis. The inflammation is caused by infection, injury, irritation, or an abnormal immune response. The inflammation makes the joint swollen, stiff, painful, warm, and reddened. Many cases of synovitis occur in toddlers and young children after infection by a virus. Doctors may prescribe rest and may treat the condition with nonsteroidal anti-inflammatory drugs (such as acetaminophen). Occasionally corticosteroids (drugs, derived from hormones, that fight inflammation) may also be prescribed. These drugs are sometimes injected into the joint. If bacterial infection is present, doctors will give the child antibiotics. Traction or surgery may be needed.

OSTEOMYELITIS

Osteomyelitis, an infection of the bone and bone marrow, usually by bacteria, occurs more commonly in children than in adults. It most often affects the long bones of the arms and legs and the bones of the spine. The infection may follow a fracture, if the bone breaks through the skin, or may be caused by bacteria that reach the bone by way of the blood. The illness typically starts abruptly, and the child complains of severe pain in the affected bone. Redness and swelling often appear over the infected area. Other symptoms may include fever, headache, chills, loss of appetite, general fatigue, and lack of use of the affected limb.

Diagnosis

Doctors diagnose osteomyelitis using blood tests, X-rays, and bone scans. To obtain a bone scan, doctors inject a radioactive substance into the child's vein that concentrates in the affected area. A computer and a camera "read" the amount of radiation given off by the area and project an image on a screen. Treatment includes high doses of antibiotic drugs, which initially may be given through a vein, and rest. The limb may require a plaster cast. With prompt treatment, osteomyelitis often clears up completely. If the condition fails to respond to antibiotics, surgery may be needed to remove infected bony tissue.

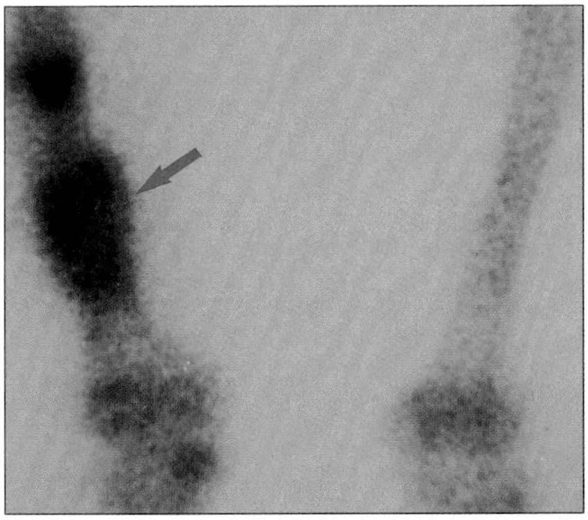

Detecting osteomyelitis
In children who have osteomyelitis, a bone scan reveals the location of the initial infection long before X-rays can show how the infection has destroyed bone tissue. The scan at right shows an area of infection (arrow) in the middle of the thighbone of a child with osteomyelitis.

Juvenile rheumatoid arthritis
The photograph below shows the characteristic features of juvenile rheumatoid arthritis in the hands of a child with the disorder. The left hand is more severely affected. The joints between the fingers exhibit spindlelike swelling, and the hands deviate outward from the wrist.

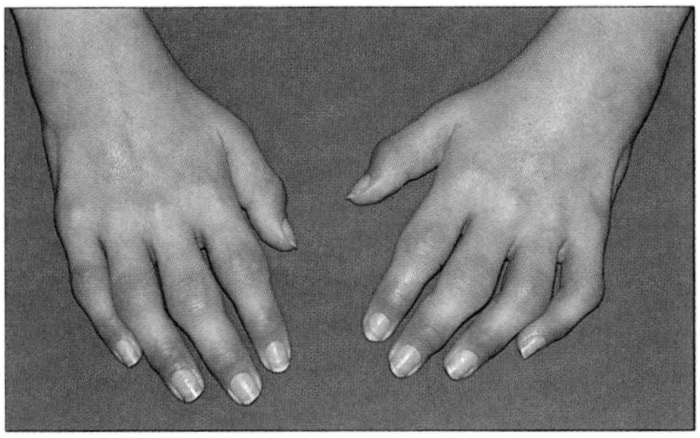

ARTHRITIS

Arthritis is pain and swelling in one or more joints, caused by inflammation. The main type of persistent arthritis in children is juvenile rheumatoid arthritis, which usually affects children under age 4. This condition can restrict growth and may leave the child with permanent joint deformities. If bacteria invade a joint from a nearby infected wound or from the bloodstream, doctors call the condition septic arthritis. Lyme disease, a bacterial infection transmitted by a tick bite, can also cause arthritis. Short-term arthritis may be caused by a virus such as the rubella (German measles) virus.

The symptoms of arthritis can develop slowly or rapidly, depending on the cause, and can affect one or more of the child's joints. The symptoms may come and go. Doctors can confirm the type of arthritis a child has through blood tests, X-rays, and bone scans.

Treatment

Each type of arthritis has a specific treatment. Doctors use antibiotic drugs to treat septic arthritis and the arthritis produced by Lyme disease. Anti-inflammatory drugs treat the symptoms of rheumatoid arthritis, but nothing can produce a cure for this type of arthritis.

VARIATIONS IN POSTURE

Children show wide variations in posture between infancy and adolescence. For example, a flat-footed baby may become a bowlegged toddler and then a knock-kneed child before growing into a graceful adolescent. These variations are normal, but if you are worried about your child's appearance, you should ask your doctor for advice. Your doctor will examine your child, first while the child is standing up and then while he or she is lying down, to detect any abnormality in posture and to check that your child's limbs are of equal size and length. These examinations help your doctor determine whether your child's posture falls outside the normal range.

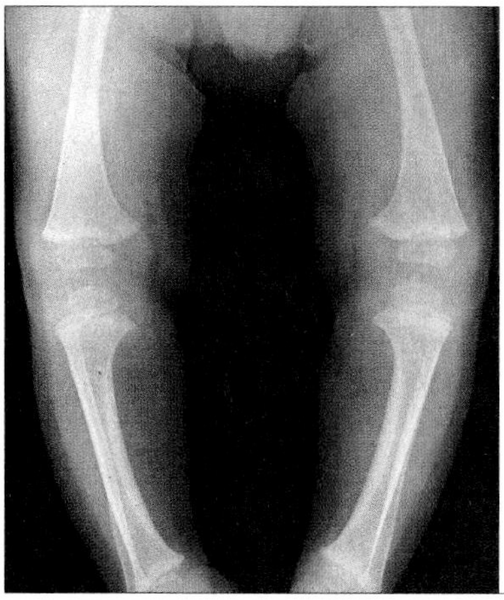

Bowlegs
Bowleggedness is an outward curving of the bones in the legs. Bowlegs are most common in children under age 2 and are a normal part of development. The curve straightens as the child grows, but you should inform your doctor if the bowing is severe or persists beyond age 6. A corrective cast or brace may be needed. In some cases, doctors perform surgery to correct the deformity.

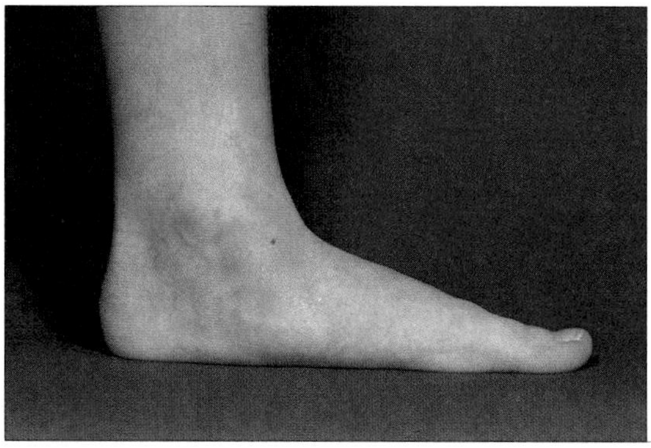

Flat feet
Doctors consider feet to be flat if they lack an arch, causing the entire sole to rest on the ground. The condition usually affects both feet. Flat feet are not a serious concern and children are normally flat-footed until age 3 or 4. After this age, you should seek treatment only if your child experiences pain. To correct flat feet, children must often wear arch supports.

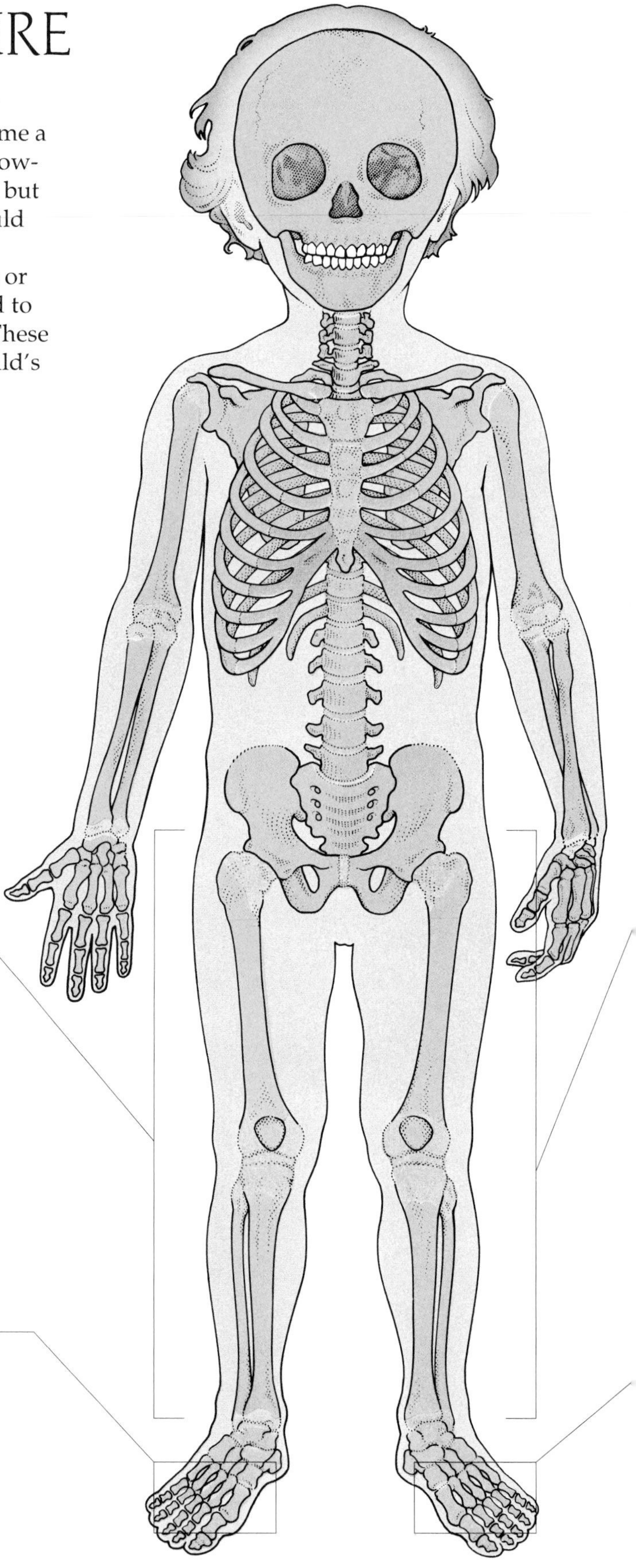

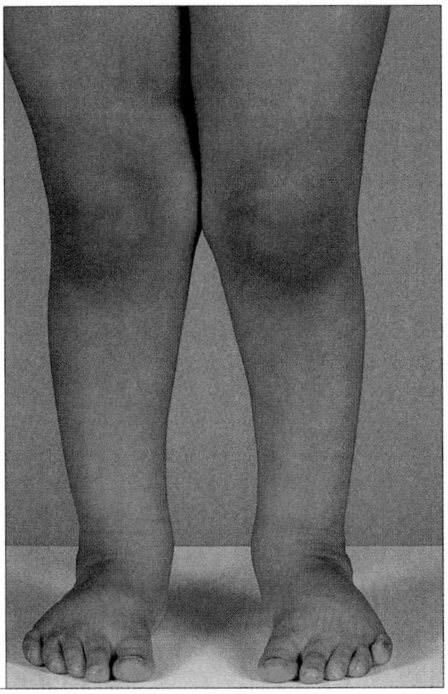

Knock-knees
Knock-knees result from an inward curving of the legs. The child's knees touch, causing the feet to lie farther apart. The condition most commonly occurs between the ages of 3 and 5. Knock-knees usually require no treatment, unless the condition persists after age 10. In rare cases, doctors may perform an operation, in which they cut and realign the shin bone, to straighten the legs. In some cases, knock-knees are caused by a disease, such as the bone disease rickets, or by a fracture.

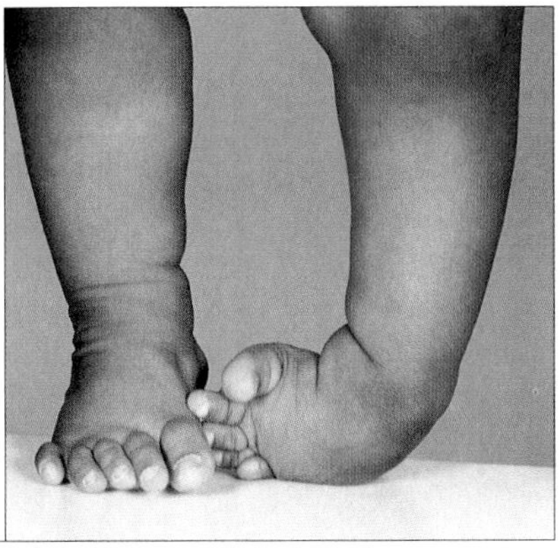

Clubfoot
Clubfoot is a birth defect in which the heel is turned inward and the rest of the foot is bent downward and inward. It is more common in boys than in girls. One or both feet may be affected. If doctors detect the condition at birth, they treat it with regular manipulation of the foot into the correct position and immobilization with strapping or a plaster cast. If the foot does not straighten after 6 months, doctors may recommend surgery.

WHAT CAN CAUSE A CHILD TO LIMP?

A limp is an uneven walk in which the child carries his or her weight more on one leg than on the other. The child may dip the pelvis to one side or fail to straighten the leg fully when placing the foot on the ground. Many children with a limp experience pain. The location of the pain sometimes helps doctors diagnose the cause of the limp. Many factors can cause a child to limp. The most common cause of a persistent limp varies by age group.

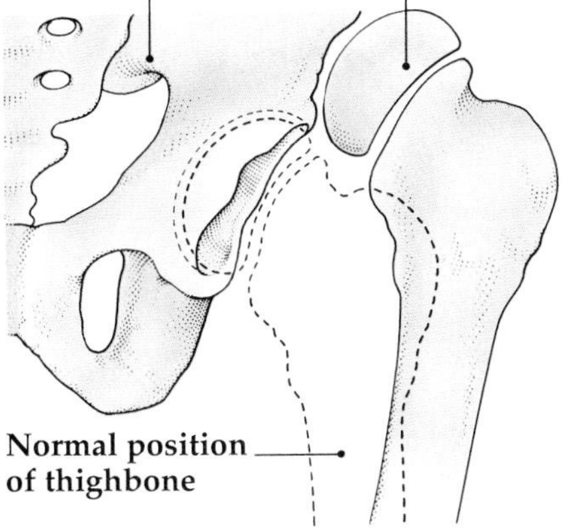

Hip dislocation
Before age 5, the most common cause of a limp is hip dislocation that is present from birth. When a hip is dislocated, the ball-like head of the thighbone slips out of the cuplike socket of the pelvis. If doctors detect the condition at birth, they apply a harness or splint to maneuver the joint back into position. If the condition is detected later, doctors use traction, realignment and casting, or surgery. If the disorder is treated early, the child usually walks normally.

Perthes' disease
Between ages 5 and 10, the most common cause of a limp is Perthes' disease, in which the head of the thighbone breaks down and softens. Doctors believe a disrupted blood supply to the bone, which can cause collapse of the hip joint, causes the disease. Perthes' disease usually affects only one hip. The condition gradually heals with rest. Some children must wear a brace. Surgery may be needed to reposition the diseased hip.

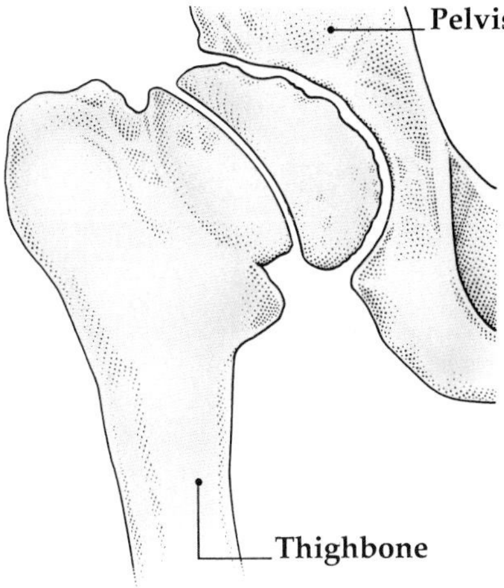

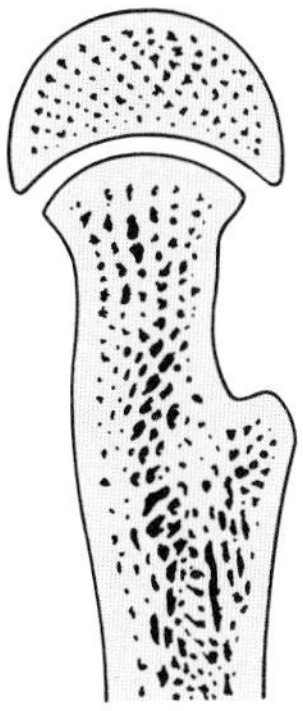

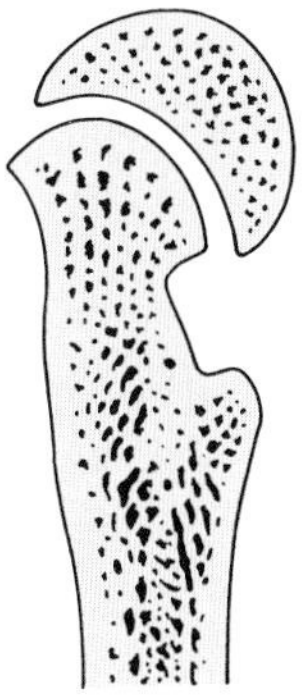

Slipped femoral epiphysis
In children between the ages of 10 and 15, the most common cause of limping is slipped femoral epiphysis, in which the upper growing end (epiphysis) of the thighbone moves from its normal position. The child tends to feel pain in the knee rather than the hip. Surgery often corrects the condition. Surgeons manipulate the displaced part of the bone back into position and secure it with metal pins.

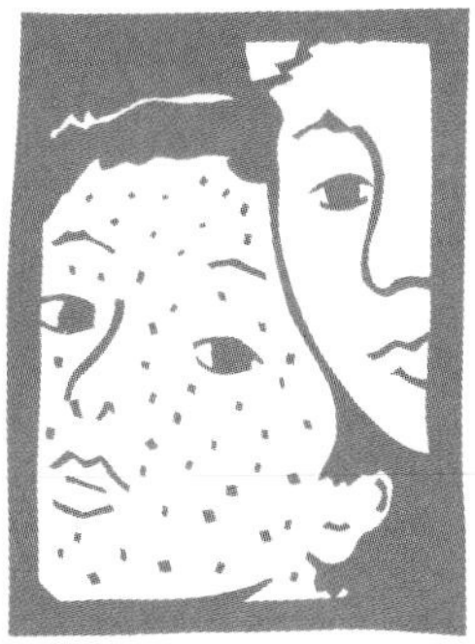

INFECTIOUS DISEASES

INFECTIOUS DISEASES occur when microorganisms, such as viruses, bacteria, or fungi, invade a child's body. Children are susceptible to infectious diseases because their immune systems have not built up much resistance to them. Most childhood infections are not serious. But certain infections can be dangerous. Immunization protects children against several serious childhood infections.

Treating a fever
A fever (a body temperature over 98.6°F) may be a symptom of infection. You can help reduce a fever by giving your child acetaminophen and plenty of fluids to drink. Do not overdress your feverish child, even if he or she is shivering. You can cool down your child's body by sponging him or her with lukewarm water.

After an initial infection, microorganisms multiply in a child's body. Doctors call this time the incubation period. During this period, the affected child may appear to be healthy but can pass on the infection to others. This means it is often difficult to prevent infection from spreading within your family.

Viruses cause most of the common childhood infections. Infections caused by a virus usually cannot be cured by antibiotic drugs, but infections caused by bacteria almost always clear up quickly and completely following treatment with antibiotics. Childhood infections tend to occur in small epidemics, spreading rapidly from child to child – especially in schools and day care centers. Certain infections, such as measles, mumps, and rubella, are now much less common than they were before immunization became widely available (see page 10).

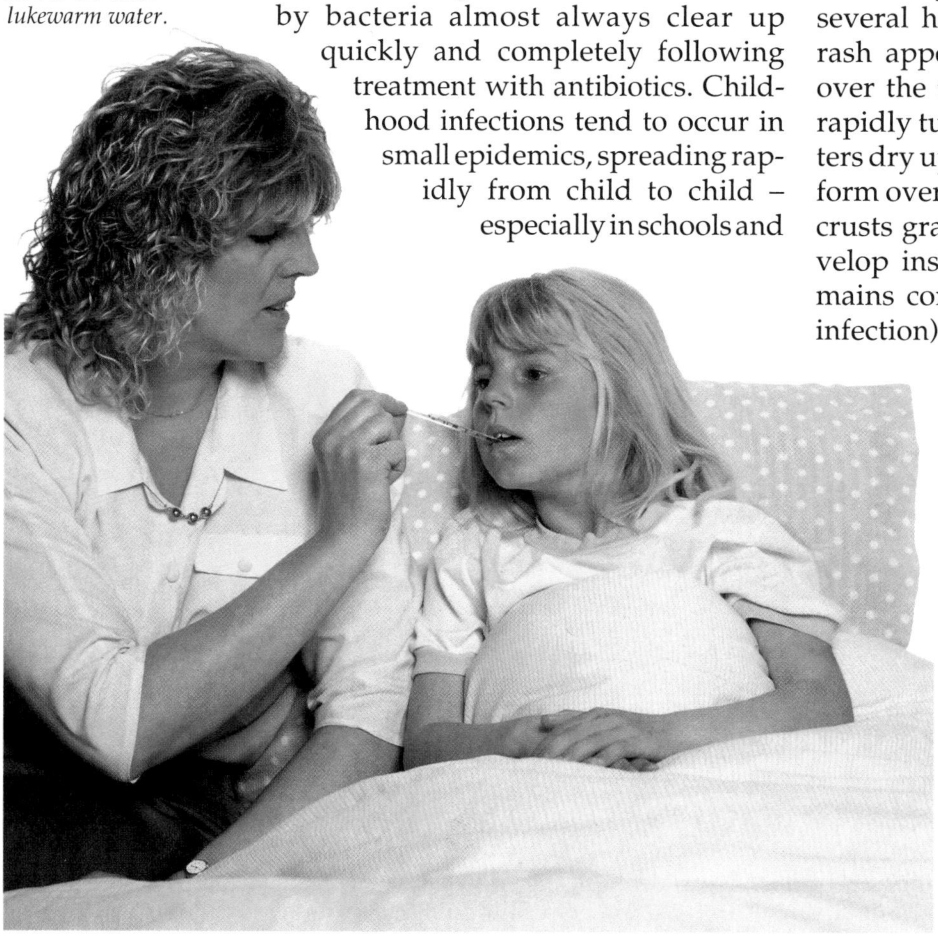

CHICKENPOX

Chickenpox is a highly contagious infectious disease, caused by a virus, with an incubation period of 10 to 21 days. The child may feel miserable and feverish several hours before the characteristic rash appears. Groups of spots appear over the trunk, starting as bumps that rapidly turn into itchy blisters. The blisters dry up within a few days, and crusts form over them. After about a week, the crusts gradually fall off. Spots may develop inside the mouth. The child remains contagious (able to pass on the infection) until scabs have formed.

Treatment for chickenpox is usually unnecessary. Calamine lotion and syrup containing antihistamine drugs may help relieve symptoms.

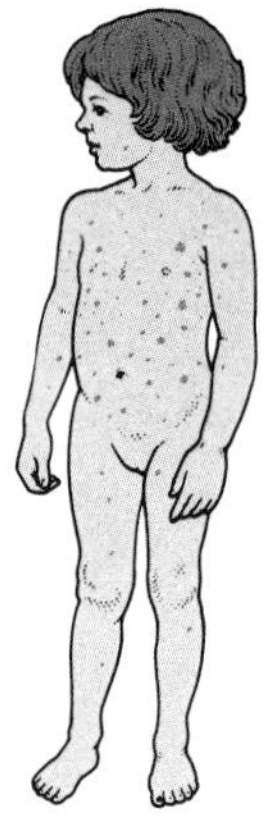

Chickenpox rash
The chickenpox rash begins as bumps that turn into blisters and then form crusted scabs. The itchy rash mainly covers the trunk but is sparse over the limbs. If your child has chickenpox, keep his or her fingernails short to help reduce the risk of further infection through scratching.

MEASLES

Measles is a highly infectious disease, caused by a virus, with an incubation period of about 10 days. Before the rash appears, the child becomes sick with a fever, cough, runny nose, and redness of the eyes. After 3 or 4 days, a blotchy rash appears, spreading down from the head to cover the whole body. The rash begins to fade after about 3 days.

No specific treatment exists for measles, other than the general measures that will keep the child comfortable. Measles can sometimes produce serious complications, including pneumonia, ear infection, and encephalitis (inflammation of the brain) that can cause permanent brain damage. If complications of measles develop, the child may need hospitalization. Doctors sometimes prescribe antibiotics if a bacterial infection occurs as a complication of measles.

To prevent infection, nonimmunized children who are exposed to someone who has measles may receive an injection of immunoglobulin obtained from the immune system of people who have already had the disease. The injection is given within 6 days after exposure.

Roseola infantum
Roseola infantum is a mild infection that most commonly affects babies under age 2. Doctors believe a virus causes the infection. The illness typically begins with a very high fever. After 3 or 4 days, the fever drops suddenly and a faint rash appears over the baby's neck and trunk. The child needs no treatment and recovers completely within 3 days.

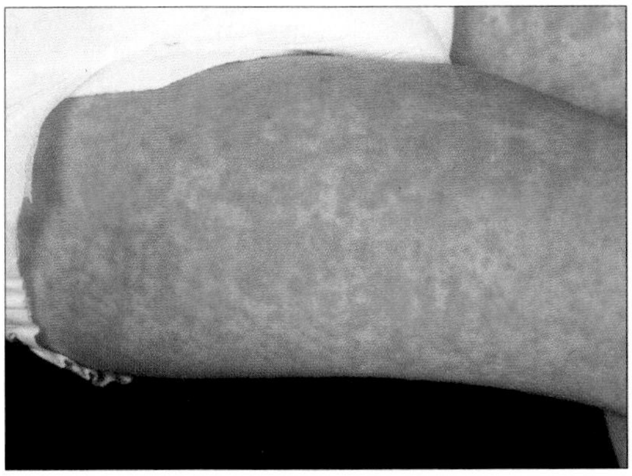

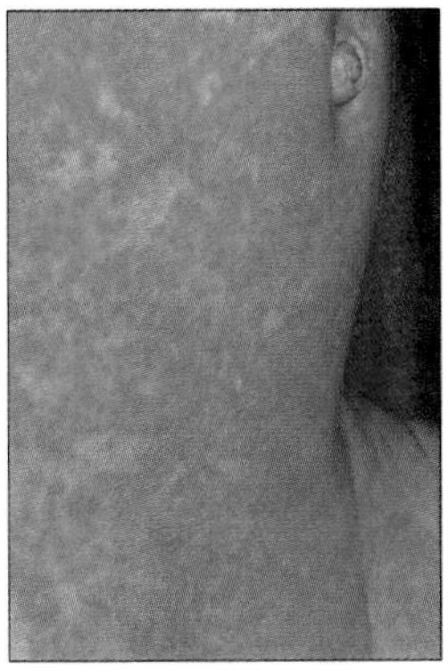

Measles rash
The measles rash does not appear until 3 or 4 days after the first signs of illness. The rash consists of flat pink spots. It usually starts on the face and then spreads over the trunk. In some children, tiny gray spots on a red base appear inside the mouth before the skin rash appears.

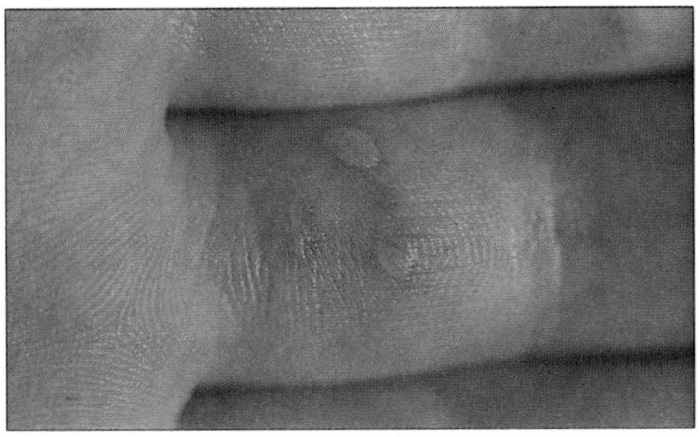

Hand-foot-and-mouth disease
Hand-foot-and-mouth disease is a fairly mild infection caused by a virus called the coxsackievirus. It produces a rash of blisters on the child's palms and soles and between the fingers. Shallow, painful ulcers develop on the tongue and elsewhere in the mouth. The rash disappears completely within a few days. No specific treatment exists, other than giving plenty of fluids and taking measures to reduce discomfort and fever.

MUMPS

Mumps is an infection, produced by a virus, that causes one or both of the salivary glands below and in front of the ears at the jaw angles to become swollen and tender. The child feels feverish and miserable and may complain of earache and difficulty swallowing. The incubation period is 2 to 3 weeks. The incidence of mumps has declined since immunization became available in 1967.

Meningitis (inflammation of the membranes that surround and protect the brain) is an uncommon complication of mumps. Meningitis can cause permanent hearing loss. Inflammation of the testicles may occur in boys who contract mumps after puberty, causing sterility. There is no specific treatment for mumps.

RUBELLA

Rubella, or German measles, is a mild infection, caused by a virus, that often goes unnoticed. It occurs most commonly between the ages of 4 and 12. After an incubation period of 2 to 3 weeks, a fine rash appears, mainly over the trunk. The child may develop enlarged lymph nodes, especially at the back of the neck and behind the ears, and may have a slight fever. No specific treatment is needed. Rubella is not dangerous in children, but if a woman contracts it during early pregnancy, the infection can cause serious abnormalities in the developing fetus.

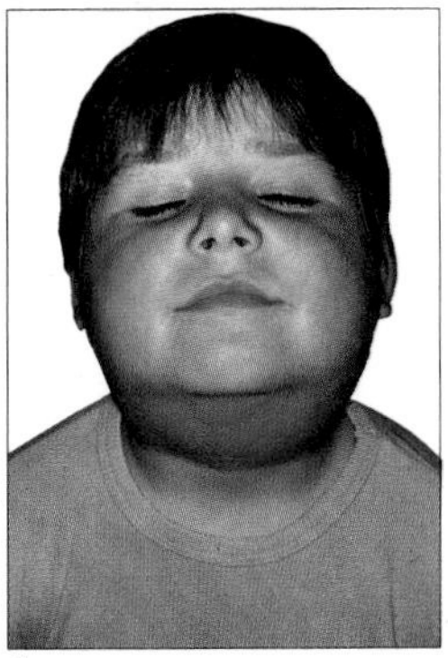

Appearance of mumps
The most obvious and characteristic sign of mumps in a child is the disappearance of the angle of the jaw, caused by firm swelling of the salivary glands in front of and below the ears. This swelling often gives the affected child a thick-necked appearance.

SCARLET FEVER

Scarlet fever is a bacterial infection caused by one of the streptococcal bacteria. It commonly occurs after a child has an untreated strep throat. Infectious droplets coughed or breathed into the air spread the bacteria from one person to another. The illness begins with fever, vomiting, and headache, followed by a widespread rash that first appears on the neck and upper part of the child's trunk. The rash appears as a red blush and gives a "sandpaper" feel to the skin.

After a few days, the rash fades and the skin starts to peel, especially on the hands and feet. If untreated, scarlet fever can cause inflammation of the kidneys or rheumatic fever (an inflammatory condition affecting the heart and other tissues). Treatment with antibiotics usually produces a rapid recovery and prevents the occurrence of rheumatic fever.

ERYTHEMA INFECTIOSUM

Erythema infectiosum is a mild infection caused by a recently discovered virus. An affected child develops a mild fever and a red rash over both cheeks, which then spreads over the child's trunk and limbs, forming a lacy pattern. The rash usually fades within a week to 10 days. Most children have no other symptoms. No specific treatment is necessary.

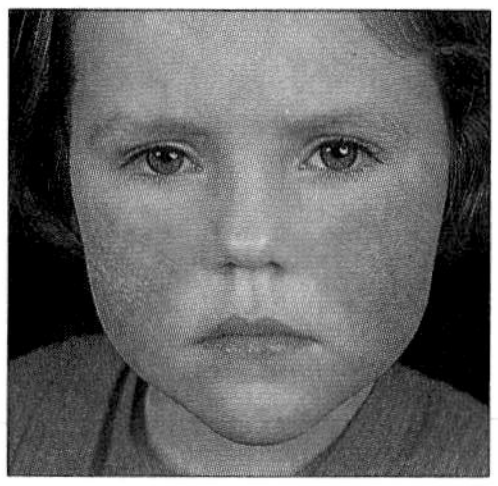

Rash of erythema infectiosum
The rash of erythema infectiosum starts on the cheeks, producing a "slapped cheek" appearance, then spreads to the trunk and limbs. The rash often appears more pronounced after a warm bath. The infection is moderately contagious.

MENINGITIS

Meningitis is inflammation of the membranes surrounding the brain and spinal cord caused by a virus or bacterium. Viral meningitis is a relatively mild condition. But bacterial meningitis can be fatal or cause brain damage. Symptoms of both kinds include fever, a severe headache, vomiting, and a stiff neck, with increased irritability and lethargy. A child with bacterial meningitis may have seizures and changes in the level of consciousness that are rare in a child with viral meningitis. Infants with meningitis usually have a bulging soft spot. Doctors treat bacterial meningitis with intravenous antibiotics in the hospital.

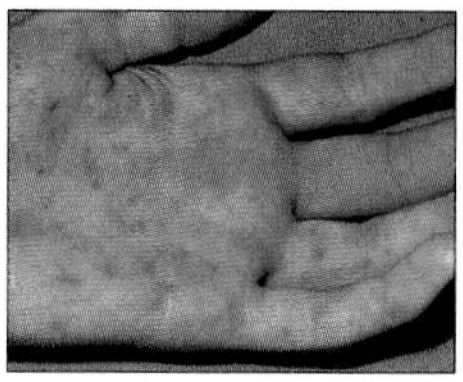

Rash of meningococcal meningitis
Children with meningococcal meningitis develop a characteristic rash. "Purpura" is the medical term used to describe the red-brown, blotchy, bruiselike appearance of this rash.

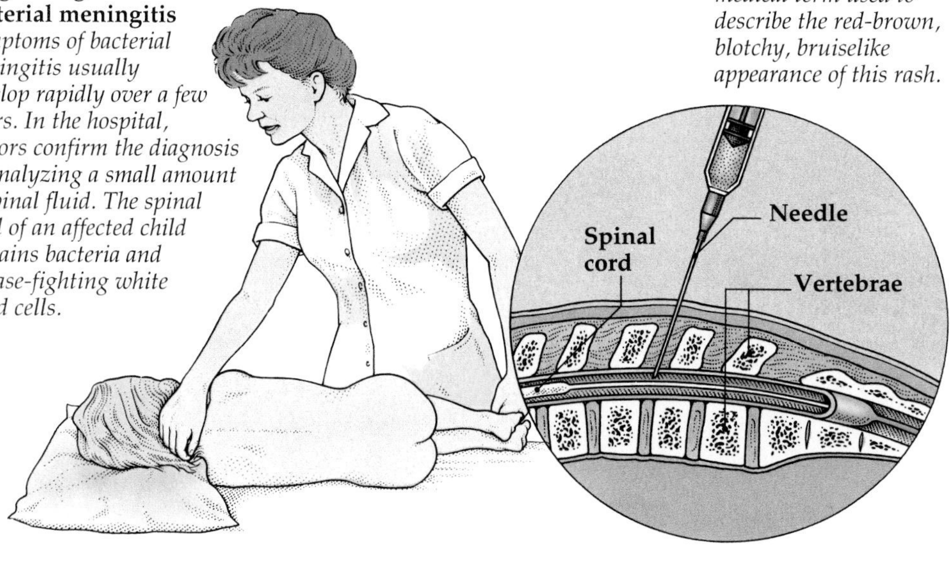

Diagnosing bacterial meningitis
Symptoms of bacterial meningitis usually develop rapidly over a few hours. In the hospital, doctors confirm the diagnosis by analyzing a small amount of spinal fluid. The spinal fluid of an affected child contains bacteria and disease-fighting white blood cells.

OTHER VIRAL RASHES

Many lesser-known viruses, such as enteroviruses, echoviruses, and coxsackieviruses, can cause an illness with a rash. These viruses usually do not produce a characteristic type of rash and are commonly misdiagnosed. The rash usually lasts for only a few days. Symptoms may include a sore throat, headache, and swollen lymph nodes. Other family members may also feel sick but may not develop a rash. No treatment is needed.

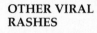

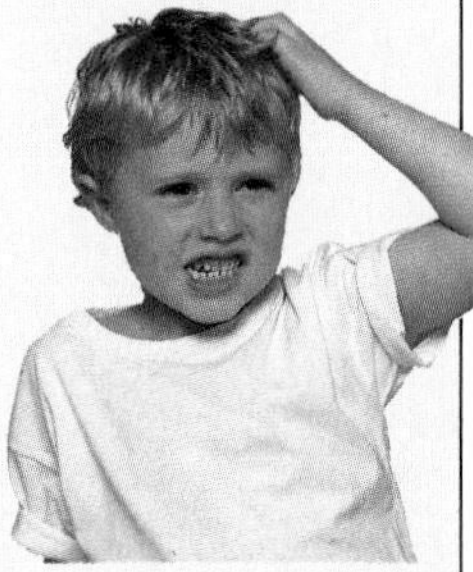

CASE HISTORY
FEVER AND A RASH

ONE MORNING, Rosie woke up with a fever, cough, runny nose, and reddened eyes. Her mother noticed that the inside of her mouth was covered with tiny grayish white spots. Rosie continued to feel sick for a few days. Then her mother noticed a blotchy red rash on Rosie's neck and behind her ears. Her mother decided to call the family doctor.

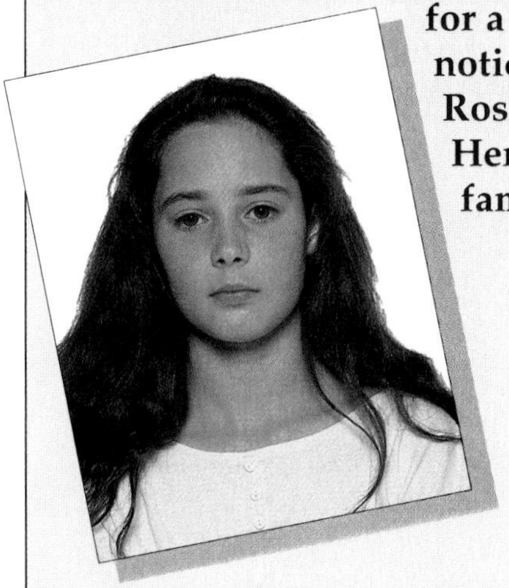

PERSONAL DETAILS
Name Rosie Alvarez
Age 13
Occupation Student
Family Rosie's parents are both healthy. Her brother Hector, aged 10, has mild asthma.

MEDICAL BACKGROUND
Rosie had her tonsils removed when she was 6 years old. Otherwise, she has had no medical problems.

THE CONSULTATION
The doctor asks whether Rosie has recently been in contact with anyone who has an infectious disease. Rosie replies that she doesn't think that she has been. The doctor learns from Rosie's medical records that she received all of her scheduled immunizations when she was 11 or 12 years old, except for her measles booster, which she should have received a year or so ago. Rosie's mother explains that Rosie was sick with a cold on the day that she was supposed to get her measles booster and then they had forgotten all about it. The doctor questions Rosie's mother about the health of her son, Hector, and learns that he has been at his cousin's house for 2 weeks but is returning the next day. Hector has been healthy the entire time.

THE DIAGNOSIS
After examining Rosie, the doctor diagnoses MEASLES, which is caused by a virus. He describes the recommendations for measles vaccination to Rosie's mother, explaining that booster injections are needed because the initial immunization may not provide lasting protection. The doctor recommends that Hector stay away from Rosie until she gets better because he could contract the disease, which can have serious complications. As an additional precaution, Hector should be given the measles booster as soon as he returns. The doctor also explains that Rosie's attack of measles will probably give her lifelong immunity and that she needs no further vaccinations.

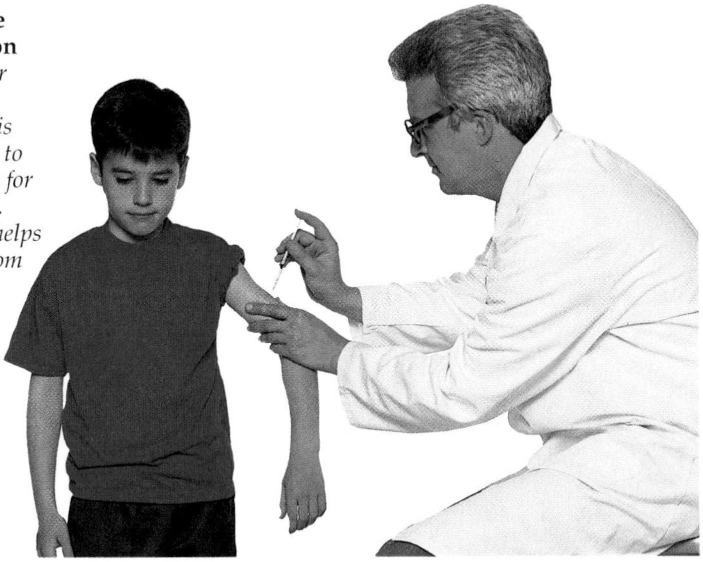

The importance of immunization
As soon as Hector returns from his cousin's house, his mother takes him to the doctor's office for a measles booster. The vaccination helps protect Hector from getting measles from his sister Rosie.

THE TREATMENT
The doctor advises Rosie to rest in bed for a few days and to drink plenty of fluids. He tells Rosie's mother to give Rosie acetaminophen (an over-the-counter aspirin substitute) every 4 to 6 hours, when needed, to help reduce her fever.

THE OUTCOME
Rosie continues to feel sick for a few days and the measles rash spreads over her entire body. Her symptoms gradually improve, until, by the 10th day of her illness, the rash has faded and she feels better. Rosie feels healthy enough to return to school the following week. Because her brother Hector received his booster injection, he remains healthy.

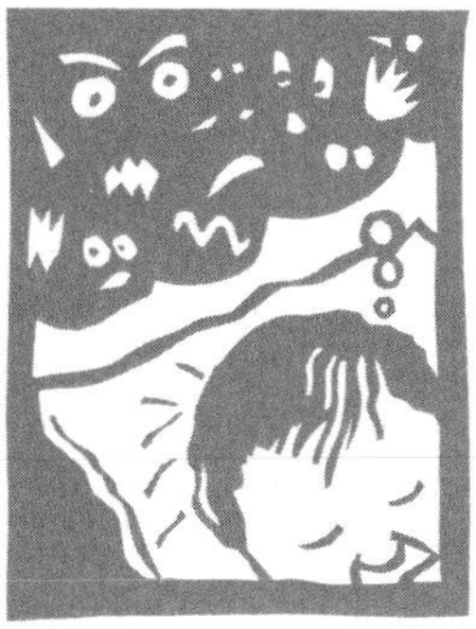

BEHAVIORAL AND EMOTIONAL PROBLEMS

CHILDREN DEVELOP emotional independence and maturity by learning how to cope with problems and interact with a variety of people. Sometimes, traumatic events – such as a death in the family – or disturbances in the developmental process can cause emotional conflict and difficult behavior. Help your child build a positive self-image by giving encouragement and support.

Coping with temper tantrums
First make sure that your child cannot get hurt or break anything and then walk away. Avoid having a confrontation with your child. Tantrums end once the child vents his or her anger. If the child resorts to physical violence, restrain the child by holding him or her. Do not hit your child.

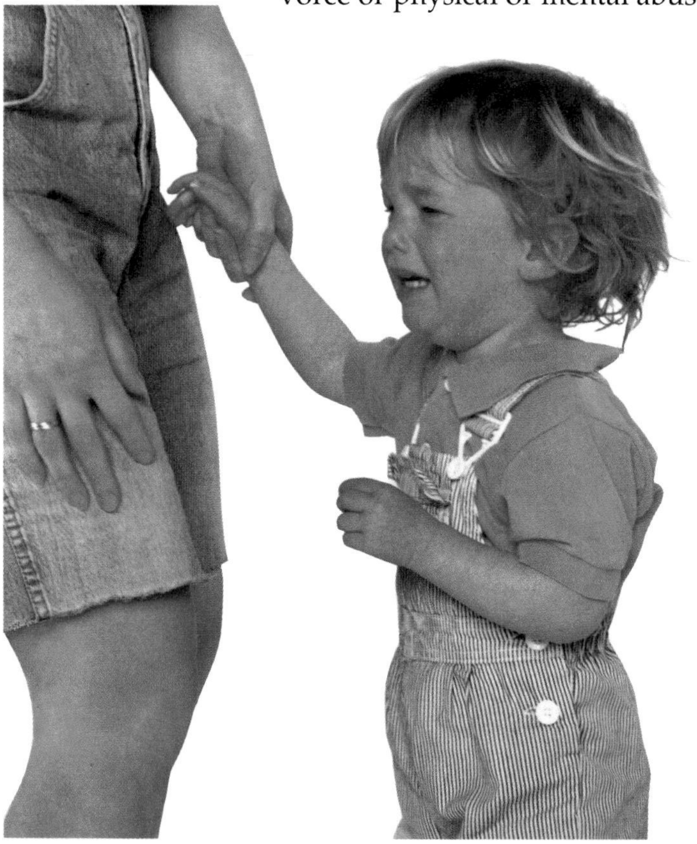

As children grow, they begin to assert themselves more and more as a means of exerting control over their environment. Although it is irritating to adults, assertiveness in a child is a natural part of his or her development. But behavioral problems can occur when the child takes this assertiveness to unreasonable extremes. Behavioral problems can also arise when a child has emotionally upsetting experiences, such as parental divorce or physical or mental abuse.

TEMPER TANTRUMS

A temper tantrum is an extreme expression of anger or frustration in a child who, temporarily, does not respond to reason. Tantrums occur most often in children aged 1 to 4 years. Although irritating, temper tantrums can help the child make the transition from dependence to increasing independence. Temper tantrums can occur any time the child does not get his or her way.

Breath holding

Some children hold their breath during a temper tantrum. Breath holding can be disturbing for parents but should not be a source of concern. If your child needs oxygen, the body's natural response to oxygen shortage will take over – the child will faint, and normal breathing will resume shortly on its own.

OTHER BEHAVIORAL PROBLEMS

Children have a strong need for love, security, and continuity in their lives. They are deeply affected by family problems, such as the divorce of their parents, the death of a close relative, alcoholism, and sexual or physical abuse. A child who experiences such events becomes confused and responds to the events by altering his or her behavior. Some

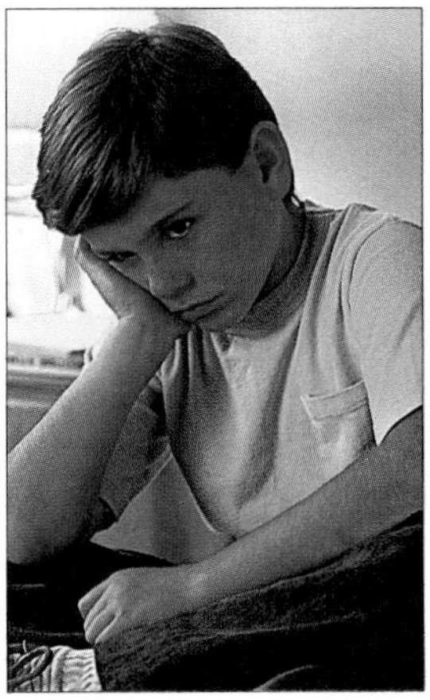

Depression
A child who has lost a parent, a close relative, or even a pet may develop depression. The child may play less and have feelings of sadness, loneliness, helplessness, and loss. An older child may become withdrawn. School performance may deteriorate. Depressed teenagers often display antisocial behavior.

children shrink into themselves. Others become angry and aggressive. Some children may begin bed-wetting at night or develop unusual sleeping or eating patterns. Although children usually outgrow these problems in time, a family can do a lot to help a child through an especially distressing period.

Anger and aggression

Children have a right to feel angry when they are provoked. But they should not feel free to act aggressively whenever they want their way. Explain to your child that physical violence is not an appropriate reaction to conflict. Talk through other options with your child, such as encouraging the child to speak up and talk about his or her problems. But do not teach your child to avoid conflict or suppress anger. These responses can lead to depression and even more violent outbursts of anger.

Bullying behavior

A certain amount of aggression in growing children is normal. Pushing and shoving often occur when children play, but if your child seems to be more violent or intimidating than necessary, or if your child regularly hits, bites, scratches, or browbeats other children, you need to teach him or her that this behavior is wrong. Look for an underlying cause for a sudden appearance of bullying behavior, such as problems in starting school or the arrival of a new baby at home. Bullying may mirror parents' relationships. Children usually treat others the way they have been treated or have seen their parents treat each other.

Stealing

Very young children take things that belong to others because they do not understand the concepts of ownership and property. But after about 6 years of age, children should know that they must not take things that do not belong to them. When older children steal, they usually hide the stolen items and lie when confronted with the facts. Some children steal on a dare from another child. Others use it as a way of attracting attention. If no reasons for theft are apparent and the child continues to steal, the entire family should consider therapy to explore the tensions and jealousies within the home. Stealing can be the child's way of expressing unconscious feelings of emotional deprivation.

Telling lies
Very young children cannot distinguish between fact and fantasy and may weave the two together when speaking. Do not discourage fantasy in young children. But encourage them to tell the truth. Explain that there are many times when people want to know exactly what has happened. Persistent lying usually indicates that the child has learned lying behavior from the parents.

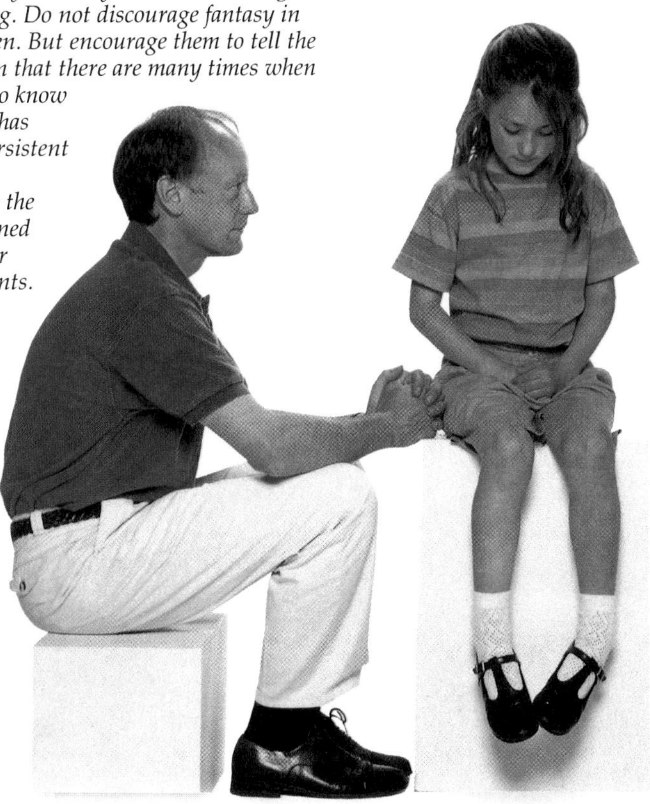

GROUND RULES

Children always test the limits of the behavioral guidelines that their parents have set for them. After establishing the rules of acceptable behavior, you should be firm in encouraging your children to follow those rules. But discipline should always be fair, reasonable, and consistent – never harsh, overly rigid, or abusive.

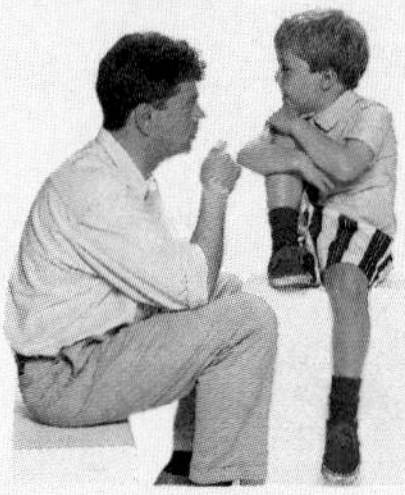

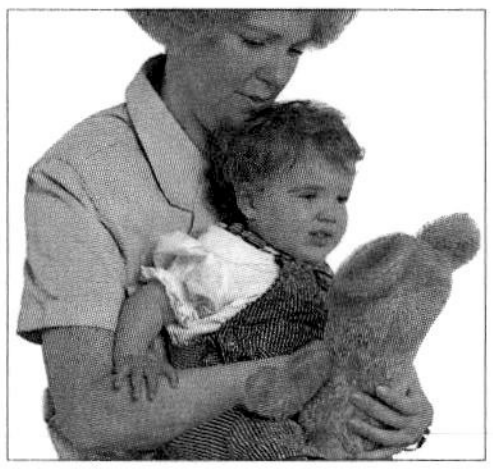

Headbanging
Between 5 and 11 months of age, some infants regularly bang their head against the side of the crib. Headbanging may occur in an infant who is teething or who has an ear infection (see page 84). Headbanging can be a way of attracting attention. To stop the behavior, divert your child's attention with soothing music or by holding him or her.

BEDTIME BEHAVIORAL PROBLEMS

Some children exhibit unusual bedtime habits that concern their parents for short periods of time. This bedtime behavior does not necessarily signal any emotional disorder. Different types of bedtime behavior occur at different ages.

Resisting bedtime

Many children, especially toddlers, resist going to bed. They may have temper tantrums or repeatedly get out of bed, insisting that they are not tired. To encourage cooperation at bedtime, establish a bedtime routine that includes a soothing bath and a story. Let your child make as many decisions as possible before going to bed, such as which pajamas to wear and which toy to take to bed, so the child can feel he or she is in control. If your child gets out of bed, immediately return him or her to the bedroom and firmly remind your child that it is time for bed. Such tactics will help your child learn to go to sleep on his or her own.

Sleepwalking

Children who sleepwalk experience partial waking from a very deep nondreaming sleep, in which they suddenly sit up, get out of bed, and walk around, while still appearing to be asleep. The sleepwalking child may perform such acts as eating, dressing, or opening doors and usually gets back into bed without help. During these episodes, the child stares straight ahead and usually does not speak. There is no need to wake a child who is sleepwalking. Gently guide him or her back to bed. Children never remember sleepwalking afterward. Minimize risks to the child's safety, such as staircases or open windows.

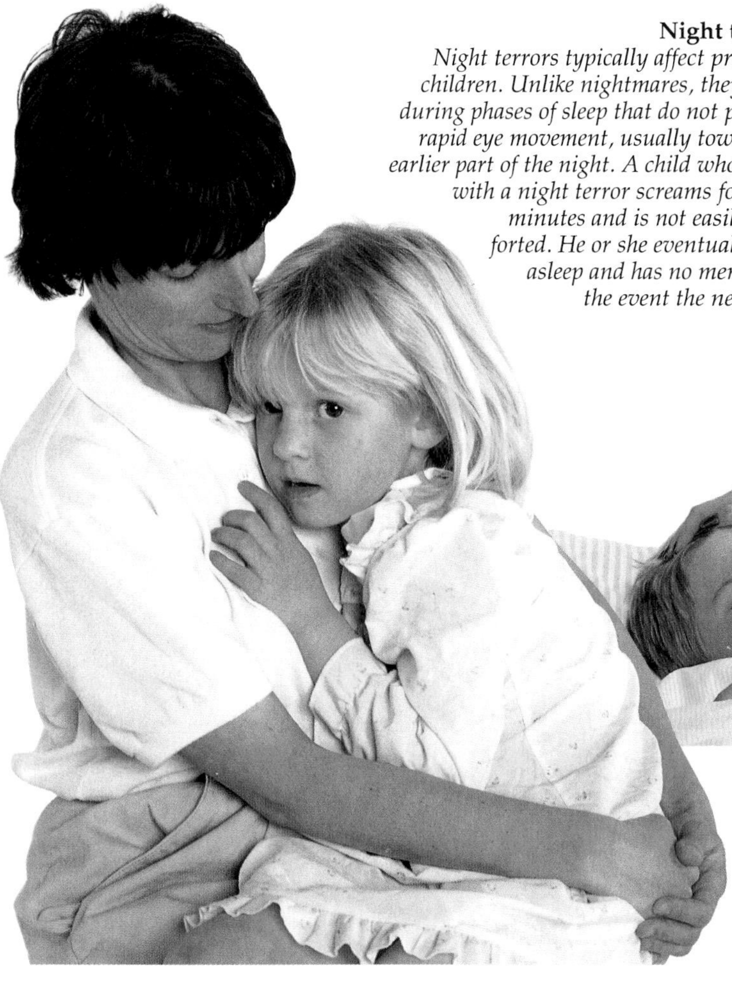

Night terrors
Night terrors typically affect preschool children. Unlike nightmares, they occur during phases of sleep that do not produce rapid eye movement, usually toward the earlier part of the night. A child who wakes with a night terror screams for a few minutes and is not easily comforted. He or she eventually falls asleep and has no memory of the event the next day.

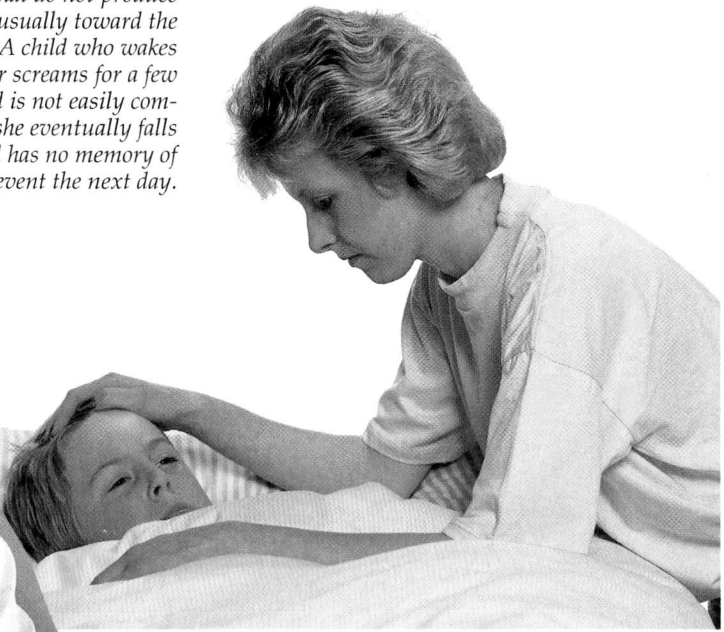

Nightmares
Nightmares are frightening, vivid dreams that commonly occur in school-age children who are about 8 to 10 years old. The child often clearly remembers the details of a nightmare upon waking. Nightmares can reflect conflicts with which the child is struggling while awake.

AUTISM

Autism is a rare condition in which a child does not develop the ability to interact socially with other people. So far, scientists have found no cause for this condition. The autistic child smiles very little, appears passive and unresponsive, and does not interact with his or her environment. Some doctors think that autism is caused by a biological problem. Others attribute it to the parents' emotional rejection of the child.

Autistic children remain isolated and solitary as they grow older. Some never learn to speak; others speak with difficulty. Autistic children sometimes have a single special skill, such as outstanding musical ability or rote memory. Most autistic children need a protected environment throughout their lives.

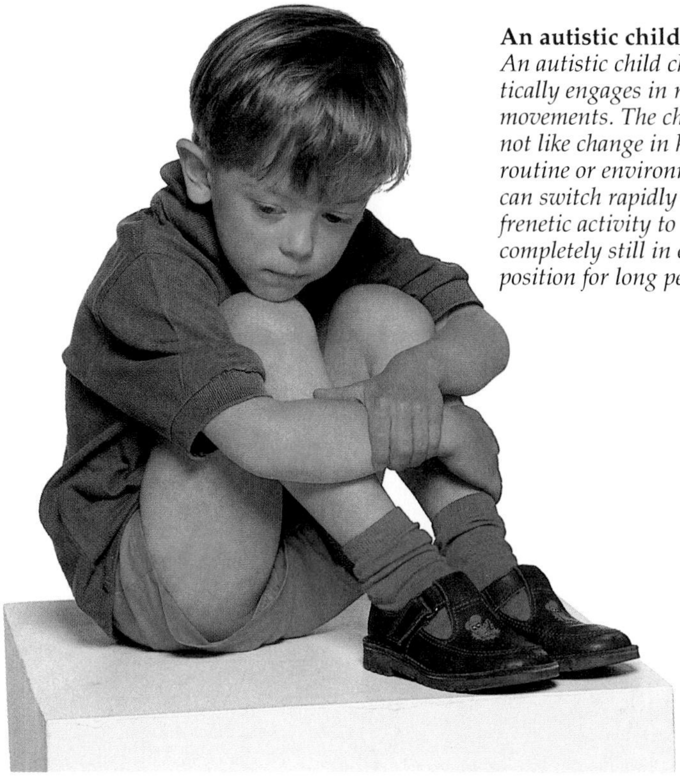

An autistic child
An autistic child characteristically engages in repetitive movements. The child does not like change in his or her routine or environment and can switch rapidly from frenetic activity to sitting completely still in one position for long periods.

ATTENTION DEFICIT DISORDER

Children with attention deficit disorder have difficulty maintaining their attention, are easily distracted, and behave impulsively. More than half of all children with an attention deficit are hyperactive. Hyperactive children are excessively energetic and demonstrate aggressive behavior. In contrast, children with an attention deficit who are not hyperactive are usually anxious and socially withdrawn. If you have a child with attention deficit disorder, the suggestions below may be helpful:

- Give structure to your child's environment by having him or her follow a regular daily routine.
- Avoid overstimulating your child, especially before bedtime.
- Do not allow your child to become overly tired. Let him or her rest after vigorous activities.
- Reward your child for successful efforts at controlling disruptive behavior and for good school performance. Set limits and enforce them by withdrawing treats and privileges.
- At home, make sure that rules are not punitive but that they encourage good behavior.
- Tackle one behavioral problem at a time.
- Make time for yourself to recoup your energies.

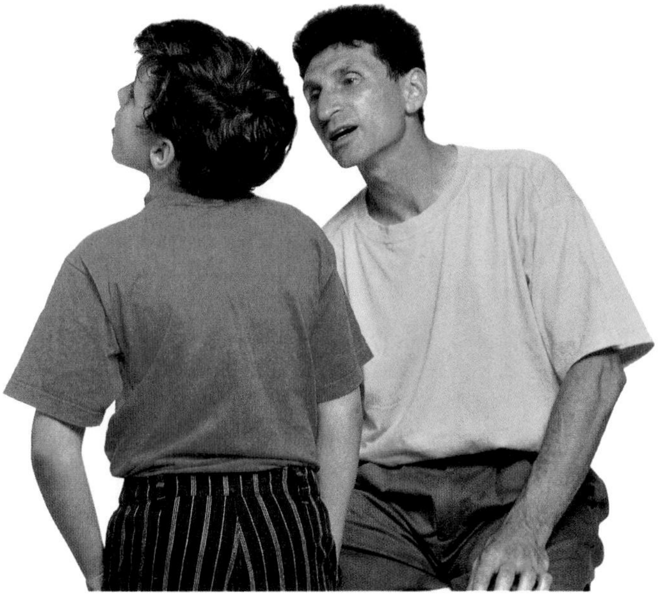

A structured environment
Children with attention deficit disorder have a short attention span and adults may have difficulty engaging them in even short conversations. Affected children often act without thinking about the consequences. They have a low tolerance of frustration and need a highly structured environment.

PROBLEMS AT SCHOOL

Most children have an occasional headache or stomachache that appears on mornings when they anticipate an activity they dislike, such as a test. In some children, these "illnesses," if they occur regularly, may signal stress about real or imagined problems that they feel unable to confront. Such children have fears about their performance in a given academic, athletic, or social situation.

Take your child to the doctor, who will perform a medical examination to make sure that the symptoms have no physical cause. Then talk with your child's teacher about aspects of school that may be causing problems for your child. Such problems could include conflict with a teacher, intimidation from another student, or even a school subject that the child dislikes. In extreme cases, a change of class or school may be the only solution to the problem.

Dislike for certain activities
Some children develop a strong dislike of certain subjects, such as mathematics, or school activities, such as gym class, because they are afraid of failure. Teach your children that each person has strengths and weaknesses and that you do not expect them to succeed in everything but that they must give the activity they dislike their best effort.

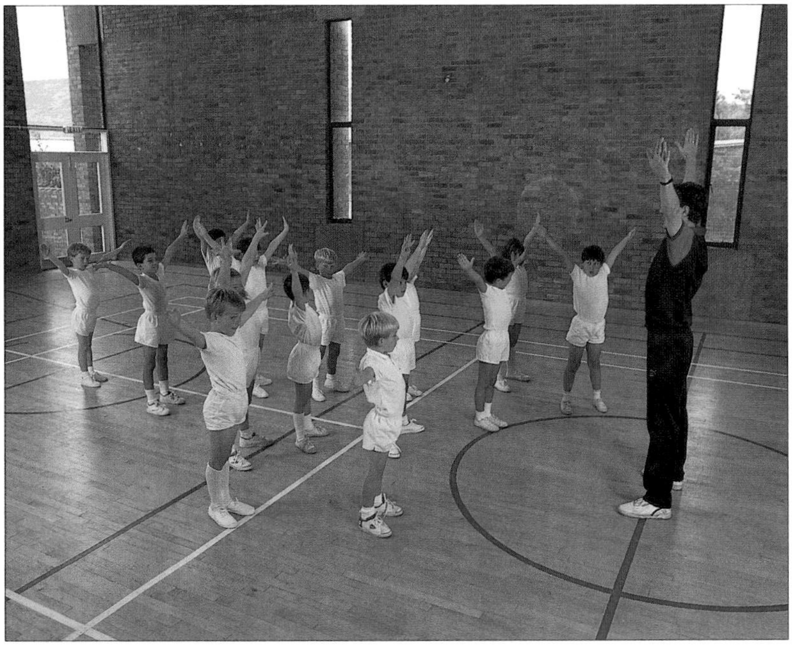

COUNSELING

If your child's behavior is a constant problem for you or his or her teachers, contact your doctor to make sure that your child has no underlying physical disorder. If no medical problem exists, your doctor may suggest counseling, either for the child who is having problems or for the entire family.

Parents should remember that asking for help carries no stigma. The best way to express concern for a troubled child is to seek professional advice. Most communities have family social service agencies, some of which are sponsored by not-for-profit groups. These agencies either have treatment services of their own or make referrals to qualified people who can help. Usually, a child meets with a social worker, a clinical psychologist, or a child psychiatrist.

Preparing for counseling
Professional counselors may test a child who has a problem not only to determine his or her intelligence level but also to record the child's reactions to a range of different situations. Counselors use the results of these tests as a starting point for therapy sessions.

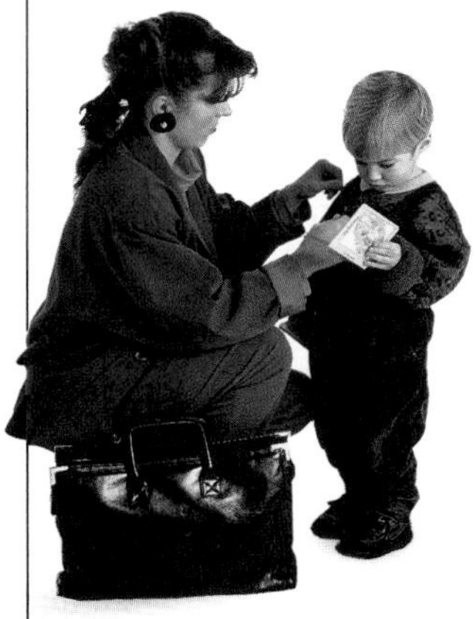

First days of school
Children may be frightened at the idea of leaving their family behind and being at school on their own. These fears subside as the child becomes accustomed to the new environment. Parents should avoid an overprotective approach that reinforces the fear of separation.

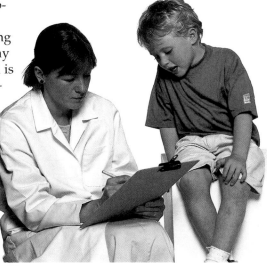

Poor performance

A child may perform poorly at school for a variety of reasons. Children may perform poorly if life at home is uncertain or chaotic. The threat of an impending divorce can lead to depression or learning difficulties. Whatever the cause, scolding and threatening do not improve a child's schoolwork and only serve to increase pressure on the child, who may already be under considerable stress. Consult a teacher about your child's capabilities and ask whether you might be expecting too much in the way of academic success. A period of extra tutoring may be all that is needed. It is also important for the child to realize that his or her worth as a person does not depend on the grades achieved. Find out if your child is experiencing any problems with other children at school or with gangs.

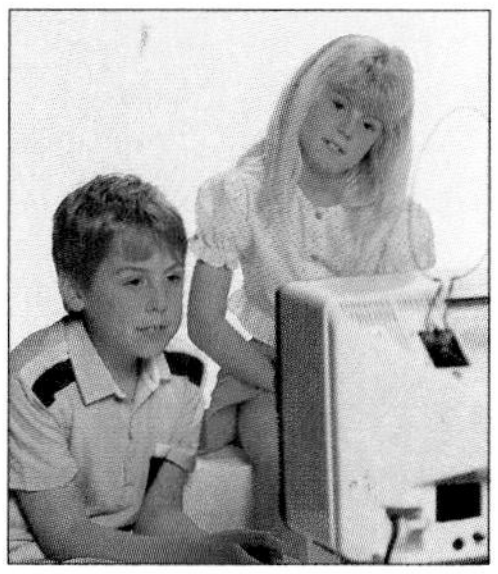

The influence of TV
Children in the US watch between 3 and 5 hours of television every day. Research has found possible connections between TV viewing and aggressive behavior, poor school performance, and the use of alcohol and other drugs in children. Eliminate violent programs from your child's viewing schedule.

Playing hooky

Skipping classes and missing school occur more frequently among adolescents than young children. In both age groups, playing hooky symbolizes running away from difficulties. Discuss the truancy with your child's teachers and a school counselor when it becomes evident.

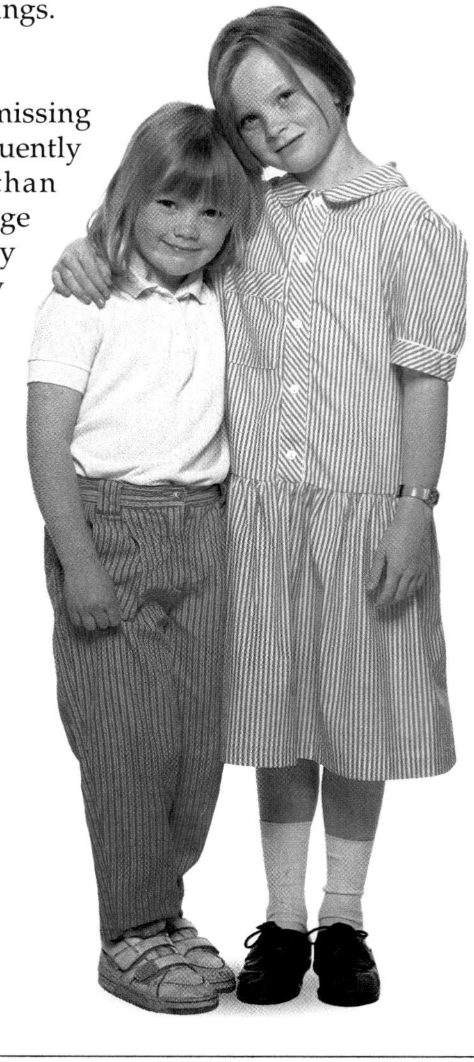

Making friends
Nurturing relationships at home foster self-esteem and make it possible for children to make friends at school. Most school-age children soon become part of a social group and choose a best friend.

ASK YOUR DOCTOR

BEHAVIORAL AND EMOTIONAL PROBLEMS

Q **My 7-year-old son is very aggressive toward younger children. Could he be taking after his father, who has a bad temper?**

A There may be many factors involved. It is important to find out what is going on in your entire family to understand your son's behavior. Your family may benefit from therapy to learn less aggressive methods of communication.

Q **When my husband was promoted, we moved to a new city. Our daughter's grades have since fallen; she has become withdrawn and refuses to talk about what is wrong. What can we do?**

A The move that symbolizes so much success to you and your husband means a new school and the loss of friends for your daughter. She needs time to adjust. Try to talk with your daughter again to find out how she feels. Then talk to her teacher and look for ways that your daughter's situation could be improved.

Q **Before my mother died, she cared for our 4-year-old son. I now work at home, but my son seems lost without his grandmother. How can I help him?**

A People of all ages who lose a loved one need about a year to recover. Assure your son of your love and answer any questions he has. Reassure him that his grandmother's death was no one's fault and that death is a natural part of life. New friends and activities might help him overcome his loss.

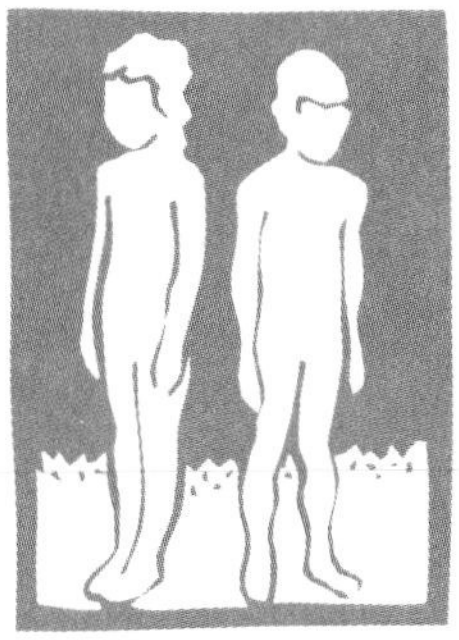

MISCELLANEOUS DISORDERS

SOME ILLNESSES, such as sore throats, affect all children. Other disorders strike only a few children, but their effects can be serious. Hormonal disorders and cancers, such as leukemia, can be life-threatening if they are not detected early. Other problems, such as infection of the lower urinary tract, are initially uncomfortable but clear up after treatment with antibiotics.

Rare medical disorders that affect only a few children include hormonal disorders, nervous system disorders, problems with the genital organs in both boys and girls, urinary system problems, and disabilities that are congenital (present from birth), such as mental retardation or cerebral palsy.

HORMONAL DISORDERS

Hormonal disorders usually affect a child's thyroid gland and pituitary gland. The thyroid gland produces hormones that regulate the body's metabolism (internal chemical processes). If the thyroid gland does not produce enough of these hormones, serious abnormalities can result unless doctors treat the deficiency early. Thyroid hormone deficiency can be present at birth or can develop during infancy. Unrecognized hormone deficiency at birth can cause irreversible mental retardation and serious growth retardation. Thyroid hormone deficiency that develops in infancy or childhood can produce such symptoms as reduced physical activity, poor appetite, a large tongue, a cool body, poor muscle tone, hoarseness, poor growth, jaundice, respiratory difficulties, and anemia.

Doctors can detect the underproduction of thyroid hormones shortly after birth with a blood test. Treatment with artificial thyroid hormones can prevent the serious abnormalities caused by thyroid hormone deficiency.

Where are the thyroid and pituitary glands? *Weighing about 1 ounce, the thyroid gland lies below the voice box. The pituitary gland is about the size of a pea and lies in a cavity inside the skull, just below the optic nerves.*

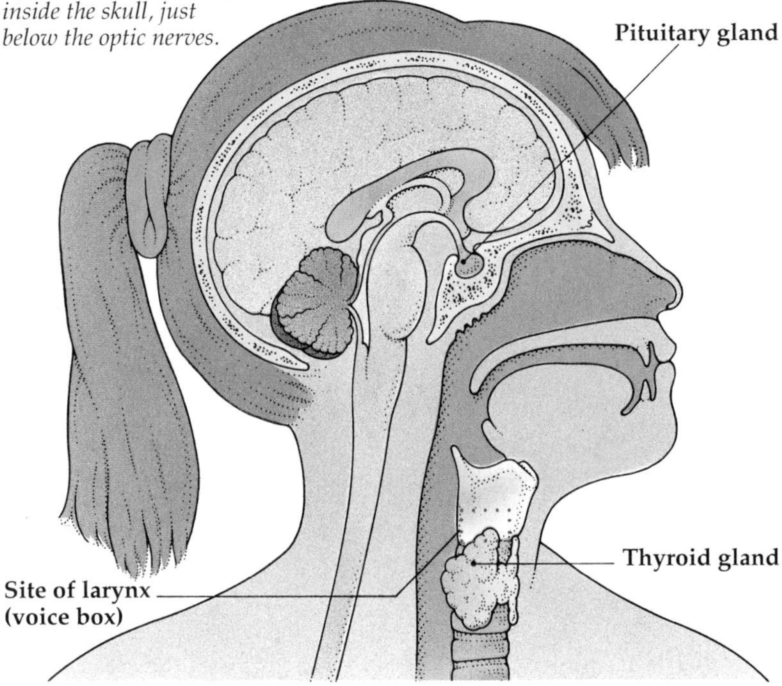

Growth hormone

Growth hormone prompts most of the cells in the body to reproduce and divide. The pituitary gland secretes growth hormone mainly during sleep. Underproduction of growth hormone causes a child's growth rate to be slowed or interrupted, leading to dwarfism if untreated. Doctors use synthetic growth hormone to treat children with this disorder. Overproduction of growth hormone is caused by a pituitary tumor. If the tumor is not removed, excessive hormone secretion causes abnormally tall stature.

DIABETES

Diabetes mellitus occurs in two main forms – insulin-dependent and non-insulin-dependent. Childhood diabetes is almost always insulin-dependent. This type is caused by the destruction of the insulin-producing cells in the pancreas. The cell destruction probably occurs when a genetically susceptible child's immune system attacks body tissues following an infection. The symptoms of diabetes are severe thirst, frequent passing of large quantities of urine, cramps in the legs and the stomach, weight loss, fatigue, and vomiting. Doctors control insulin-dependent diabetes with a structured diet and daily injections of insulin.

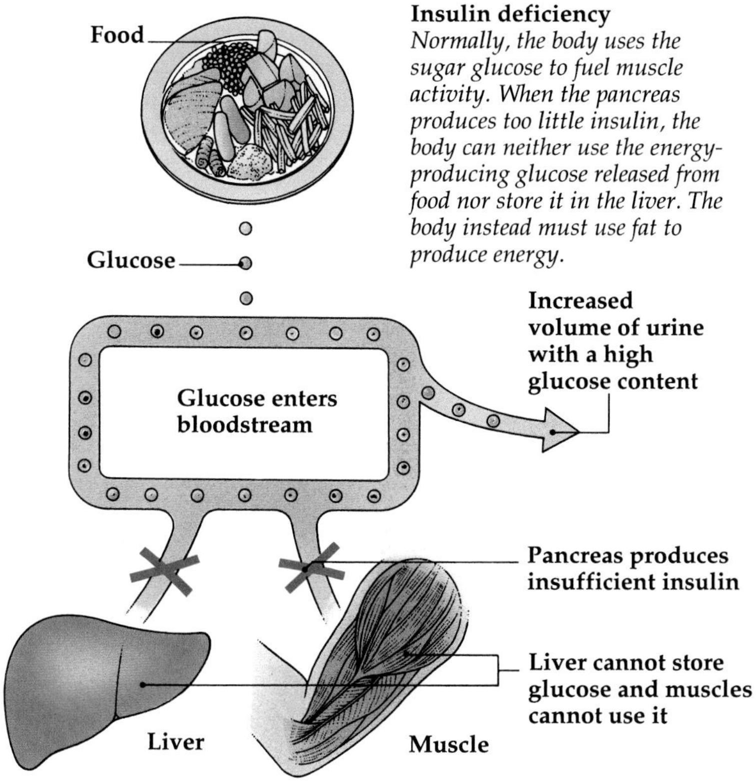

Insulin deficiency
Normally, the body uses the sugar glucose to fuel muscle activity. When the pancreas produces too little insulin, the body can neither use the energy-producing glucose released from food nor store it in the liver. The body instead must use fat to produce energy.

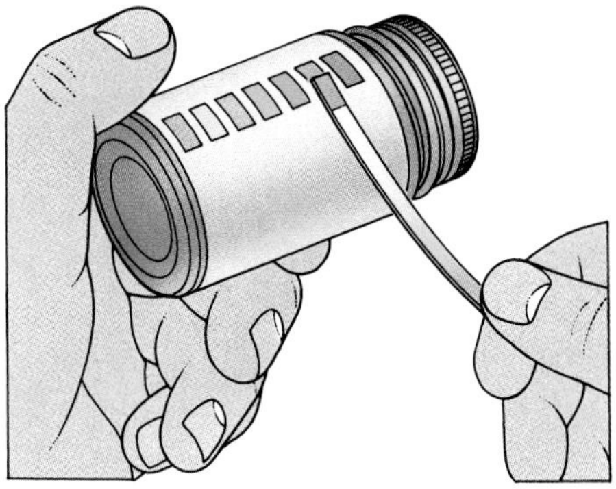

Monitoring blood sugar levels
Some older children with diabetes monitor the glucose levels in their own blood indirectly by measuring the amount of glucose in their urine. The child dips a chemical strip into a sample of urine and compares the color the strip produces to a color scale.

LEUKEMIA

Leukemia is a cancer that affects the cells that produce blood. Abnormal white blood cells proliferate in the bone marrow, blocking the production of red blood cells, platelets (which help the blood to clot), and normal white blood cells. Leukemia can occur at any time during childhood but is most likely to appear around the age of 4.

A child with leukemia tires easily and may have fever, pain in his or her bones, and spontaneous bruising. Lymph nodes swell in the neck, armpits, and groin. The liver and spleen enlarge. An affected child becomes anemic and bleeds from various parts of the body, especially the nose. The cancerous white blood cells may not show up in a blood test but will appear in a bone marrow sample.

Treatment

More than half of all cases of the most common type of leukemia, acute lymphoblastic leukemia, are curable. Doctors treat this type with anticancer drugs and corticosteroid (inflammation-fighting) drugs. Bone marrow transplantation has proved successful in some cases.

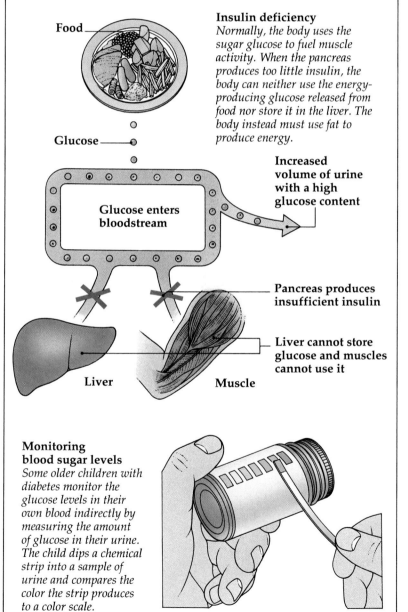

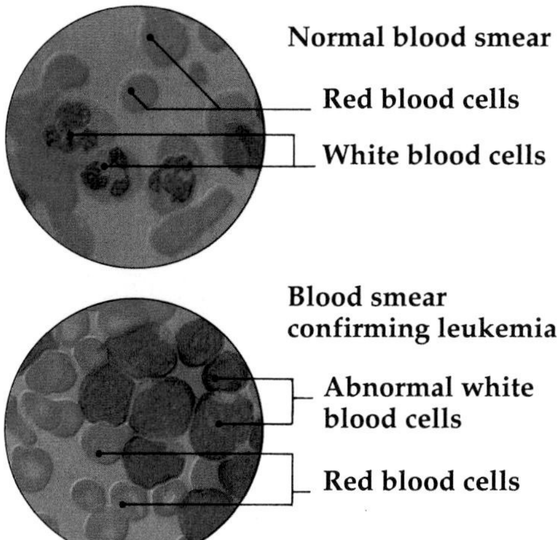

Leukemia
Bone marrow affected by leukemia produces large numbers of abnormal white blood cells. Rapid multiplication of these cells impairs the production of normal white blood cells, platelets, and red blood cells, which are gradually crowded out and replaced.

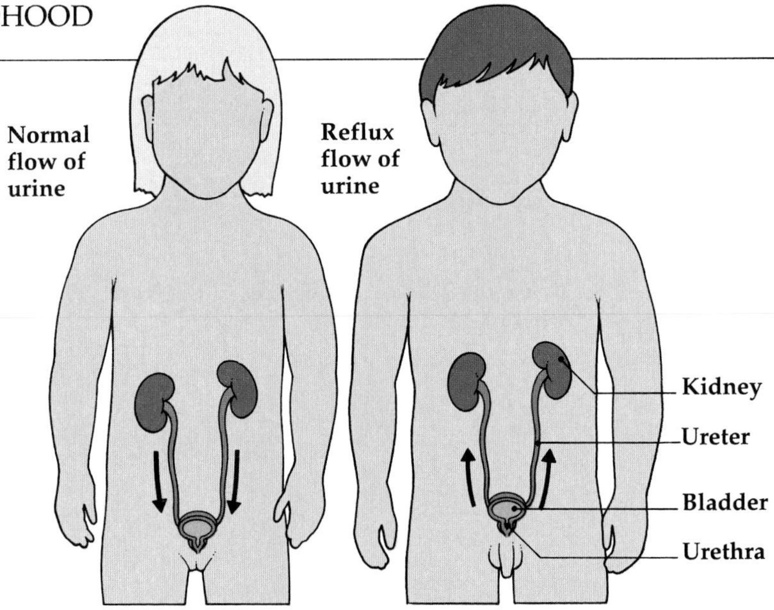

URINARY SYSTEM PROBLEMS

Bacteria can enter the urethra, the tube through which urine passes out of the body, and ascend to the bladder, causing a urinary tract infection. Poor hygiene, an uncircumcised penis, or sexual activity can cause a child to be more susceptible to urinary tract infections. A child with a bladder infection has a fever, has pain during urination, and frequently urinates. The symptoms of severe urinary tract infection include fever, cloudy or red urine, and burning pain when urinating. Back pain, high fever, and chills indicate that infection has spread from the urinary tract into the kidneys. Doctors treat urinary tract infections with antibiotics.

If a child has more than one infection of the bladder or the ureters (urine drainage tubes connecting the kidneys to the bladder), the doctor may need to investigate whether there is an obstruction or other abnormality affecting the child's urinary system, such as vesicoureteral reflux (see above right).

Nephritis

The most common cause of nephritis (inflammation of the kidneys) in children is an immune system reaction to an infection that has occurred elsewhere in the child's body. For example, a child may develop nephritis about 3 weeks after the onset of a skin infection or sore throat caused by streptococcal bacteria (strep throat). The child develops fever, loss of appetite, and high blood pressure and passes only small quantities of bloody urine. Fluid accumulates in all parts of the child's body. Children under 6 years old are most susceptible to nephritis.

GENITAL PROBLEMS IN GIRLS

Many girls experience genital itching. Possible causes include urinary tract infection; pinworms; or foreign objects in the vagina, such as toilet paper. The low level of sexual hormones present in a young girl may make her more vulnerable to infection of the vagina (the muscular passage that connects the neck of the uterus with the external genitalia).

Vulvovaginitis

Inflammation of the vagina and the vulva (the external, visible part of the female genitals) is known as vulvovaginitis. The skin becomes red and sore and the girl experiences pain when urinating. Girls should wear cotton underwear to prevent recurrence of the condition.

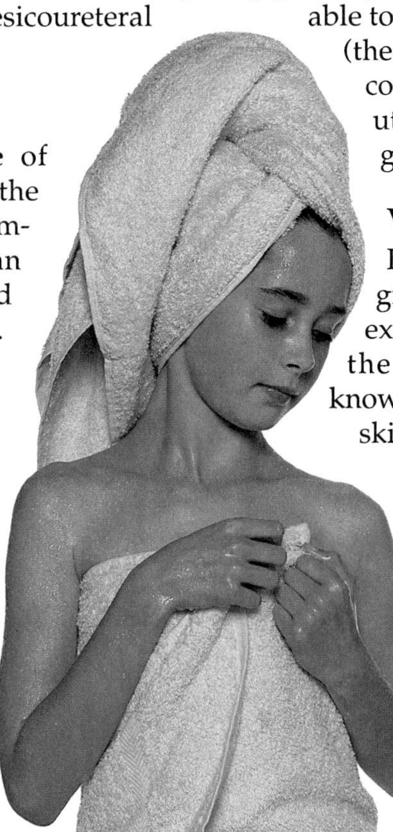

Hygiene and vaginitis
A girl who has vulvovaginitis should wash her vulva daily with clean, warm water. She should not use antiseptics, soaps, shower gels, or bubble bath. Be sure to rinse detergent thoroughly from your daughter's laundered underclothes.

Reflux of urine
Urine may pass back up the ureters if there is an abnormality at the junctions between the ureters and the bladder. Doctors call this condition vesicoureteral reflux. If not treated, it can damage the kidneys.

WARNING

Genital herpes and warts, chlamydial infection, and gonorrhea can all cause vaginal itching, discharge, or pain. If these infections occur in a girl before puberty, a strong possibility of sexual abuse exists. Take the girl to a doctor immediately and inform the proper authorities of the suspected abuse.

GENITAL PROBLEMS IN BOYS

The testicles (male sex organs that, in an adult, produce sperm and the male sex hormone testosterone) usually descend into the scrotum, the pouch that hangs below the penis, by the time a baby boy is born. If not, they descend before 1 year of age. Testicles that remain in the abdomen (undescended testicles) do not produce sperm, although they still produce sex hormones. Surgery is needed to correct this condition because cancer and infertility are more likely to occur in males with undescended testicles.

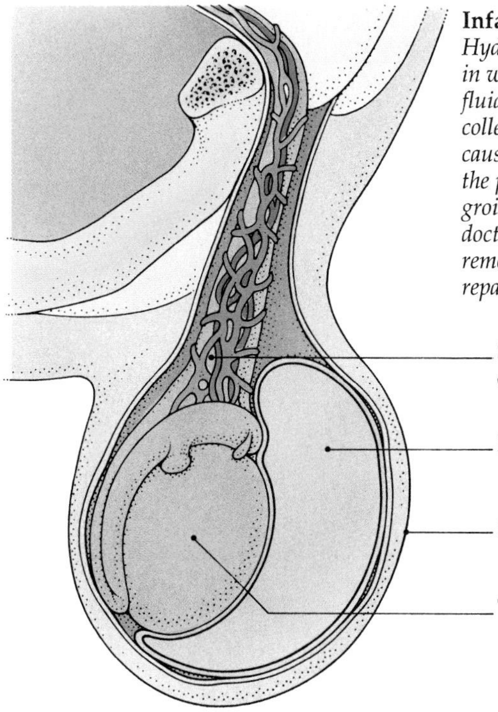

Infantile hydrocele
Hydrocele is a painless condition in which clear, amber-colored fluid from the spermatic cord collects around a testicle and causes swelling. It may signal the presence of a hernia in the groin area. If a hernia is present, doctors perform surgery to remove the hydrocele and repair the hernia.

Twisting of the testicles

Twisting, or torsion, of the spermatic cord (which moves relatively freely in the body) is a disorder that can affect boys at any age. The boy affected has a sudden, intense pain in his genitals, which is accompanied by nausea and vomiting. The affected testicle becomes tender and appears higher than normal, and the scrotum becomes swollen. Immediate surgery is needed to avoid permanent damage to the testicle.

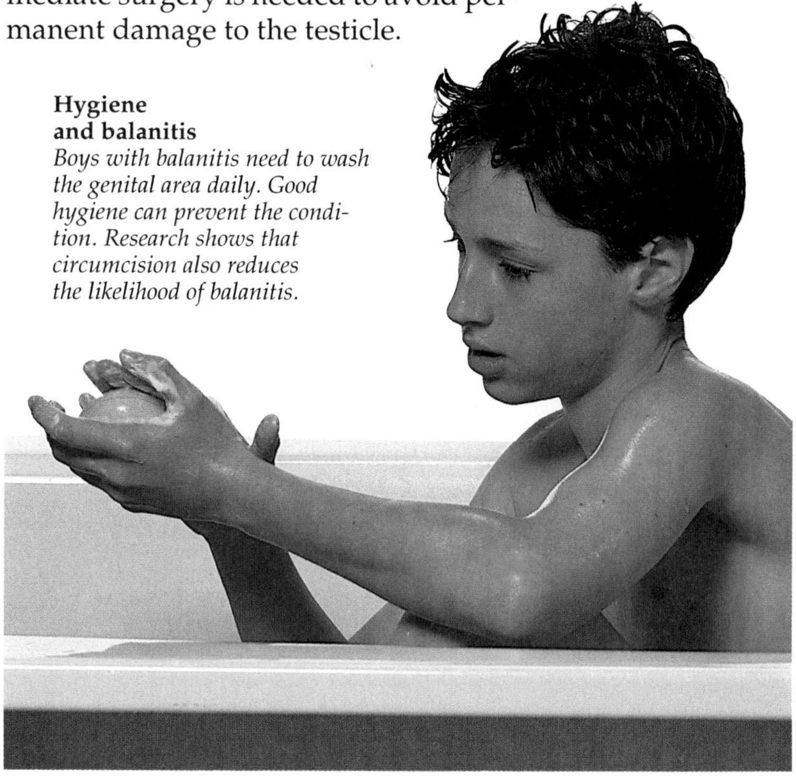

Hygiene and balanitis
Boys with balanitis need to wash the genital area daily. Good hygiene can prevent the condition. Research shows that circumcision also reduces the likelihood of balanitis.

Balanitis

Inflammation of the head (glans) of the penis is known as balanitis. The foreskin, if present, sometimes also becomes inflamed and itches intensely. Balanitis is usually caused by poor hygiene, which sets the stage for infection by bacteria or fungi. A boy can prevent or relieve most cases of balanitis by washing daily with warm water, but antibiotic or antifungal creams may also be needed.

Tight foreskin

It is fairly common for the foreskin of a boy's penis to be tight and difficult to pull back from the glans (head) until he is about 3 years of age. Do not force the foreskin back. If the boy experiences difficulty urinating or develops an infection, he may need circumcision.

If a tight foreskin is pulled back over the glans, the glans will swell because the veins that transport blood out of the area become compressed at the same time that the arteries are providing more blood. A doctor may need to return the foreskin to its normal position. The doctor may recommend circumcision so that the problem does not recur.

HEAD INJURIES AND DISORDERS

You should consider any childhood head injury or disorder to be potentially serious. Take your child to your doctor as soon as you detect the condition to rule out the possibility of brain damage. Parents of children with conditions such as migraine headaches or epilepsy can help their children most by learning the facts about their child's condition and responding appropriately when episodes occur.

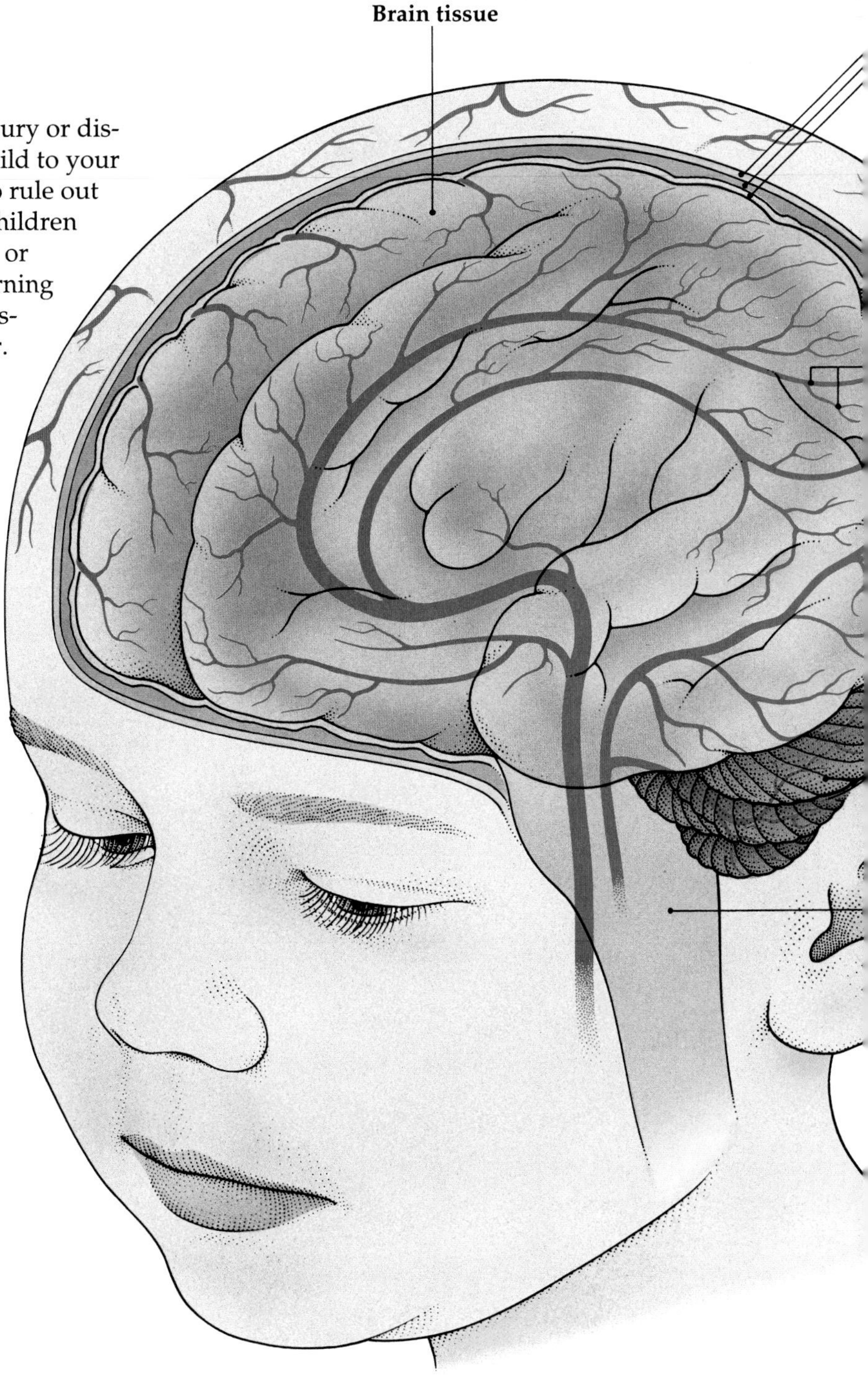

Migraine
The symptoms of migraine include severe headache, nausea, and vomiting and may also include visual disturbances and sensitivity to light. Doctors think migraine attacks are caused by abnormal changes in the diameter of blood vessels in the scalp and brain. Effective treatments are available, so you should consult your doctor.

Headaches
Headaches can represent a child's reaction to anxiety, tension, family discord, and emotional upset. Sinus infection also commonly causes a headache. Very few headaches indicate serious physical problems. But a brain tumor can cause headaches. A child with severe, recurring headaches should be taken to a doctor, who will evaluate and treat the headache appropriately.

Open head injuries
Doctors describe head injuries as "open" if they involve fractures of the skull that expose the brain and render it susceptible to infection. Children with open head injuries should be taken to the hospital emergency department immediately.

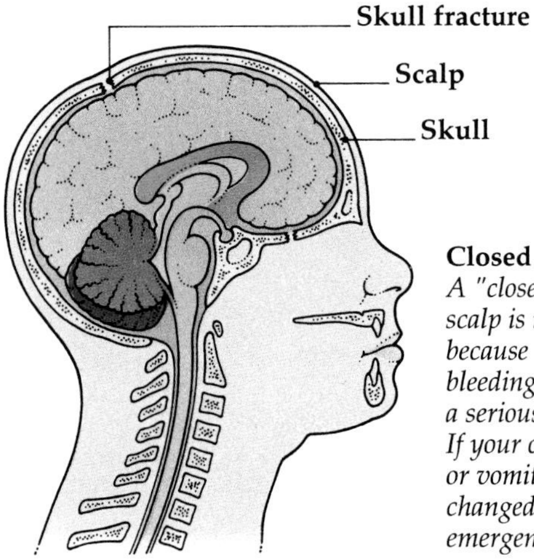

Closed head injuries
A "closed" head injury, in which the scalp is intact, may not seem serious because there is no wound or visible bleeding. But a skull fracture (see left) or a serious brain injury may have occurred. If your child has lost consciousness, or vomited or his or her behavior has changed, take him or her to the hospital emergency department immediately.

Febrile seizures
A rapid rise in body temperature can cause a febrile seizure (uncontrollable jerking of the limbs caused by a fever). Such seizures most commonly occur in children aged 6 months to 5 years. Most children who have had a febrile seizure never have another. If your child has a febrile seizure, call your doctor.

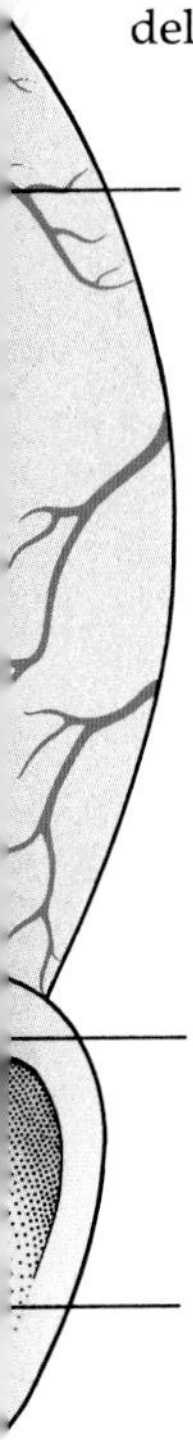

Meninges

Bacterial meningitis
The term bacterial meningitis refers to inflammation of the meninges (the membranes surrounding the brain) caused by bacterial infection. Bacterial meningitis can cause brain damage and lead to epilepsy, deafness, or significant developmental (motor and mental) delay (see MENINGITIS on page 104).

Blood vessels

Viral meningitis
A virus can cause inflammation of the meninges; viral meningitis may arise as a complication of measles or mumps. Symptoms include fever, irritability, and a stiff neck. A doctor must evaluate a child with meningitis to rule out bacterial meningitis, the more serious of the two types. Viral meningitis needs no specific treatment because the disease resolves on its own.

Cerebellum

Brain stem

Encephalitis
Inflammation of the brain tissue, caused by viral or bacterial infection, is known as encephalitis. The herpes simplex virus can cause encephalitis, as can certain viruses spread by insect bites. Antiviral drugs are effective in treating herpes simplex. Although there are no known cures for the other viral infections that cause encephalitis, recovery often occurs without treatment.

WARNING

You should take your child to your doctor after any head injury that causes loss of consciousness, no matter how brief. Unconsciousness for more than a few minutes may signal a brain injury. Your doctor should assess your child's condition.

EPILEPSY

A sudden, abnormal discharge of uncontrolled electrical activity in the brain causes an epileptic seizure. A major, or grand mal, seizure can be alarming to an observer because the person's entire body convulses. The person having the seizure often remembers nothing when the episode is over. The mildest form of epilepsy is the absence seizure (petit mal). During a petit mal seizure, which can last from a few seconds to half a minute and can occur hundreds of times a day, the child's attention "switches off," but he or she can continue an activity, such as bicycling.

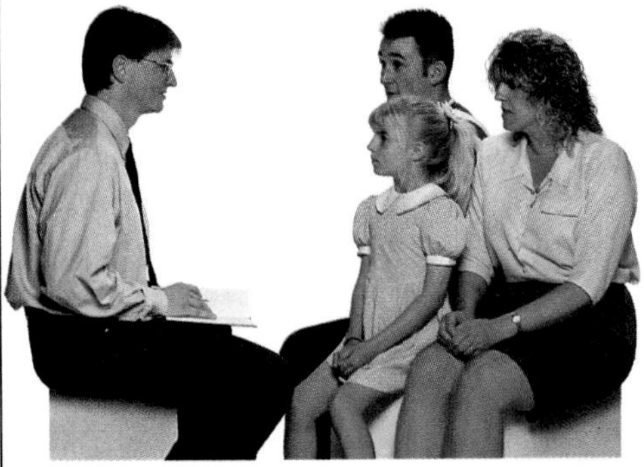

Understanding epilepsy
A child who has epilepsy may encounter misunderstanding or negative feelings some people have about the disorder. To help minimize these effects, talk to your doctor to learn all you can about your child's condition. Make sure your child understands that epilepsy is a medical disorder that does not affect intelligence or psychological status. Offer plenty of support.

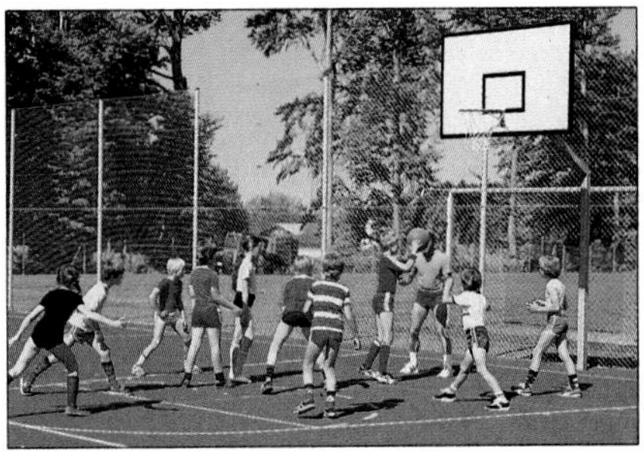

Encouraging a full life
Resist the urge to be overly protective of a child with epilepsy. A child with epilepsy needs to know that he or she is not different from other children in most respects. Encourage your child to engage in any activities that interest him or her unless your doctor advises against them.

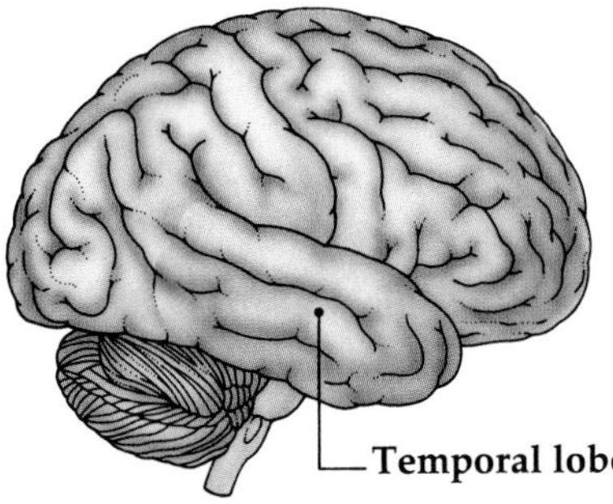

Partial seizures
Partial epileptic seizures affect only a small part of the brain, usually the temporal lobe, which controls perception of sounds, smells, and tastes. A person experiencing a temporal lobe epileptic seizure may have strange perceptions: an often unpleasant taste in his or her mouth, or abdominal pain.

Abnormal brain waves
Recordings made of brain waves during an epileptic seizure show disordered electrical activity.

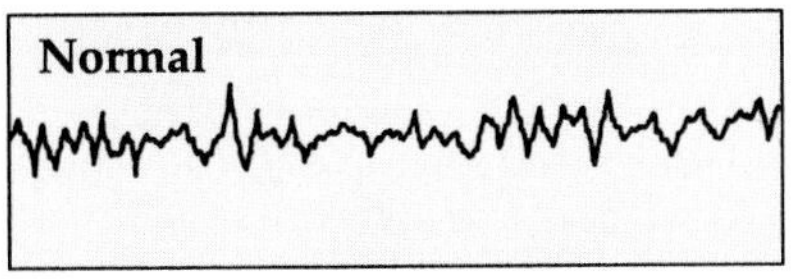

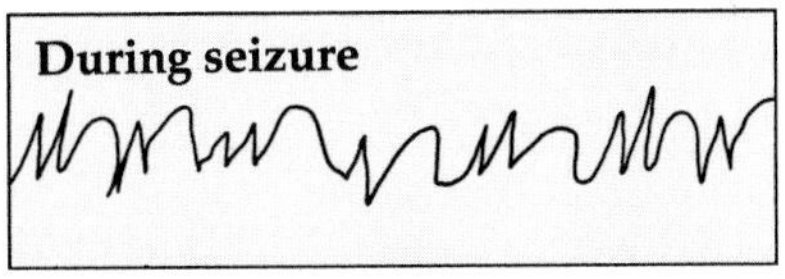

CASE HISTORY
FEVER AND SEIZURE

BRIAN IS A HAPPY toddler. One afternoon, he became fussy and tearful. He refused to eat or drink and felt hot to the touch. The next morning, Brian had a cough and a high fever. His mother wrapped him in blankets to help him "sweat it out." Suddenly, Brian's eyes rolled back. His body became stiff, then relaxed. His limbs jerked for a minute and then became still. Brian's mother immediately called an ambulance.

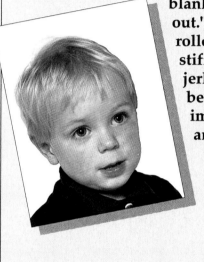

PERSONAL DETAILS
Name Brian Hope
Age 2
Family Parents and older sister are all healthy.

MEDICAL BACKGROUND
Brian is a healthy child who was born after a normal full-term pregnancy. His development has been normal and he walks and talks well.

THE CONSULTATION
By the time the ambulance reaches the hospital, Brian seems to have recovered. His mother explains to the doctor exactly what happened. The doctor takes detailed notes about the seizure and what preceded it. She examines Brian thoroughly, checking his throat, eyes, lymph nodes, ears, chest, and reflexes. She takes his temperature and checks his neck for stiffness, which is not evident. The doctor also draws a sample of Brian's blood and obtains a sample of fluid from around his spine.

THE DIAGNOSIS
The doctor tells Brian's mother that Brian has had a FEBRILE SEIZURE, which is common in children between the ages of 6 months and 5 years. She says that Brian's problem began with a sudden ear infection and that the infection caused a fever that increased when his mother wrapped him in blankets. The doctor assures Brian's mother that her son has not had an epileptic seizure and that such attacks usually do not increase the chances of epileptic seizures in the future. She explains that there is no reason to believe that this attack has caused brain damage.

THE TREATMENT
To bring down Brian's temperature, the doctor gives him a dose of acetaminophen (an aspirin substitute) and then sponges his body with lukewarm water. The doctor also treats the ear infection with antibiotics. She tells Brian's mother to keep Brian's bedroom no warmer than 67°F. She says that Brian should wear little or no clothing and that he needs only a cotton sheet on his bed until the fever subsides.

THE OUTCOME
Brian's mother is relieved that Brian does not have a serious disorder. Although he has a few more ear infections later during his childhood, Brian never has another febrile seizure. Because of this episode, his mother has learned how to keep his temperature from rising too high when he has a fever by sponging his body with lukewarm water and dressing him in minimal clothing.

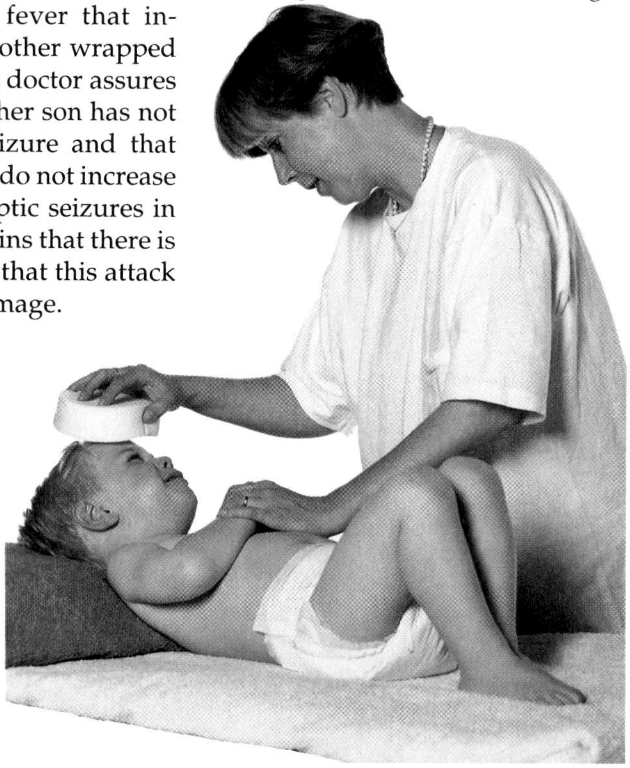

Sponging to reduce fever
The doctor tells Brian's mother that the next time Brian has a fever, she should sponge his face and neck and the insides of his arms and his legs with lukewarm water. As long as the room is warm, Brian's mother can leave his body slightly damp so that evaporation will cool down his body.

CEREBRAL PALSY

Cerebral palsy is a general term used to describe a group of central nervous system disorders caused by damage to the brain before birth, during birth, or after birth (up to 9 years). Such brain damage impairs the coordination between the child's nervous and muscular systems. Some causes of cerebral palsy are unknown, but known causes include an inadequate oxygen supply to the fetus, bleeding in the uterus, infection in the mother that affects the fetus, incompatibility between the blood groups of the mother and the fetus, malformation of the fetus, genetic disorders, alcohol and other drug use, premature birth, and complications during birth. After a baby is born, several factors can cause cerebral palsy, including meningitis or encephalitis (see page 117), injury, or ingestion of a toxic substance, such as lead.

Spasticity of the limbs

Most children with cerebral palsy have a condition called spasticity or spastic paralysis of the limbs. Their muscles are tightly contracted, making controlled movements difficult or impossible. The legs, for instance, have a tendency to "scissor" if the child tries to walk. In severe cases, all four limbs are affected and defects of vision, hearing, and speech are present. Some children have involuntary writhing movements.

Caring for affected children

Caring for a child with cerebral palsy is physically and emotionally demanding for his or her parents and care givers. Some parents find themselves unable to provide the constant attention and care the child needs and place the child in a facility that provides professional care. Many children with cerebral palsy are mentally retarded, but some display normal or high intelligence. Children who are only mildly affected by the disorder can lead nearly normal lives.

TYPES OF SPASTIC MUSCLE WEAKNESS

Children affected by spasticity from cerebral palsy fall into three distinct categories.

Hemiplegia
Hemiplegia means that the limbs on only one side of the body are affected, with the arm usually more affected than the leg.

Quadriplegia
Quadriplegia means that all four limbs are equally affected. The child is also usually severely mentally retarded, although mental retardation can occur with any type of spastic muscle weakness.

Diplegia
Diplegia means that all four limbs are affected, with the legs more affected than the arms.

MENTAL RETARDATION

The signs suggesting that a child may be mentally handicapped include slow physical and emotional development and physical incoordination. Delays in speech and walking can be caused by mental handicap. Some children are only mildly affected by retardation, but others are profoundly disabled.

Although the potential of a child who is mentally handicapped is limited, comprehensive care (including physical, occupational, and speech therapies) and training can bring slow but steady progress. Often, the family can care for the child at home, with support and counseling provided by professionals.

MENTAL HANDICAP

The intellectual development of a mentally handicapped child stops prematurely, so the child's mental age is usually lower than his or her chronological age. Causes include rubella (German measles) during pregnancy, genetic disorders, and brain damage from injury or exposure before birth to alcohol or other drugs.

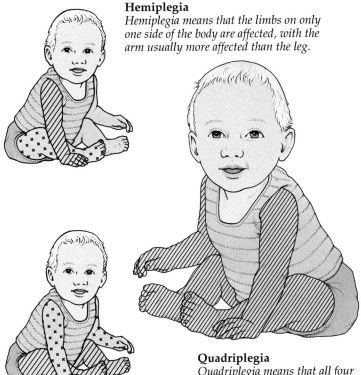

CHAPTER FIVE

ADOLESCENCE

ADOLESCENCE SPANS the years between childhood and adulthood, a stage of life roughly corresponding to the teenage years. Adolescence begins at puberty with the onset of body changes that lead to physical and sexual maturity. The physical changes of adolescence are accompanied by the development of emotional maturity, which combine to produce an independent adult who has a clear idea of his or her own identity.

Many teenagers have difficulty adapting to the rapidly occurring physical and sexual changes of puberty. They feel self-conscious about their developing bodies, unhappy about their perceived imperfections, and anxious about anything that sets them apart from their peers. They also have to come to terms with their newly awakened and powerful sexual feelings and must gradually learn how to form, and maintain, sexual relationships. At this stage, some teenagers may also begin to question their sexual orientation, becoming aware that their sexual feelings are stronger toward members of their own sex than toward those of the opposite sex.

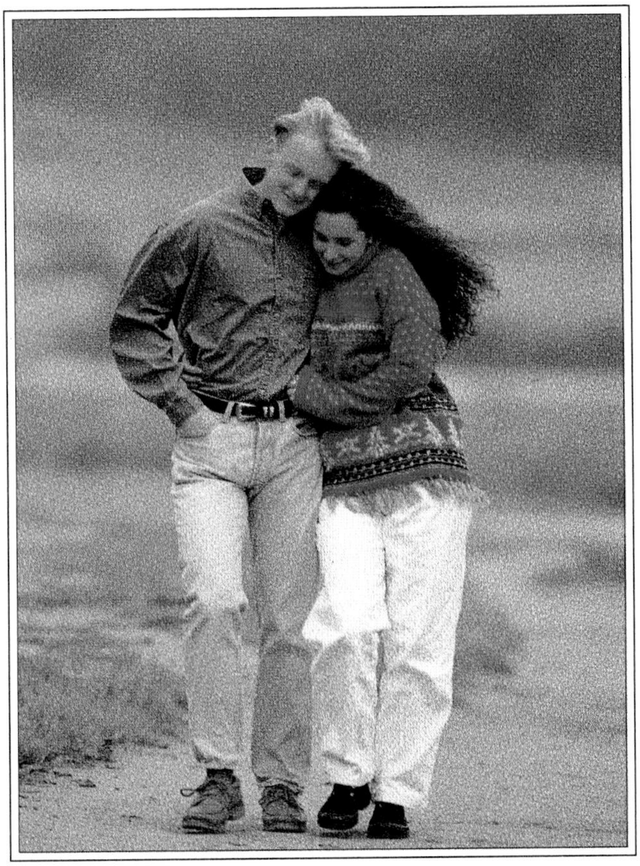

The complex transition from childhood to adulthood rarely runs smoothly. During these years, parents increasingly expect their adolescent children to behave like adults, while still often treating them like children. Adolescents strive for independence but at the same time need parental support and approval. In the process of forging an identity apart from the family, teenagers often adopt attitudes and opinions that oppose those of their parents. Teenagers begin to look for approval from their peers rather than from their parents. But most teenagers turn to their parents for advice about important decisions that will affect their future, such as where to go to school and how to get their first job.

Much friction between parents and teenagers arises over how much independence a teenager should have and how soon it should be granted. Although girls usually become self-sufficient and see themselves as adults sooner than boys do, parents frequently perceive a daughter as especially vulnerable and may attempt to place strict curbs on her freedom. Eventually, parents have to learn to let their children go. On the other hand, many of today's children stay financially dependent on their parents long after they have become emotionally independent, especially if the children go to college. For most adolescents, these years mark a child's final separation from the family. They also signify the beginning of a new relationship within the family, in which parents and children can relate to each other as adults.

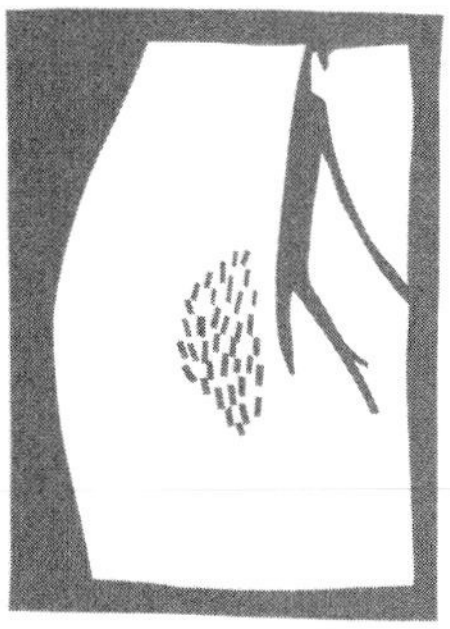

PUBERTY

THE TERM PUBERTY describes the hormonally determined physical changes that lead to sexual maturity and also drive the emotional changes of adolescence. Puberty usually occurs between the ages of 10 and 15 in both sexes, although girls tend to enter puberty at a slightly younger age than boys. The physical changes that take place are usually completed in 3 or 4 years.

During puberty, a child's body changes into its adult form. The sexual organs become mature so that reproduction can occur. Secondary sexual characteristics develop, such as facial hair in boys and breasts in girls.

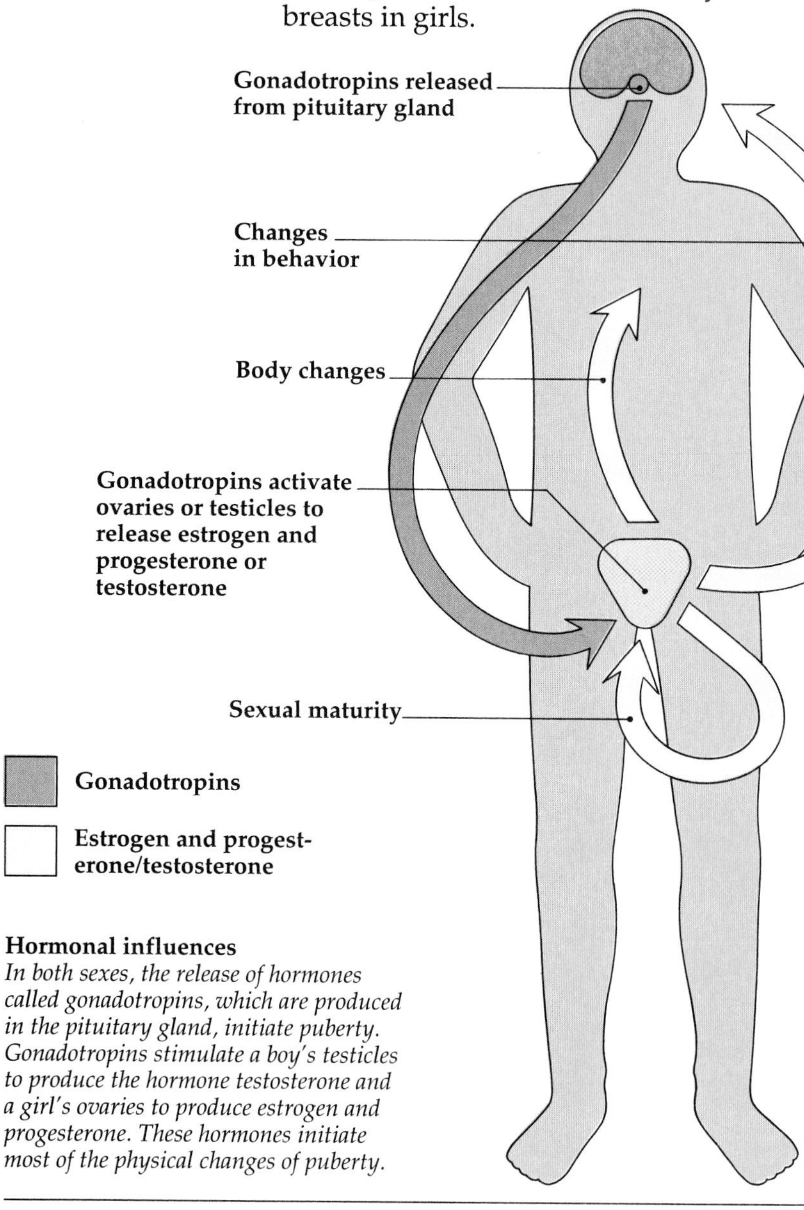

Hormonal influences
In both sexes, the release of hormones called gonadotropins, which are produced in the pituitary gland, initiate puberty. Gonadotropins stimulate a boy's testicles to produce the hormone testosterone and a girl's ovaries to produce estrogen and progesterone. These hormones initiate most of the physical changes of puberty.

PHYSICAL DEVELOPMENT

Although all adolescents of the same sex follow the same pattern of development during puberty, the age at onset and rate at which these physical changes occur vary enormously. Teenagers often worry because their bodies are developing more slowly or more quickly than those of their friends. They usually feel reassured when they learn that the physical development of puberty is continuous and that once the first signs appear – the growth spurt in boys and the budding of the breasts in girls – the rest of the changes will follow in time. A teenager in whom puberty begins late usually catches up with his or her peers by the age of about 16 for girls and 18 for boys.

Growth rate

In both sexes, puberty accompanies a sudden increase in the rate of growth. Boys begin this growth spurt later than girls and, because boys have about 2 more years of steady growth than do girls, they are generally taller than girls when they reach adulthood.

The speed of growth during puberty often makes adolescents feel awkward and uncoordinated. For example, an adolescent boy's feet and hands are often disproportionately large because they become adult-sized before the boy reaches his adult height.

Changes in boys during puberty
The principal changes that occur in boys during puberty are the enlargement of the sex organs, widening of the shoulders, deepening of the voice, and growth of facial and body hair.

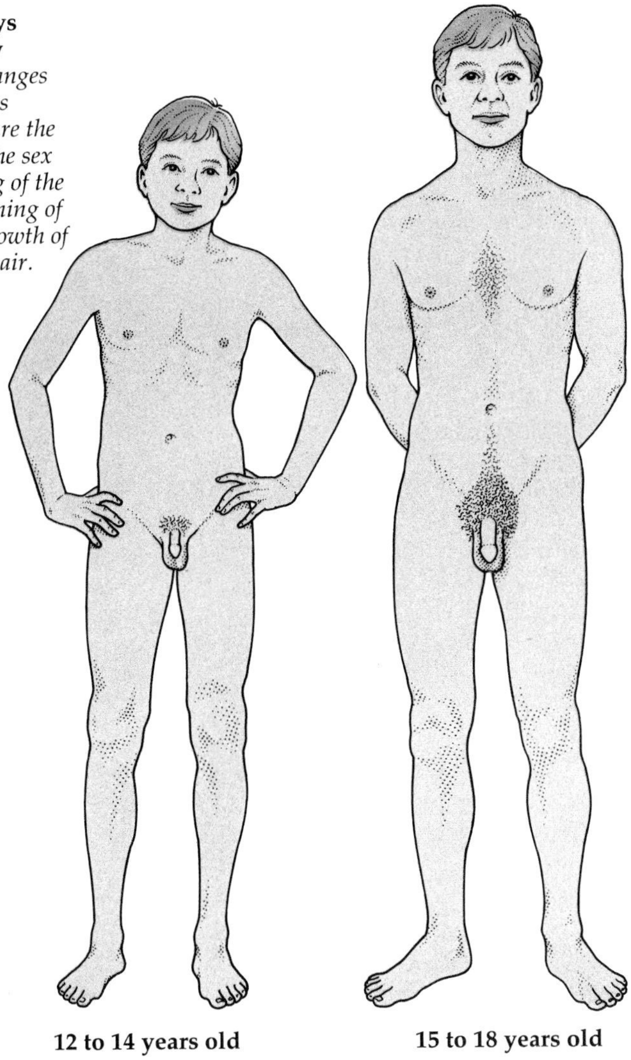

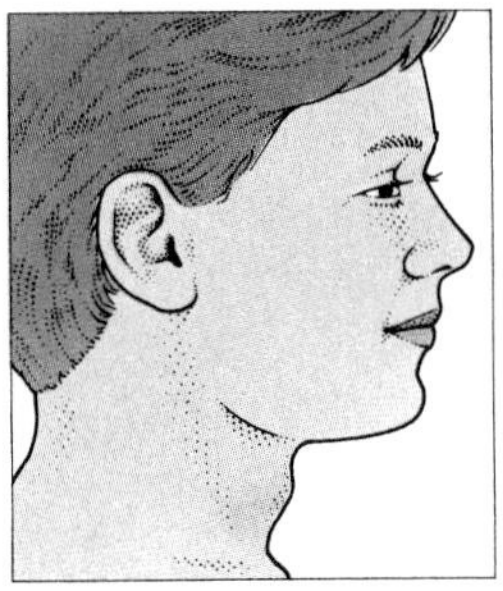

Voice changes in adolescence
The voices of both adolescent boys and girls change with the enlargement of the voice box (larynx), but the change is more dramatic in boys. The cartilage that surrounds the voice box may protrude, forming what is known as an "Adam's apple."

Body odor

During adolescence, the sweat glands in the armpits and around the genitals, called the apocrine glands, start to function. To prevent unnecessary concern about body odor, teach your adolescent child that he or she will need to wash the armpits and genital area every day. Deodorants should be used only on the armpits and never on or near the sensitive skin of the genitals.

Body hair

Both boys and girls begin to develop pubic and underarm hair during puberty. Under the influence of the male hormone testosterone, boys begin to develop facial hair, hair on the chest, underarm hair, and hair that grows up from the pubic area toward the navel. Under the influence of the female hormones estrogen and progesterone, adolescent girls develop underarm hair and an inverted triangle of pubic hair.

PUBERTY IN BOYS

Boys start the growth spurt that signals the onset of puberty at about the age of 12. The fastest growth tends to occur at about age 14, when a boy may grow as much as 6 or 8 inches in 2 years. A boy's body weight can double during adolescence because of the increases in height and muscle growth. Teenage boys are slighter than adult men and continue to broaden until they are about 25. Growth stops between 18 and 20 years of age.

Sexual maturity

Most boys show signs of sexual development by the time they are 14 and are sexually mature by age 17 or 18. Under the influence of the hormone testosterone, the genitals start to enlarge at age 11 or 12 – first the testicles and scrotum and then, about a year later, the penis. The production of semen begins as soon as the testicles start to enlarge, but a boy does not usually have his first ejaculation until about 2 years later. If a boy's penis or testicles have not started to enlarge by the age of 14, talk to your doctor.

Pubic hair first appears around the age of 11 or 12; underarm and facial hair become visible between ages 13 and 15. Hair grows from the abdomen up to the chest and on the chest itself.

Teenage boys often ejaculate during sleep. So-called "wet dreams" can embarrass or concern a boy who does not expect them. Erections, and sometimes ejaculations, occur automatically during dreaming (whether or not the dream is erotic). Because a period of dreaming usually occurs just before awakening, most boys awaken with an erection in the morning. The morning erection disappears when the boy urinates.

PUBERTY IN GIRLS

Girls begin puberty and the accompanying growth spurt earlier than boys – at about the age of 10. This means that, for a time, girls are heavier and taller than their male peers. Girls reach their adult height by the age of 15 or 16. A girl's body weight doubles between the ages of 10 and 18. This increase in weight is caused by the rapid jump in height and by the natural deposits of fat that give the female body its curved appearance.

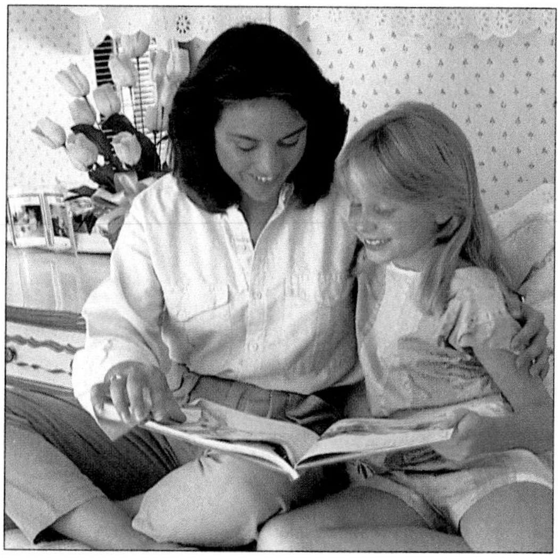

Preparing girls for womanhood
Young girls often feel uncomfortable about their bodies and need reassurance that the changes they are experiencing are normal. Mothers should discuss the physical changes of puberty with their daughters before the girls have their first period.

Sexual maturity

Most girls show signs of sexual development by the time they are 13 and reach sexual maturity by age 16. Under the influence of the female hormone estrogen, a girl's nipples start to enlarge at about the age of 10. Breast development is a common first sign of puberty, although the appearance of pubic hair occurs first in one in three girls. Underarm hair begins to grow a little later than pubic hair.

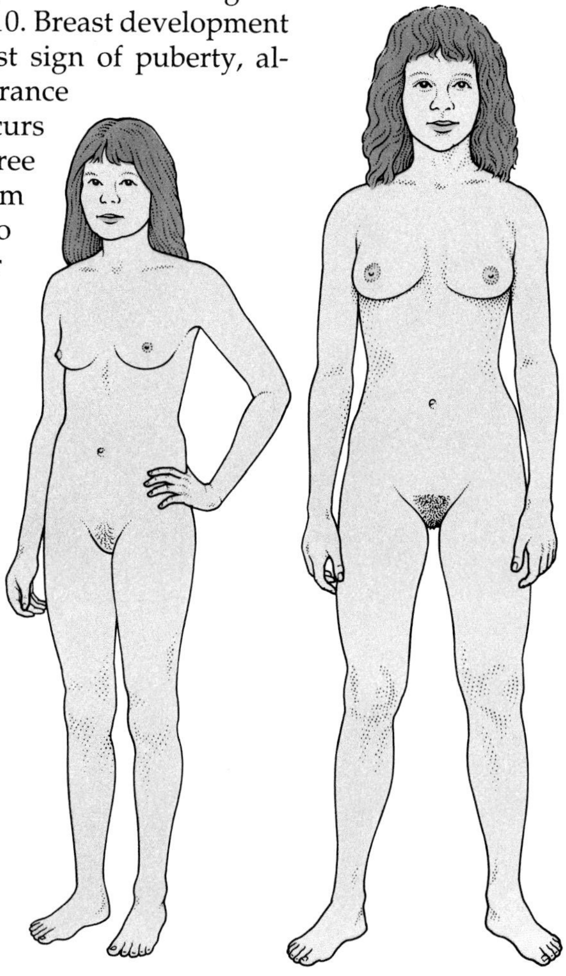

Changes in girls during puberty
The principal physical changes that occur in girls during puberty are the development of breasts, the growth of pubic and underarm hair, widening of the hips, enlargement of the uterus, and the onset of menstruation.

10 to 12 years old **15 to 16 years old**

Menstruation

The onset of menstruation is usually one of the last changes of puberty. Menstruation begins about 2 years after the breasts have started to develop and always after the growth spurt. A girl probably will not start to menstruate before she has reached a weight of 100 pounds.

About a year after menstruation begins, the vagina starts to produce a clear or white discharge, which is normal. Ovulation does not occur until a girl's periods have become regular – usually about 18 months after they begin. But it is safest to consider a girl to be fertile as soon as she begins to menstruate.

Call your doctor if your daughter's breasts do not develop by the time she is 13, or if her periods have not started by age 16. Very rarely, a hormonal problem delays pubertal development.

EMOTIONAL EFFECTS OF PUBERTY

Puberty can be a very confusing time for an adolescent. A teenager's fragile self-esteem can easily shatter at the first sign of disapproval by a peer. A common cause of depression in adolescents is rejection by a boyfriend or girlfriend. Some teenagers have more serious problems to deal with. In 1988, a survey found that 45 percent of eighth- and 10th-grade

THE MENSTRUAL CYCLE

Once a teenage girl has reached sexual maturity, her ovaries release an egg each month. Unless fertilization takes place, the lining of the uterus is shed, causing the bleeding known as menstruation. The entire cycle lasts between 24 and 35 days; the average is 28 days. The length of the period of bleeding varies from 1 to 8 days; the average is 5 days.

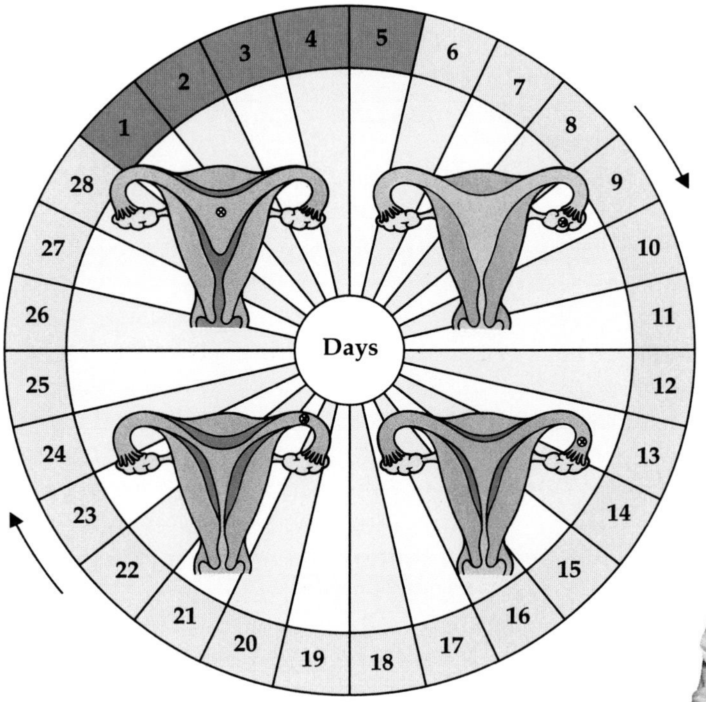

students in the US had problems at home that they felt unable to solve. Thirty-four percent had considered suicide and 14 percent had attempted it. If your teenager displays any of the common symptoms of depression, including episodes of uncontrolled crying or anger, antisocial behavior, withdrawal from social or family activities, changes in weight or sleep patterns, or difficulties in school, try to help him or her resolve the problem. If the depression persists, your doctor can determine whether your child is a candidate for counseling.

It is normal for some boys to become more aggressive during puberty than before because of the rise in levels of the male hormone testosterone. But extreme or disruptive behavior in either sex, whether at home or at school, can be a sign of depression. Such an adolescent may need professional help.

Early development

Some children reach puberty earlier than others. There may be an advantage to developing early, especially for boys. Boys who are bigger and stronger than their peers often have more self-confidence than smaller boys.

The advantages of being an early developer are not so clear-cut for girls. Girls who begin puberty early may feel self-conscious as they tower above their friends. Sexually mature girls are often still children emotionally and psychologically and may want to remain that way for a while longer. Their adult appearance can provoke interest from the opposite sex when they are unprepared to cope with it. Menstruation, too, may be a jarring signal that they are leaving childhood behind. You should give your early developer plenty of support and understanding and assure her that her friends will catch up in time.

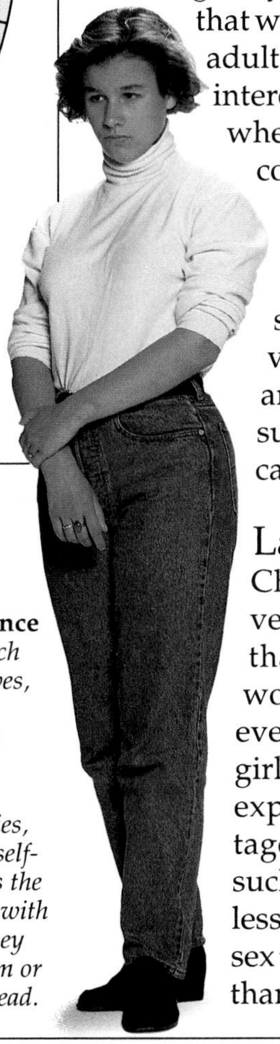

Low self-confidence
Teenagers judge each other, and themselves, by appearances. Teenagers are often self-conscious or embarrassed about their changing bodies, which affects their self-confidence. Discuss the changes of puberty with your child before they occur to prepare him or her for what lies ahead.

Late development

Children whose physical development lags far behind that of their friends may wonder whether they will ever catch up. Both boys and girls who develop late may experience some disadvantages in physical activities, such as sports, and may feel less attractive to the opposite sex than their peers. More boys than girls are late developers.

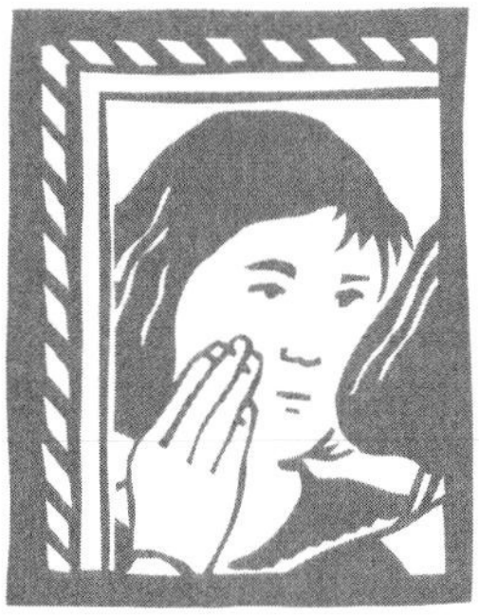

AN ADOLESCENT IN THE FAMILY

HAVING AN ADOLESCENT in the family can bring turbulent and difficult times for many households. While children are young, parents maintain control of the family. But during the teenage years, the balance of power shifts as the adolescent becomes increasingly independent. Parents have to learn to adapt to this change as their children mature into self-reliant individuals.

Friendships
Adolescents, especially during the early teenage years, have a powerful need to be "one of the crowd." Teenagers loosen family ties and friends begin to play a much larger role in their lives. Teenagers reinforce their sense of belonging by wearing similar hairstyles and clothes and by liking the same music.

Conflict between an adolescent and his or her parents usually develops because the adolescent's increasing independence seems to defy what the parents believe is best for the child. The adolescent wants more freedom, but the parents want to keep the adolescent safe. The adolescent wants to make decisions, but the parents feel that decisions about the adolescent are still their responsibility. Although many parents want to retain as much control of their children as possible, they need to realize that some degree of independence is essential if the teenager is ever to separate from the family and establish his or her own identity.

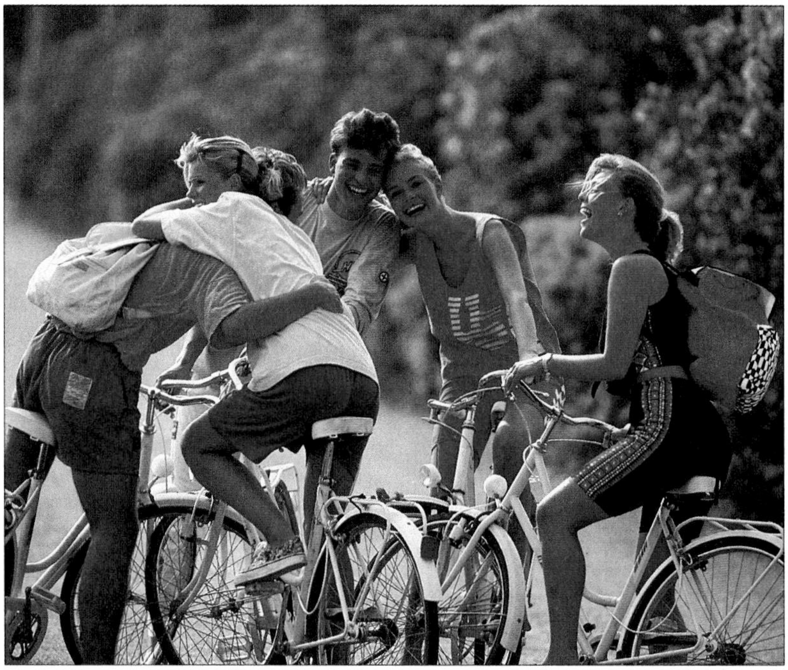

COMMUNICATING WITH ADOLESCENTS

Adolescence is a time for experimenting and testing limits. Many parents have difficulty communicating with their teenage children, who seem to challenge or disregard every word they say. Most parents also worry about the extent to which their adolescent children will experiment with cigarettes, alcohol, and other drugs. Parents may also find it difficult to accept the fact that their child is developing sexual relationships.

Building self-confidence

During their teenage years, adolescents are attempting to build a sense of identity and self-esteem. Their self-confidence is often fragile, so it is important for parents to encourage their efforts and praise their achievements. Show interest in what your children are doing and let them know that you appreciate and respect them for who they are. Encourage them to express and discuss their opinions and to develop their own values.

Despite an adolescent's defiant attitude toward parental authority, parental approval matters to teenagers. Parents should avoid teasing, sarcasm, or criticism. A parent who, without thinking, calls a teenager clumsy or stupid may not realize how deeply such comments can hurt a sensitive adolescent.

Family rules

Parents need to make it clear to their adolescent children that they must obey certain rules to impress on them that certain kinds of behavior are unacceptable. Generally, it is best to keep the rules to a minimum and to confine them to issues that you feel strongly about or that you think can affect your teenager's safety. After all, your ultimate aim is to teach your teenager to become responsible for himself or herself, not to blindly follow the rules you make for him or her.

Negotiating responsibilities

Most teenagers respond best when parents approach conflicts as problems to be solved rather than as battles to be won. Negotiation always works better than confrontation – it usually means that both sides make concessions, and one side has not "won" while the other side has "lost." A teenager is more likely to cooperate if you make decisions together.

Accept the fact that you eventually have to relinquish some responsibility to your adolescent children. Stand firm in the areas in which you intend to keep control, such as how late they stay out at night, and negotiate those areas in which they can take responsibility, such as how neat they keep their rooms and how they spend their own money. Let your teenage children make some decisions, even though you suspect that they will probably make some mistakes.

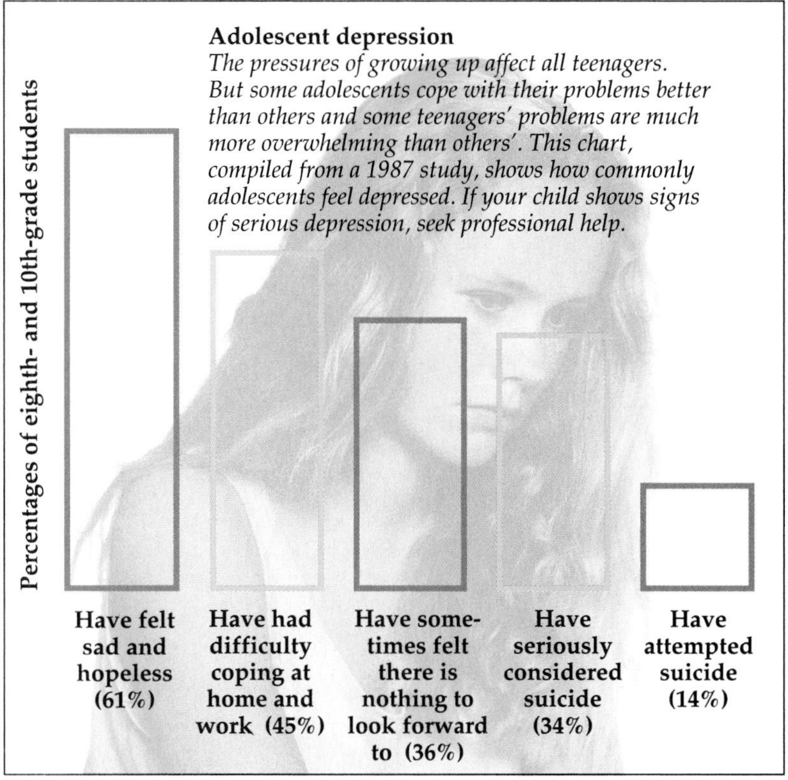

Adolescent depression
The pressures of growing up affect all teenagers. But some adolescents cope with their problems better than others and some teenagers' problems are much more overwhelming than others'. This chart, compiled from a 1987 study, shows how commonly adolescents feel depressed. If your child shows signs of serious depression, seek professional help.

Positive reinforcement

Take opportunities to acknowledge your teenager's achievements and good behavior. Even the most rebellious teenager needs parental approval, and positive reinforcement helps to encourage constructive behavior. Remember that you will never make a teenager behave in a certain way without his or her cooperation.

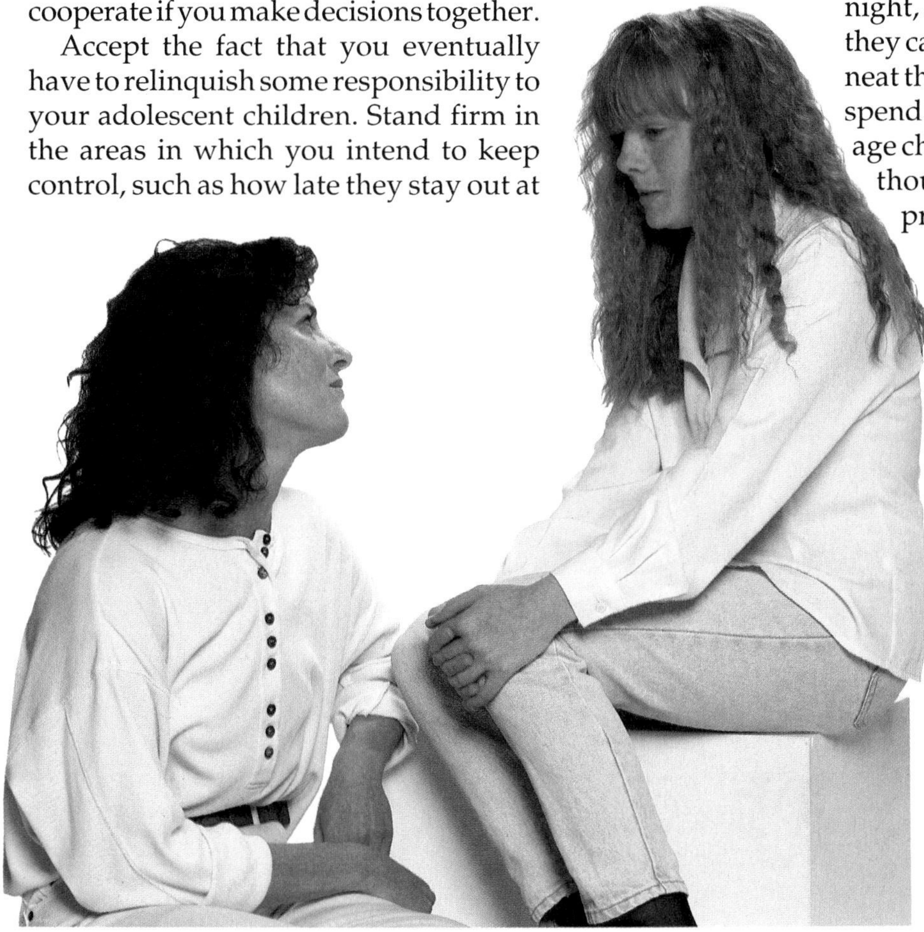

Listening
Make time to sit down and talk to your teenager about his or her interests and problems. Listening is a way of showing your teenager that what he or she thinks and says is important and that you are trying to understand and appreciate his or her point of view.

COMMON HEALTH PROBLEMS OF ADOLESCENCE

Appearances are extremely important to teenagers and few are secure enough to believe that their friends like them for themselves. They know that appearance plays a role in the way their peers judge each other. Most adolescents are intensely self-conscious about their rapidly changing bodies and acutely aware of any real or imagined physical defects. These concerns may seem trivial to a parent, but they are extremely important to a teenager. These two pages list common health problems that concern adolescents.

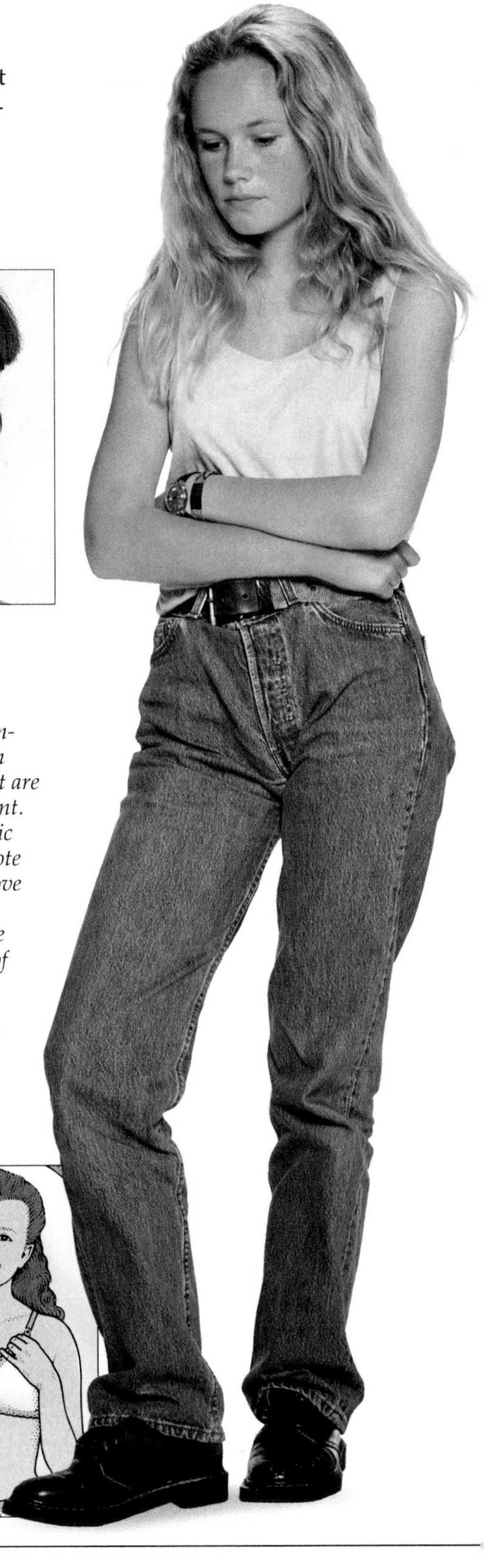

Acne
Acne, inflammation of the hair follicles and adjacent oil-producing glands in the skin, tends to appear on the face, neck, shoulders, and chest. Mild acne responds well to over-the-counter skin preparations that contain benzoyl peroxide. Severe cases respond to daily treatment with antibiotics, taken by mouth or applied to the skin. Treatment with the female hormone estrogen can be effective in females.

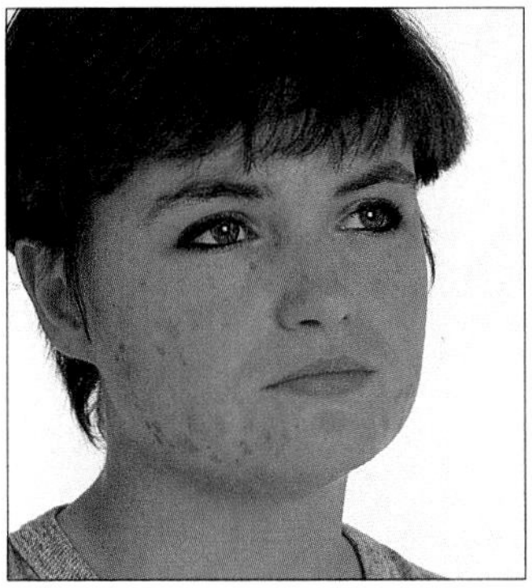

MENSTRUAL PROBLEMS

Girls who are smaller or thinner than average may start menstruating later than others. Call your doctor if your daughter has not begun her periods by age 16. Pain is not usually a problem during a girl's first few periods, but if your daughter does have cramps, rest and the application of a heating pad or hot water bottle can ease them. If these measures do not help, ask your doctor about medication, such as ibuprofen or other painkilling drugs. For about the first 18 months after a girl has started to menstruate, her periods may be irregular. Gaps of 2 to 3 months between periods are quite normal. Suggest to your daughter that she mark her periods on a calendar so that she can identify an emerging pattern.

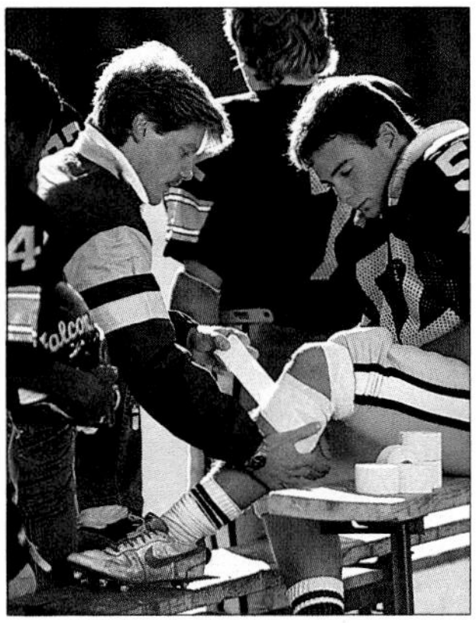

Sports-related injuries
Sports-related injuries are common. Weight lifting can strain bones, muscles, and joints that are still developing in an adolescent. Some teenage boys use anabolic steroids (hormones that promote muscle development) to improve athletic performance. Doctors strongly oppose their use. Side effects include accumulation of fluid in body tissues; damage to the testicles, liver, and adrenal glands; and increased fat levels in the blood.

Breast development
Hormonal changes prompt breast development. Teenage girls are often self-conscious about the size of their breasts. They also worry that their breasts are not growing evenly. Uneven breast development is normal and may continue into adulthood. Some boys may be alarmed by breast swelling during puberty. A boy needs to be reassured that such swelling will disappear when his hormones settle down.

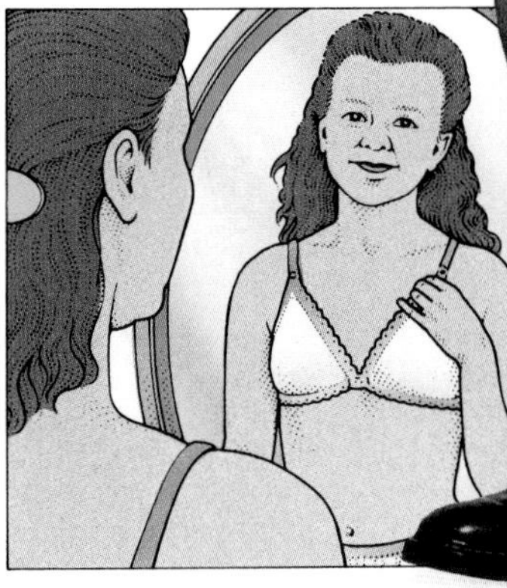

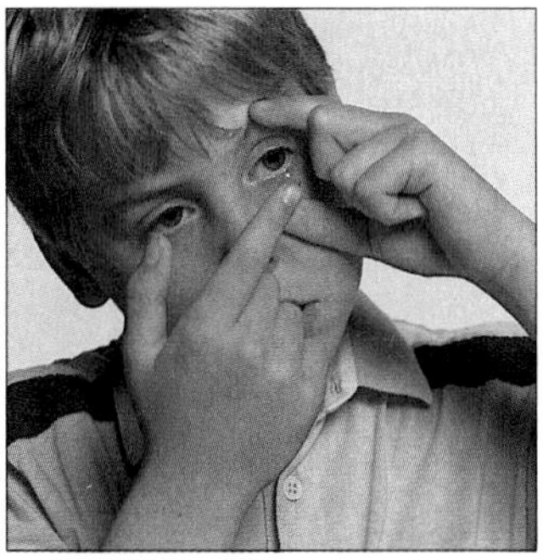

Defective eyesight
Adolescents don't want to look different from their peers in any way. Teenagers sometimes feel awkward when they have to wear eyeglasses to correct vision. If contact lenses can correct the teenager's vision, they may solve the appearance problem and boost the teenager's self-confidence.

Irregular teeth
Orthodontic treatment, a means of repositioning crooked teeth using pressure exerted by braces, can improve a teenager's appearance. Early adolescence, when the teeth and jaw are still growing, is a good time to begin treatment, which can last for up to 20 months. The dentist adjusts the braces every 3 to 6 weeks. Then the child wears a retainer for several months.

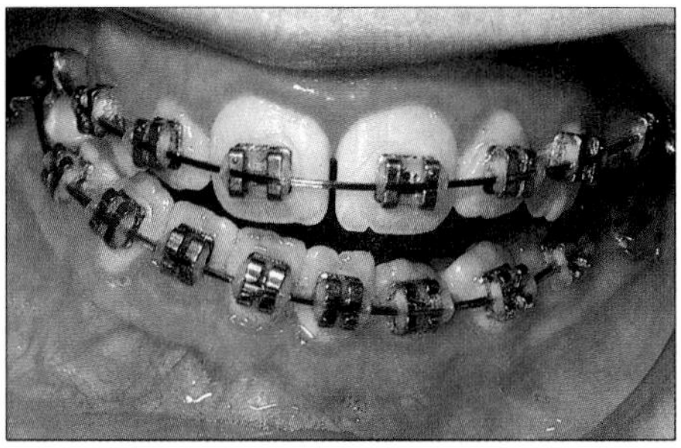

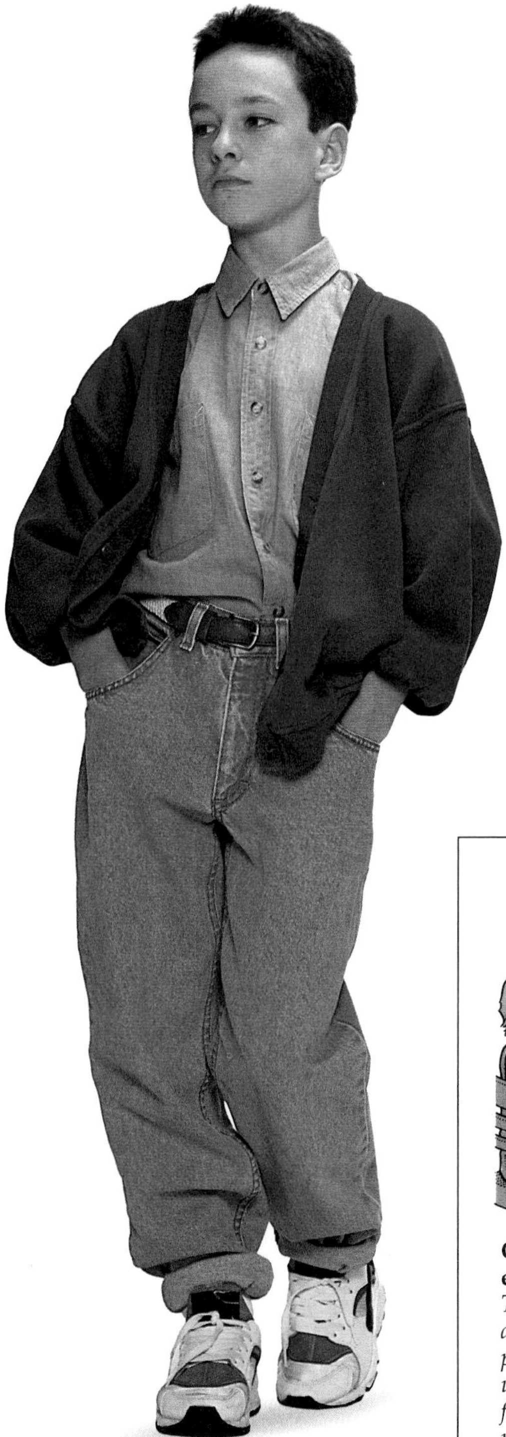

Awkwardness with members of the opposite sex
A teenager may feel increasingly awkward and uncomfortable with members of the opposite sex, even those he or she has known for years, especially if the teenager feels self-conscious about his or her appearance.

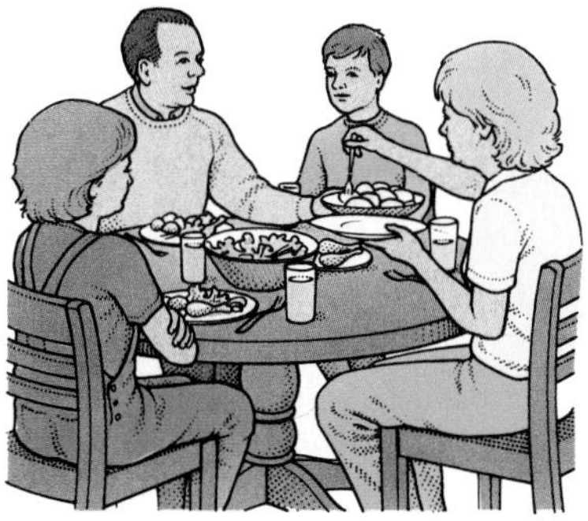

Overcoming eating disorders
Teenagers with eating disorders need medical and psychiatric treatment. Doctors usually prescribe group and family counseling, along with modification of the adolescent's eating habits. Parents may find it difficult to initiate treatment because the adolescent usually denies having an eating disorder. In severe cases, the individual may need to be hospitalized.

EATING DISORDERS

The incidence of two eating disorders, anorexia nervosa and bulimia, is increasing among teenage girls. The disorders rarely occur in boys.

◆ An adolescent with anorexia nervosa claims to be too fat and diets even when emaciated. She may exercise excessively. Menstrual periods usually stop. Anorectics are typically high-achieving perfectionists who excel in school. Complications of anorexia include hair loss, brittle nails, constipation, and heart problems that can be fatal.

◆ The adolescent with bulimia binges on huge quantities of high-fat, sugary foods and then purges her body by self-induced vomiting. Many also use laxatives, diet rigorously, or fast to offset the effects of binging. The constant vomiting can produce erosion of the teeth by stomach acid, rupture of the esophagus, and dehydration.

PRESSURES OF ADOLESCENCE

An adolescent must adapt to the physical changes that happen during the transition to adulthood, and also the pressures exerted by parents, peers, and the popular culture. Parents pressure them to do well in school, to take responsibility within the family, and to act maturely. Peers push them to conform and become one of the crowd, or risk being ostracized and ignored. A teenager's behavior signals unity with his or her peers, and teenagers often feel pressured to be rebellious against parental authority.

GANG INVOLVEMENT

Adolescents who are surrounded by poverty, poor schools, high unemployment, and weakened family and community structures may turn to gangs. Gangs reinforce their group identities by wearing certain colors, using hand signals, displaying gang-related graffiti, and engaging in violent initiation rites. The availability of guns, coupled with intense gang rivalries, sometimes leads to disabling or fatal gunshot injuries. Most gang members are boys, but female gangs are on the rise. Factors that tend to encourage gang membership include illiteracy and lack of skills, the lack of a sense of future, feelings of invulnerability, and learning disabilities.

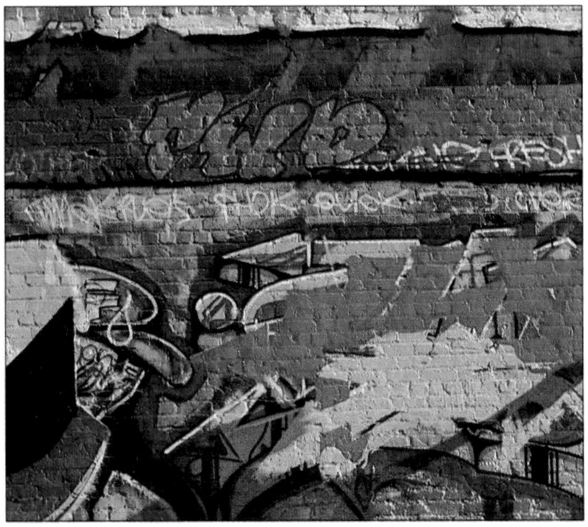

The spread of gangs
Once found only in large cities, gangs are now spreading into suburban areas and small towns, primarily to sell drugs. Gang-related graffiti is often the most apparent sign of gang activity in an area.

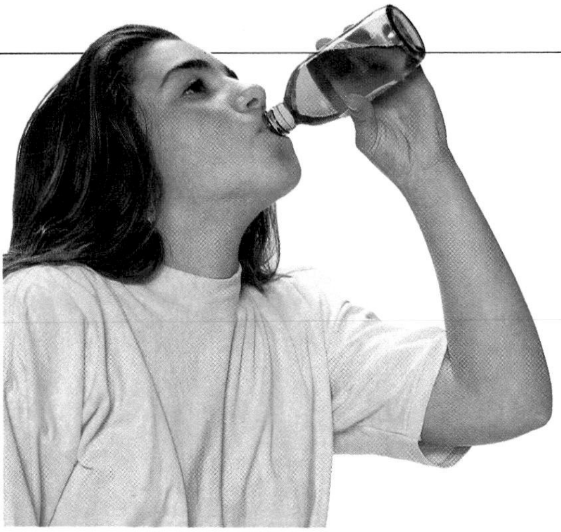

Alcohol and accidents
Deaths and injuries from automobile accidents, falls, drownings, and injuries caused by diving into shallow water occur much more commonly among adolescents who have been drinking alcohol. About half of all adolescent drivers involved in motor-vehicle accidents have been drinking.

ALCOHOL

Although it is illegal to sell alcohol to people under 21 years old, teenagers in the US obtain and drink more alcohol than ever before. Young people are more likely to drink alcohol excessively if their parents do so or if the parents rigidly oppose alcohol consumption. Responsible parental drinking provides a healthy model for a child to emulate.

SMOKING

An adolescent's decision to smoke cigarettes greatly depends on the smoking habits of those around him or her. Many adolescents think smoking gives them a sophisticated image. Others see smoking as a sign of rebellion or as a way to lose weight. Adolescent girls are starting to smoke at increasingly early ages, and girls are more likely than boys to continue smoking. People who have not started to smoke cigarettes by the age of 21 usually never begin to smoke.

Discuss the serious health risks of smoking with your children. The best way to influence your child not to smoke is not to smoke yourself.

RESISTING ALCOHOL

Help your children to resist the social pressure to drink alcohol:

- ◆ Teach them that nonalcoholic drinks are socially acceptable.
- ◆ Do not drink in front of your children to cope with your problems or drink to excess at home.
- ◆ Encourage them to seek friends who do not drink and activities that do not involve drinking.
- ◆ Do not buy alcohol for a son or daughter under 21. Parents are legally responsible for the actions of their children who drink alcohol.
- ◆ Teach them not to drink alcohol if they intend to drive and never to ride with someone who has been drinking.

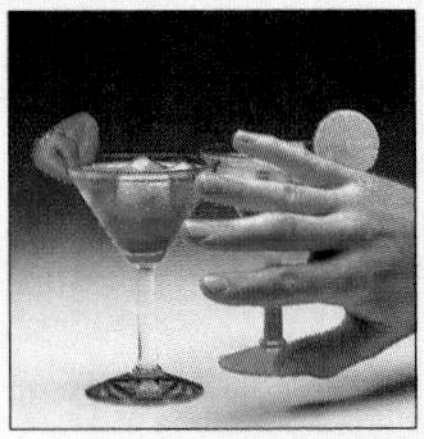

CASE HISTORY
FALLING GRADES

MARY HAD ALWAYS been a high achiever in school, but recently her grades had started to fall. She had also found a new group of older friends. Her parents worried that she might be taking drugs. One day, Mary's father noticed that a bottle of whiskey was missing from his liquor cabinet and that many of the other bottles were depleted. He suspected that Mary might have an alcohol problem.

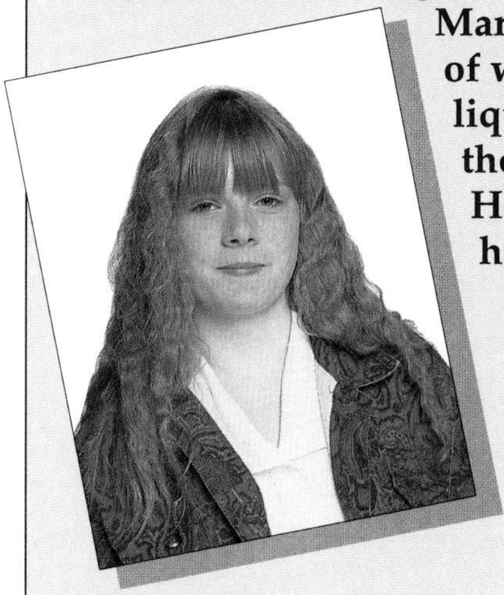

PERSONAL DETAILS
Name Mary Proctor
Age 15
Occupation Student
Family Mary's parents are both lawyers. Her mother is in good health. Her father regularly drinks heavily.

FAMILY BACKGROUND

Mary's parents have high hopes for her. Her upbringing has been strict, but Mary has recently distanced herself from her parents. During the past few months, Mary and her parents have often argued about the time she spends with her older friends and her rebellious behavior. Mary's parents suspect that she may be abusing alcohol and neglecting her studies. They make an appointment with her school counselor.

AT SCHOOL

Mary's counselor confirms that Mary's behavior has become increasingly antisocial, uncooperative, and unpredictable. He suggests that Mary obtain counseling from a specialist who deals specifically with adolescent problems.

COUNSELING

During counseling, Mary confesses that she feels she can never live up to her parents' expectations. She says that her parents treat her like a child and that associating with an older crowd is her way of showing them how grown up she is. But Mary admits that having older friends has been very stressful. She feels pressured to take drugs and to become sexually active. She says that drinking alcohol helps her loosen up and feel like part of the group. But Mary now finds she can't face going to school unless she has a drink. The counselor suggests that the family see a doctor who specializes in alcoholism and other addictive disorders. Mary and her parents agree to do so.

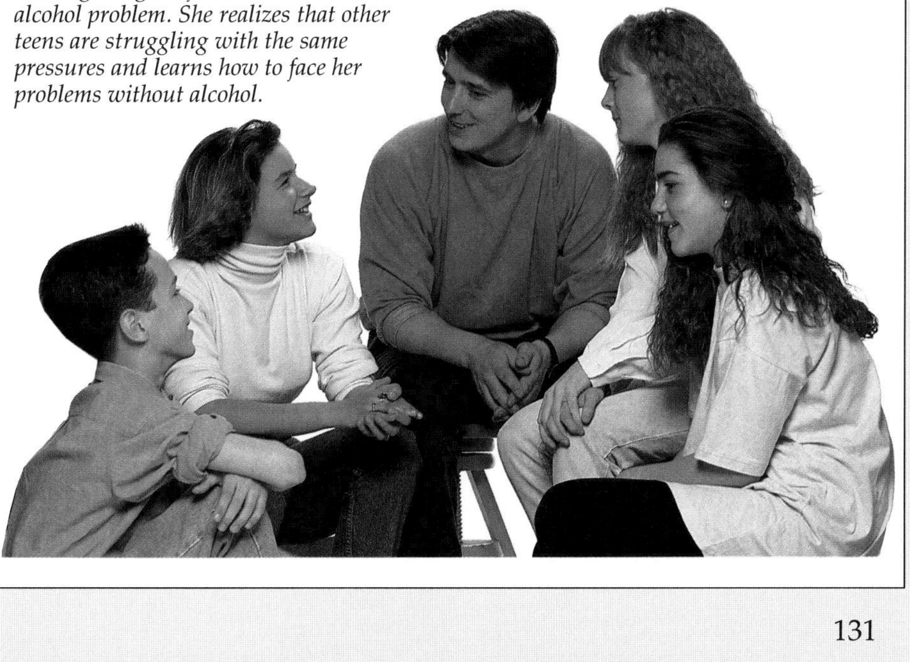

Support and encouragement
Mary attends a weekly support group meeting designed for adolescents with an alcohol problem. She realizes that other teens are struggling with the same pressures and learns how to face her problems without alcohol.

DIAGNOSIS AND TREATMENT

The addiction specialist examines both Mary and her father and diagnoses ALCOHOLISM. He looks for any alcohol-related health problems and, finding none, refers them to an ongoing treatment program. Mary and her father are not in the same treatment program, but the two programs work together to ensure that Mary and her father support each other.

THE OUTCOME

With the help of her treatment program and her doctor, Mary has not had an alcoholic drink for several months. She feels better than she has for some time, is working hard at school, and spends more time with friends of her own age.

DRUG ABUSE

Many teenagers experiment with drugs, especially stimulants, such as amphetamines or cocaine, or cannabis (marijuana or hashish). Boys are more likely to try any form of drug than are girls. Adolescents usually abuse drugs or become drug dependent to relieve or forget personal or social problems.

To prevent your child from turning to drugs as an escape, help your child face his or her problems. Confronting and dealing with problems as they come up will give your child confidence in coping with life so he or she can withstand the temptation to use drugs.

Helping an addicted adolescent

An addicted adolescent must first recognize that he or she has a serious problem and must want to give up the addiction. He or she needs to enter a drug treatment program willingly or the treatment will not work. The child needs your support

SIGNS OF DRUG ABUSE

Listed below are common signs of drug abuse. But teenagers who do not use drugs may occasionally show some of these signs, so do not jump to the conclusion that your teenager is a drug abuser. Check carefully before making accusations. Be alert for:

- Altered sleeping patterns
- General lethargy, drowsiness, or sleepiness
- Sudden mood swings
- Changes in appetite
- Unusual irritability or aggressiveness
- Loss of interest in school, friends, and hobbies
- Lying and excessive secrecy
- Unexplained shortage of money or the sudden disappearance of expensive possessions or money

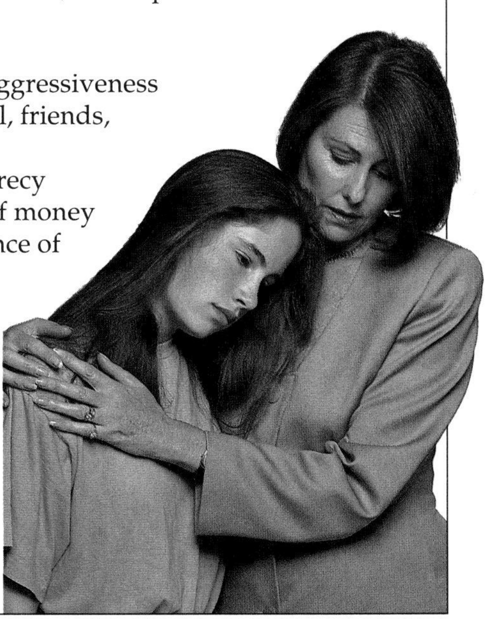

Do not withhold your love
Although you do not approve of your adolescent's use of drugs, show that you still love him or her. Encourage your child to seek prompt treatment in a drug treatment program.

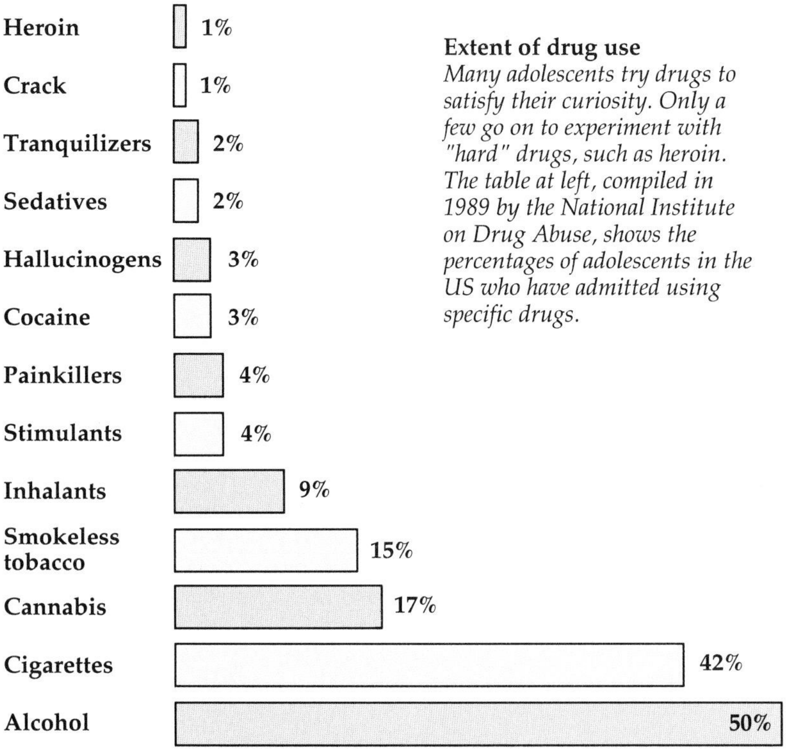

Percentage of 12- to 17-year-olds who have used substances

Extent of drug use
Many adolescents try drugs to satisfy their curiosity. Only a few go on to experiment with "hard" drugs, such as heroin. The table at left, compiled in 1989 by the National Institute on Drug Abuse, shows the percentages of adolescents in the US who have admitted using specific drugs.

and the support of a therapist, who will try to help the adolescent deal with the problems that made him or her turn to drugs. If your child is to remain drug free, he or she must find new interests and make radical changes in his or her life-style. Family members may also need to make difficult changes.

TEENAGERS AND SEX

Today's adolescents are more sexually experienced than their parents were at the same age. By age 17, 75 percent of boys are sexually active; 75 percent of girls are sexually active by age 19. Most teens say they are not promiscuous.

Parental guidance

As a parent, you must learn to accept your growing children's sexuality. You also need to teach your children about their sexuality so that they can make informed choices about sex. Teenagers need guidance in coping with their powerful sexual feelings. Encourage teenagers to wait until they are older before having sex so they can form a mature, loving relationship with a partner. If you are too embarrassed to talk to your children about sex yourself, ask a school counselor, your doctor, or another adult who is close to your children to talk to them for you. Make sure your children know about the risks, such as sexually transmitted diseases, that are inherent in sexual relationships. Teach them about the important responsibilities that surround a sexual relationship, including the possibility of conceiving a child. Discuss reliable methods of contraception to prevent pregnancy. But remind them that abstinence is the only way to ensure absolute protection against pregnancy and sexually transmitted disease.

SEXUALLY TRANSMITTED DISEASES IN TEENAGERS

- Three million teenagers contract a sexually transmitted disease, such as a chlamydial infection, every year.
- The incidence of gonorrhea is highest among females aged 15 to 19.
- One in four sexually active teens will contract a sexually transmitted disease before graduating from high school.
- Human papillomavirus (HPV) rates are as high as 46 percent among adolescent females. HPV causes genital warts and can increase a female's risk of cervical cancer.
- Forty percent of all teenagers are unable to recognize common symptoms of sexually transmitted diseases.

CONTRACEPTION

About 50 percent of adolescents do not use contraception the first time they have sexual intercourse. Teenagers often find it embarrassing to buy contraceptives. But if your adolescent has made the decision to have sex, he or she needs contraception. The advice that you give to your teenagers about contraception must be practical and positive. Remind them that becoming a parent too soon will radically alter their future. Some parents fear that the information they give to adolescents about contraception will encourage them to be promiscuous. No evidence exists that this assumption is true.

Condoms

Condoms offer protection against an unwanted pregnancy, especially when used with a spermicide. They also help protect against sexually transmitted diseases. By using a condom, a boy can fulfill his responsibility for contraception. Condoms are not as effective as the contraceptive pill, but their availability and convenience may encourage more consistent use than other methods of contraception. Latex condoms protect against HIV (human immunodeficiency virus), the virus that causes AIDS (acquired immunodeficiency syndrome), but condoms made of natural materials do not.

Contraceptive pill

The contraceptive pill is a very reliable method of preventing pregnancy. It does not protect against AIDS or sexually transmitted diseases. Ask your doctor if the pill is the most suitable contraceptive method for your daughter. Other reliable forms of contraception exist, including the diaphragm and cervical cap.

MASTURBATION

Masturbation is the most common form of adolescent sexual activity. If you have negative feelings about masturbation, try not to communicate them to your children. They may become anxious or feel guilty about a normal, harmless part of their sexual development. Explain that masturbation is a normal step toward adult sexual development.

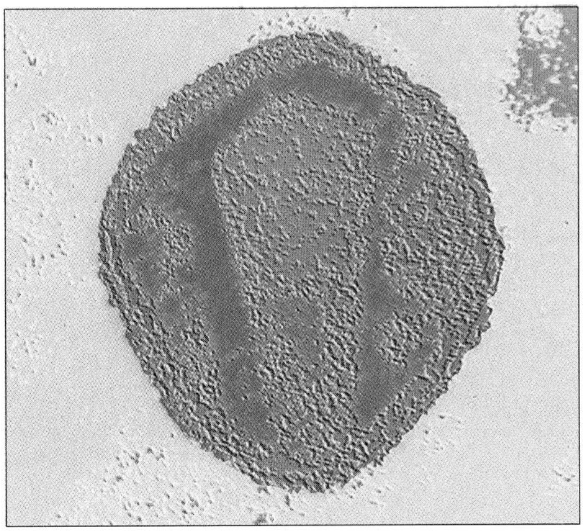

Teenagers and AIDS
Adolescents who engage in unprotected sexual intercourse put themselves at increased risk for infection by HIV, the virus that causes AIDS. Infection with the AIDS virus (see left) has increased by 70 percent in teenagers during the last few years. AIDS is now the sixth leading cause of death in people 15 to 24 years old.

TEENAGE PREGNANCY

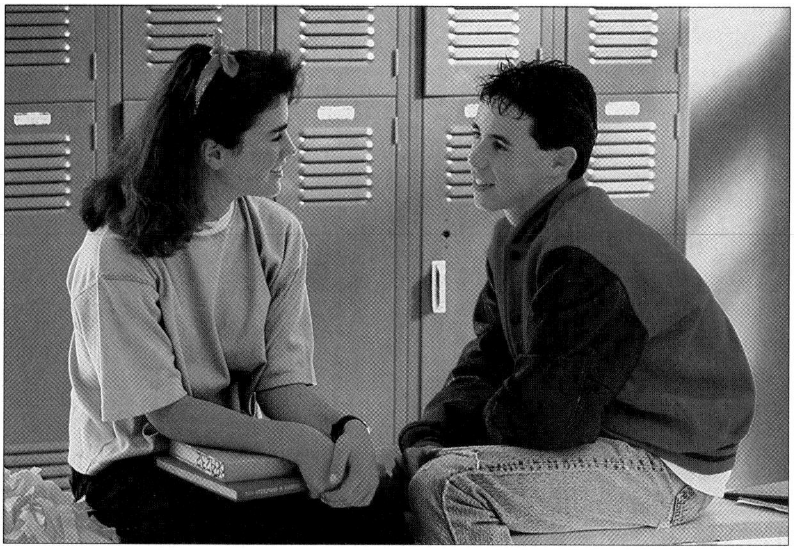

Over 1 million teenage girls become pregnant every year in the US. Most of these pregnancies are unintentional. Girls and boys are physically able to become parents long before they are emotionally mature enough for parenthood. To help prevent teenage pregnancy, parents need to advise their children about the risks and responsibilities of sexual activity. If your daughter becomes pregnant, she will be terrified of telling you about it. Let her know that she can look to you for help even though you are upset by the consequences of her behavior. Take your daughter to your doctor so that he or she can confirm a suspected pregnancy. Carefully consider and discuss the options your daughter has and the impact that this decision will have on her future. Abortion and adoption are options available to her. If she decides to carry the fetus to term, your daughter will need prenatal care from the first weeks of pregnancy. Pregnancy and childbirth carry medical risks, especially for an adolescent girl who may be afraid to seek medical care. Talk to your daughter's teachers to make sure she can stay in school before and after she delivers the baby.

Responsibilities and risks
Both boys and girls need to understand the responsibilities and risks that surround a sexual relationship. Parental guidance about sexuality helps them act responsibly.

HOMOSEXUALITY

Many adolescents question their sexual identity when they find themselves attracted to a friend or teacher of the same sex. For most of these adolescents, such attraction is a stage through which they pass. But others experience it as the beginning of an awareness that their orientation is homosexual. Statistics show that about 5 to 10 percent of adolescents are aware that they are homosexual. Although gay and lesbian adolescents may experience emotional turmoil as they encounter the social stigma attached to homosexuality, their orientation is a normal variant of sexual behavior, not a disorder. Doctors do not yet know the origins of homosexuality. Parents of homosexual adolescents need to communicate to their children that they accept them for who they are. Support groups can give families the courage they need to face the prejudice they often encounter.

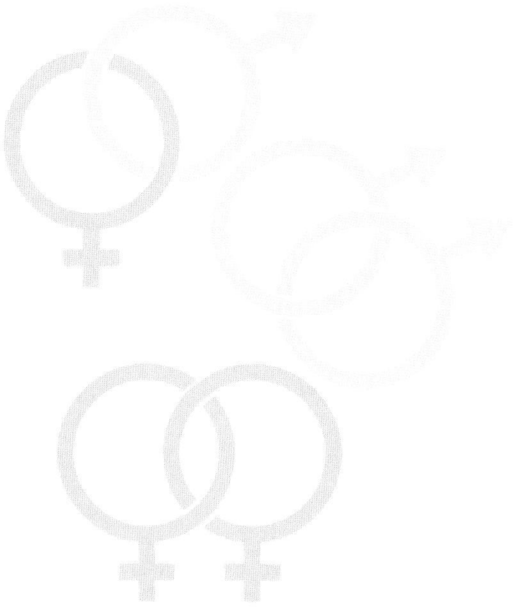

Medical risks
Male homosexuals are at increased risk of contracting HIV, the virus that causes AIDS. The risk of HIV infection and sexually transmitted diseases rises as the number of sexual partners increases. The use of latex condoms protects against transmission of these diseases.

DATE RAPE

The sexual inexperience of some adolescent girls can make them targets of rape on dates. The incidence of date rape is increasing. Teach your adolescent boy that forceful aggression is never acceptable with a sexual partner. Make sure your teenage girl knows that she has the right to say "no" under any circumstances.

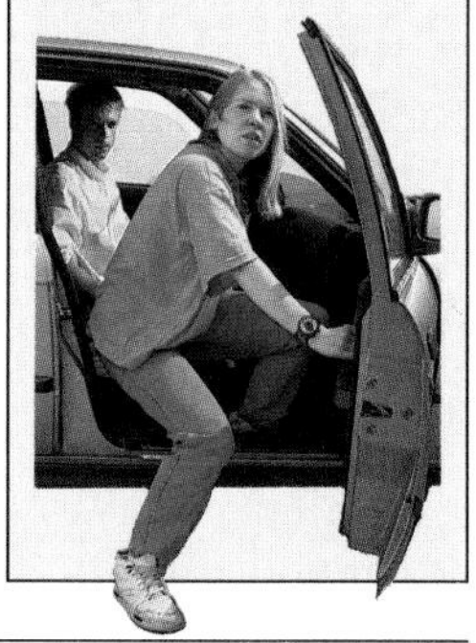

CASE HISTORY
FATIGUE AND A SORE THROAT

CHRISTI HAD ALWAYS been a bright and active student, but she had been feeling tired and depressed and had lost interest in school during the last couple of weeks. Christi's mother attributed these symptoms to Christi's recent breakup with her boyfriend. During the last week, Christi developed a sore throat, fever, headache, and swollen glands in her neck. Christi's mother decided to call the family doctor.

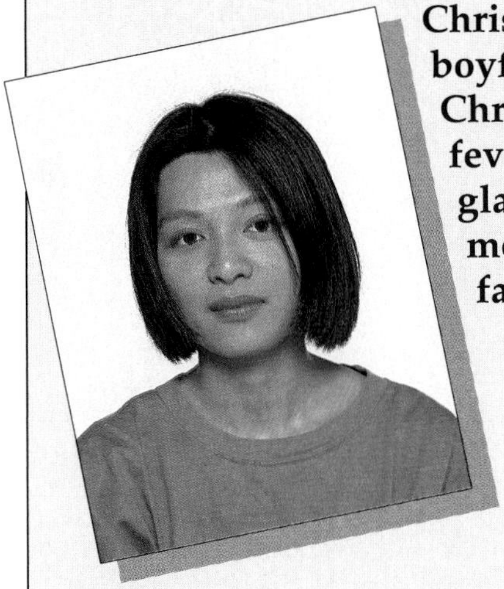

PERSONAL DETAILS
Name Christi Chang
Age 15
Occupation Student
Family Christi is an only child. Her father has high blood pressure; her mother is healthy.

MEDICAL BACKGROUND
Christi had chickenpox as a young child. She has received all of her scheduled immunizations.

THE CONSULTATION
The doctor listens while Christi describes her symptoms. After examining Christi, the doctor suspects that Christi may have a viral infection that is common among teenagers. The doctor explains that blood tests are needed to confirm this possibility and takes a sample of Christi's blood for analysis.

THE DIAGNOSIS
The results of Christi's blood tests confirm the doctor's suspicions. Christi has contracted the viral disease INFECTIOUS MONONUCLEOSIS, which the doctor has identified from the characteristic appearance of Christi's white blood cells and the presence of certain antibodies (proteins produced by white blood cells in response to foreign proteins in the body) in the blood sample. Some call mononucleosis the "kissing disease," but it can also be spread by nonintimate contact. Its peak incidence occurs around ages 15 to 17.

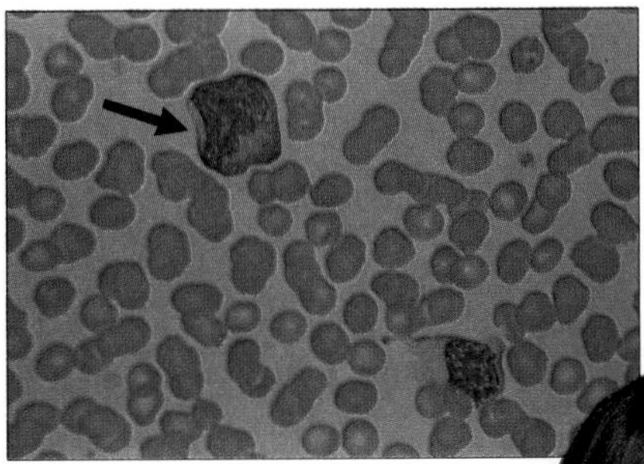

Examining Christi's blood
The doctor examines a smear of Christi's blood under a microscope. Some of Christi's white blood cells, called lymphocytes, look abnormal. The presence of such cells (see arrow above) helps the doctor establish the diagnosis.

THE TREATMENT
The doctor explains that no specific treatment exists for infectious mononucleosis and reassures Christi that, although she may feel tired and listless for a while, her symptoms will gradually improve during the next few weeks. She recommends the aspirin substitute acetaminophen to help relieve Christi's aches, sore throat, and fever and tells Christi to rest as much as possible until her condition improves. The doctor specifically warns Christi to avoid exercise and sports for at least 6 weeks or her liver and spleen could be damaged. She should also avoid kissing or very close contact with other people during this time to prevent the spread of the infection. The doctor asks Christi to return in a few weeks for a follow-up appointment so that she can check on her recovery.

THE OUTCOME
After a few days, Christi's sore throat and fever disappear, but she continues to feel tired. After 3 weeks, she feels well enough to return to school. At her follow-up appointment, Christi tells the doctor that she found it hard to concentrate during the first few days at school but that she is now beginning to feel like her old self again. The doctor tells Christi to rest anytime she feels she has overextended herself.

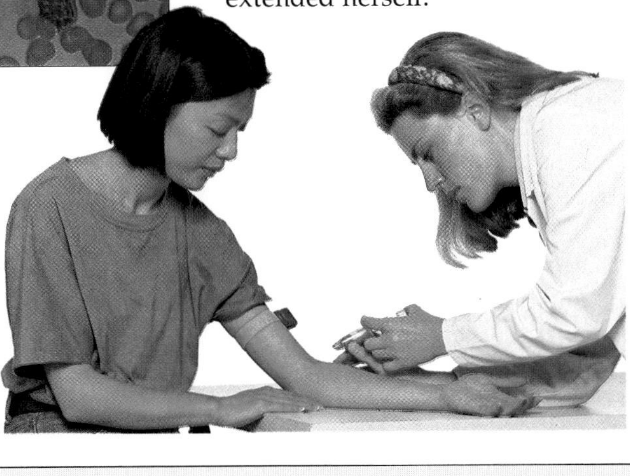

CHILD ABUSE

The term child abuse refers to any form of serious physical, emotional, or sexual mistreatment or neglect of a child. The abuser is usually a parent, step-parent, or other care giver. Child abuse occurs at all socioeconomic levels, although it appears to be more common in underprivileged groups. Abused children sustain not only physical injury but also emotional damage. Between 2 and 4 million children are abused or neglected each year in the US, and about 4,000 children die annually from the effects of child abuse.

Most nonaccidental injuries in children are inflicted by an adult who has an unrealistic expectation of the child and who has entirely lost control of his or her anger. Children under 3 years old are at the greatest risk of physical abuse, because at this age they are very demanding but are too young to respond to reason. Factors that reduce a parent's capacity for self-control, such as alcohol or emotional disturbance, increase the likelihood of child abuse.

REPEATED PHYSICAL ABUSE

Premeditated, repeated abuse of children is rare. When it does occur, it is usually a sign that a parent has a severe emotional disorder. The parent's abusive behavior is often a repetition of the cruel treatment he or she received as a child.

Repeated abuse can cause multiple fractures, damage to internal organs, and even death. Physical abuse is often accompanied by deliberate neglect, when the parent makes no attempt to feed, clothe, or supervise the child adequately. In adulthood, an abused child often becomes an abuser of his or her own children.

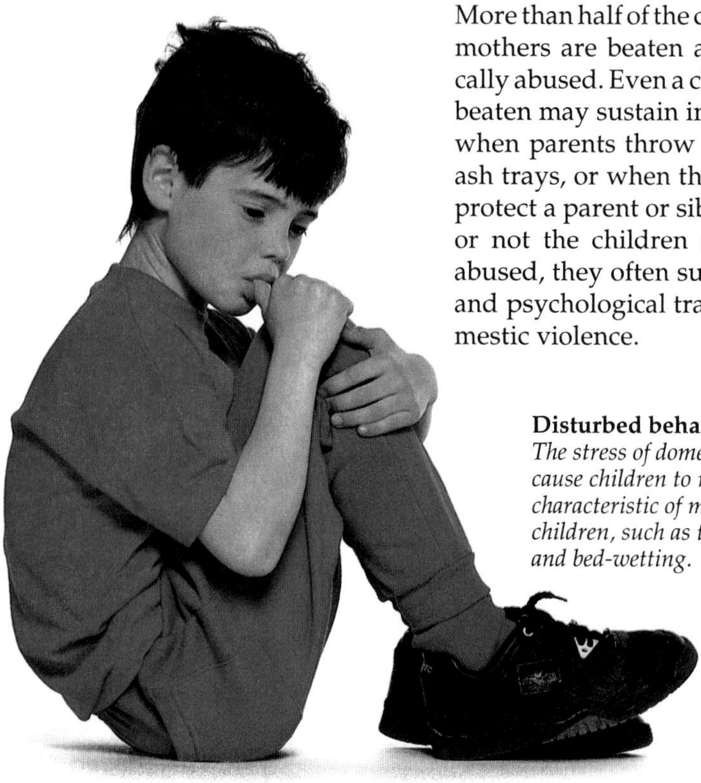

Disturbed behavior
The stress of domestic violence can cause children to revert to behavior characteristic of much younger children, such as thumb-sucking and bed-wetting.

DOMESTIC VIOLENCE

Each year, 2 million women in the US are beaten by their partners. More than half of the children whose mothers are beaten are also physically abused. Even a child who is not beaten may sustain indirect injuries when parents throw items, such as ash trays, or when the child tries to protect a parent or sibling. Whether or not the children are physically abused, they often suffer emotional and psychological trauma from domestic violence.

FAMILY RISK FACTORS

A number of family circumstances can increase the risk of child abuse:

- One or both parents have been abused.
- The parents' relationship is breaking down or the child is the product of a previous relationship.
- The parents are very young.
- The child needs special care, as does a disabled child.
- The parents have financial and/or housing problems.
- The parents have no relatives or friends to whom they can turn for relief or support.

Psychological effects

Children may not witness violence occurring in the home, but they are almost always aware of it. Children of abused mothers are denied the kind of home life that fosters healthy development. They may be deprived of adequate nutrition and rest because their eating and sleeping habits are disrupted by shouting and fighting. These children often have stress-related physical ailments, such as headaches, vague abdominal pain, ulcers, and rashes.

Children from violent homes constantly fear injury to their mothers and themselves. They experience depression and feel guilty about loving or hating their abuser. Children exposed to family violence blame themselves for causing the conflict and feel powerless to stop it.

Children from violent homes may be overly aggressive and difficult to control, or they may be abnormally passive and withdrawn. Domestic

BREAKING THE CYCLE OF VIOLENCE

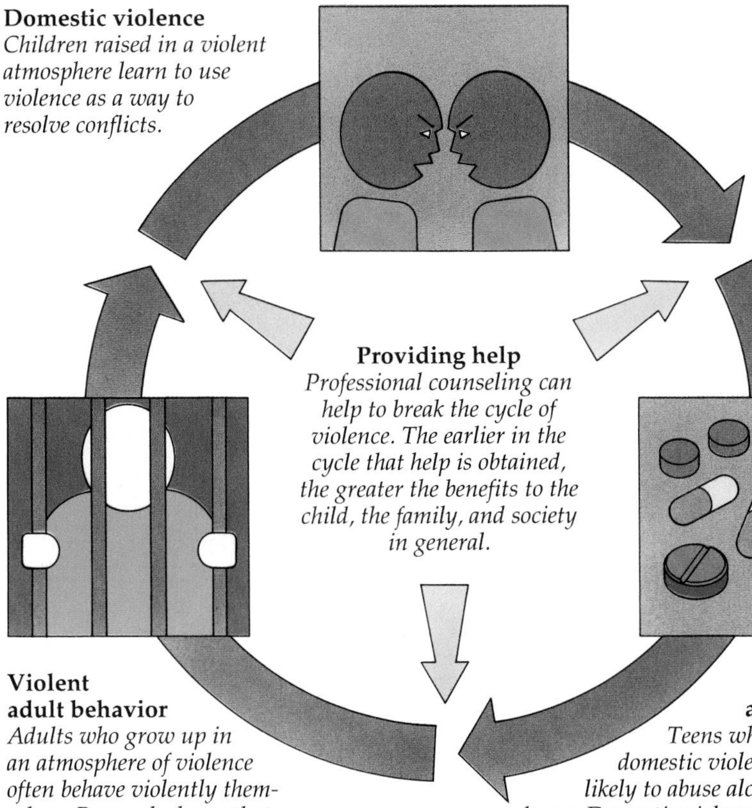

Domestic violence
Children raised in a violent atmosphere learn to use violence as a way to resolve conflicts.

Troubled adolescence
Teens who experience domestic violence are more likely to abuse alcohol or other drugs. Domestic violence contributes to the problems of teenage runaways and teenage homelessness.

Violent adult behavior
Adults who grow up in an atmosphere of violence often behave violently themselves. Research shows that most convicted criminals were raised in abusive homes.

Providing help
Professional counseling can help to break the cycle of violence. The earlier in the cycle that help is obtained, the greater the benefits to the child, the family, and society in general.

violence often prevents children from concentrating at school and from doing homework, drawing them down into an ever-worsening spiral of underachievement.

NEGLECT

Neglect of a child's physical and emotional needs may arise from an inability of the parents to understand those needs. Intentional neglect of the child is usually a sign that the parents have severe emotional problems. Neglected children are usually smaller than average or undernourished. Their skin and hair are often in poor condition, and they may develop rashes in areas of the body where dirt collects.

Sometimes a parent fulfills a child's physical needs but ignores the child's emotional needs by withholding support, guidance, affection, or stimulation. A child who is emotionally abused may fail to thrive and exhibit slow development as well as a lack of normal emotional responses. Such a child usually attains a normal weight and becomes more responsive when placed with alternative care givers who are more caring.

SEXUAL ABUSE

Girls are the most frequent victims of sexual abuse, although boys are also at risk. Most cases of sexual abuse involve a parent, close relative, or family friend who takes advantage of a child's innocence and affection. The abuser usually conducts the abuse in secrecy and makes the child fearful of what would happen if he or she revealed the abuse. Adults should never ignore a child who claims to have been sexually abused. Tell the child that what happened was not his or her fault. Take the child to a doctor, who will conduct a physical examination and may refer the child to a psychotherapist who specializes in such abuse.

SIGNS OF SEXUAL ABUSE

Sexual abuse can produce physical signs and changes in speech or behavior. Speak to the child gently to find out whether abuse has occurred. Signs include:

◆ Sexual explicitness in conversation, drawings, or play.
◆ Signs of a sexually transmitted disease, such as a discharge or a sore on the genitals.
◆ Recurrent urinary tract infection.
◆ Injuries of the genitals or anus.
◆ Sudden unexplained changes in behavior.
◆ Recurrent sleep problems, including nightmares, and bed-wetting or bed-soiling in an older child.
◆ Unexplained problems at school, including truancy.
◆ Low self-esteem or feelings of worthlessness in older children.
◆ Loss of trust in family or friends.
◆ Feelings that the body is "dirty."

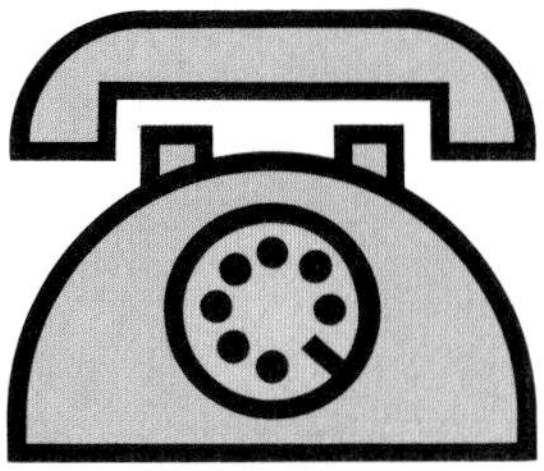

Taking action
If you suspect that a child is being abused, contact your doctor, local social service agency, or police department. To protect the child, authorities may remove the child from the home while investigations are being conducted. Whenever possible, the family is kept together and given appropriate professional support and guidance.

GLOSSARY OF DISORDERS

This glossary gives a brief description of a number of disorders occurring in children or adolescents that are not covered elsewhere in this volume.

A

Apnea, sleep
A prolonged pause in the breathing of an infant, usually during sleep. In mild cases, breathing stops for only 10 to 15 seconds. Apnea usually occurs in premature infants.

B

Brain tumor
A new growth of tissue, either benign (noncancerous) or malignant (cancerous), occurring in or around the brain. Brain tumors may cause headaches, unexpected projectile vomiting, clumsiness, behavior changes, seizures, paralysis, and other symptoms. The tumors are rare but require immediate treatment to minimize brain damage and to save the child's life. Brain tumors are the most common tumors, outside blood-forming tissues, in children.

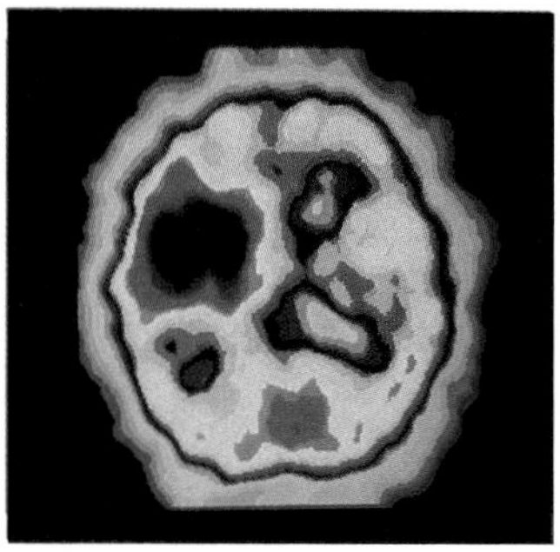

PET scan of the brain
Doctors use imaging techniques, such as positron emission tomography (PET) scanning, to obtain cross-sectional images of the brain. The image above is a color-enhanced PET scan that shows the presence of a brain tumor (large red and black area).

Bronchiolitis
A viral infection of the bronchioles (smaller airways of the lungs) that affects infants and toddlers, producing a cough, wheezing, and rapid breathing. Affected infants may need hospitalization.

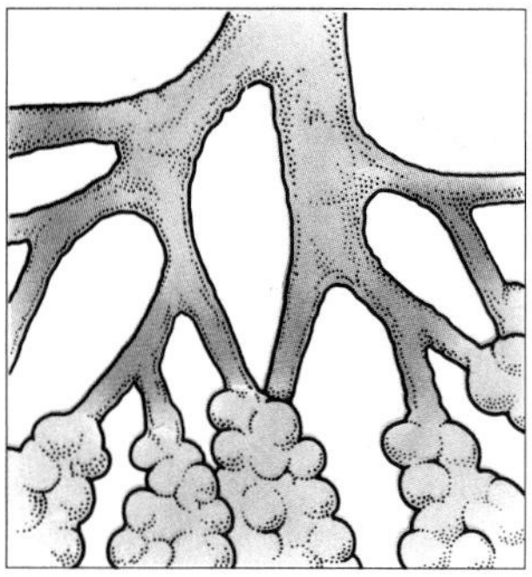

Bronchiole infection
The airways begin as a single tube (trachea) that branches first into two bronchi and then into smaller tubes called bronchioles. Infected bronchioles become inflamed, causing breathing difficulties.

C

Chondromalacia patellae
A painful condition of adolescence that usually occurs in girls in which the cartilage behind the kneecap becomes inflamed. Pain occurs when the person flexes the knee, especially during activities such as climbing stairs. A prescribed exercise program usually clears up the condition.

Coarctation of the aorta
Localized narrowing of the aorta, the main artery of the body. The narrowing causes elevated blood pressure in the upper part of the body and reduced blood pressure in the lower part. The condition is present at birth.

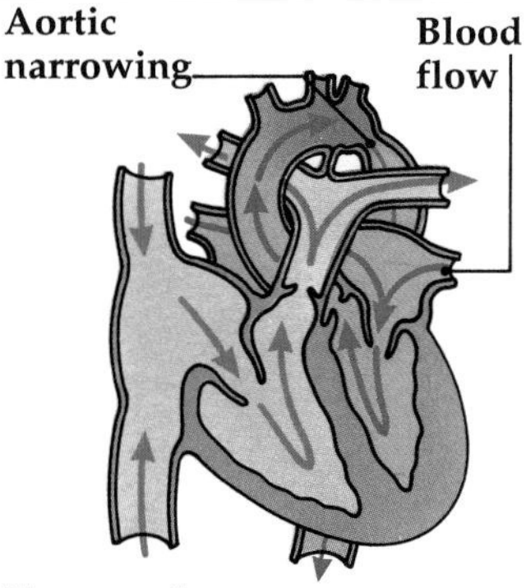

Narrowed aorta
Coarctation of the aorta (narrowing of the body's main artery) causes an uneven distribution of blood to the upper and lower parts of the body. It affects about one in 2,000 babies.

Congenital adrenal hyperplasia
A genetic disorder characterized by a hormone imbalance that causes masculinization in females at birth (sometimes with ambiguous genitalia) and early puberty in males. Some forms of this disease cause dehydration and failure to thrive. Doctors treat this disorder with hormones and screen for one form of the disease in newborns with a routine blood test.

Coxa vara
A hip deformity in which the neck of the thigh bone (femur) lies at a smaller-than-normal angle to the bone's shaft, causing shortening of the leg and a limp.

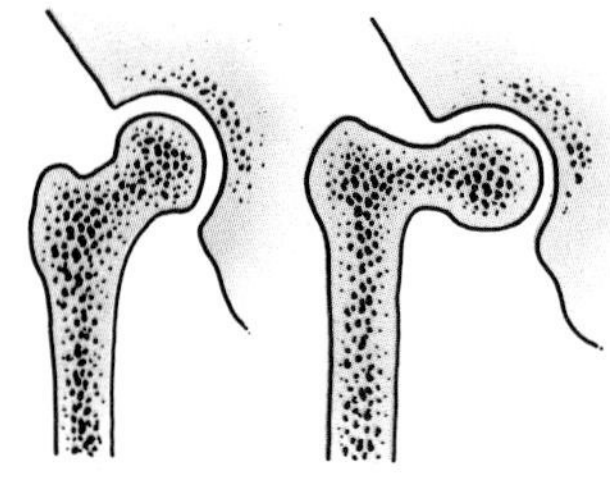

Normal hip **Coxa vara**

Craniosynostosis
A condition, present at birth, in which the skull is abnormally small. The premature fusion of the bony plates that form the skull prevents normal skull growth.

Cushing's syndrome
A condition, more common in girls than boys, caused by overproduction of steroid hormones from a tumor in the adrenal glands or from long-term treatment with corticosteroid drugs. Characteristic features of Cushing's syndrome include fat deposits in the face, neck, and trunk; muscle wasting; weakness; facial hair; and acne. A pituitary tumor can also bring about the disease.

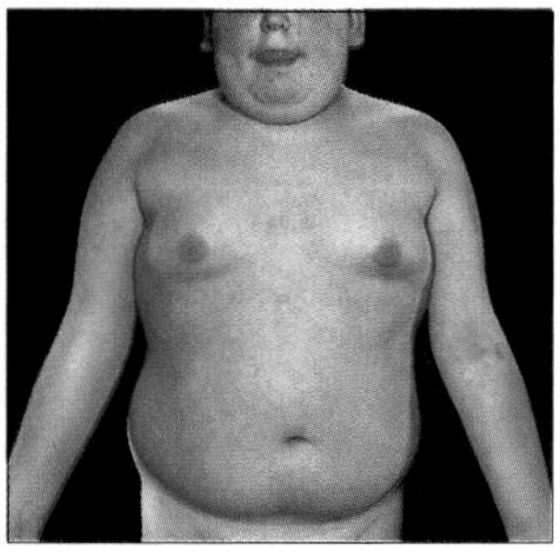

Characteristic appearance
Children with Cushing's syndrome tend to appear obese because of fat deposits in the trunk, but muscular wasting causes their arms and legs to appear thin.

D

Diabetes insipidus
Impaired water-reabsorption by the kidneys caused by inadequate production of a pituitary gland hormone or kidney insensitivity to the hormone. Symptoms include a massive output of urine.

Down's syndrome
A disorder, also called trisomy 21, caused by an additional chromosome 21 in a person's cells and featuring widespread bodily abnormalities, including a small skull, a flattened bridge of the nose, sloping eyes, a large tongue, and short fingers. Children with Down's syndrome have some degree of mental retardation and a high incidence of heart defects.

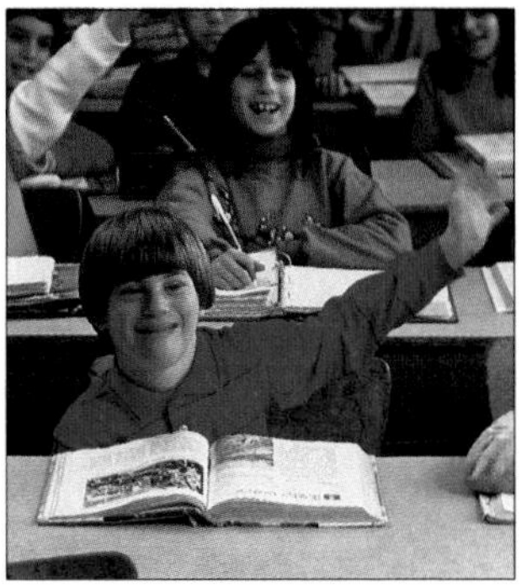

Learning abilities
The severity of mental retardation in children with Down's syndrome varies. Some affected children need special education classes. But mildly affected children may attend regular schools.

E

Erb's palsy
A form of paralysis, affecting the upper arm muscles but sparing the small muscles of the hand, caused by injury during childbirth to the nerve roots in the lower part of the neck.

Ewing's sarcoma
A malignant (cancerous) bone tumor, usually affecting a long bone or a pelvic bone. The condition is more common in adolescent boys over 15 and causes pain, swelling, fever, and an increase in the number of white blood cells. The tumor responds to chemotherapy and radiation therapy but often recurs. Amputation may be needed.

F

Funnel chest
A deformity in which the breastbone is deeply hollowed and the front ends of the ribs are curved inward. The deformity is somewhat evident at birth but becomes progressively worse during childhood.

G

Giardiasis
An illness caused by intestinal infection with a type of single-celled animal parasite. Contaminated water or food spreads the parasite. Common in tropical countries, it is also found in the US, where outbreaks have occurred among children who attend day care centers. Symptoms of giardiasis include severe diarrhea, intestinal gas, nausea, and loss of appetite.

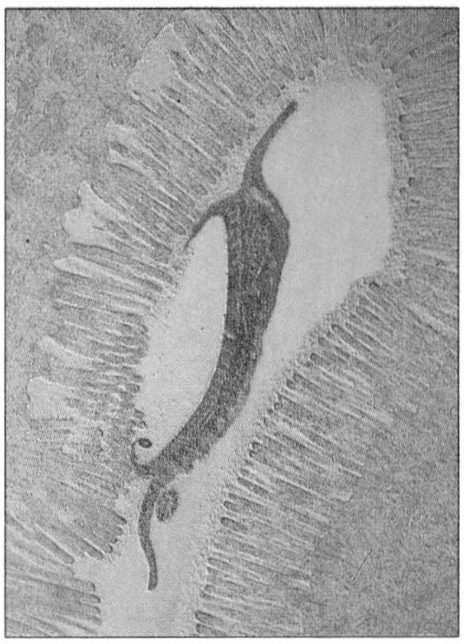

A single-celled parasite
Symptoms of the illness giardiasis usually develop several days after infection by the single-celled parasite Giardia lamblia. *The photograph above shows the organism* Giardia lamblia *(in green) attached to the microscopic fingerlike projections (villi) that line the human small intestine. The parasite absorbs the fluid contained in the lining of the small intestine and interferes with the absorption of nutrients from food.*

H

Hemolytic disease of the newborn from Rh incompatibility
Excessive destruction of the red blood cells of a fetus or newborn infant. The condition usually stems from Rh factor incompatibility, a blood group incompatibility in which the immune system of an Rh-negative mother recognizes proteins in the blood of an Rh-positive fetus as foreign. Antibodies formed in the mother cross the placenta and destroy the baby's red blood cells. The disease is now rare because mothers usually receive an injection to inhibit their immune response to the baby's proteins.

Hemolytic-uremic syndrome
A rare disease of young children in which red blood cells and platelets (blood cells that help the blood form clots) are broken down prematurely in the blood vessels throughout the body. This process causes kidney damage and an inability to produce urine (kidney failure).

Hemophilia
An inherited bleeding disorder caused by an absence of the blood-clotting protein factors VIII or IX. Affected children are almost always males. Bleeding may occur spontaneously or after minor injury. Joints are commonly affected. Hemophilia can be controlled by injections of the deficient blood-clotting factor.

Hypospadias
A defect that is present at birth in which the urine tube (urethra) opens on the underside of the penis, sometimes so near the root of the organ that fertility can be impaired. The defect occurs in about one in 300 male babies. Surgery can correct the condition.

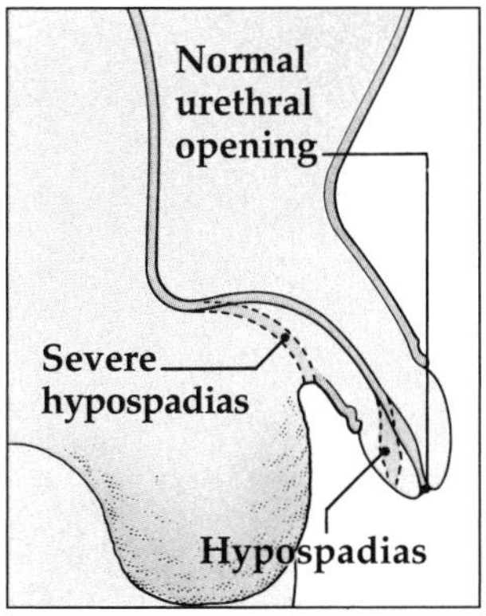

Hypospadias
Hypospadias varies in severity. All but the mildest forms require surgical treatment.

I

Idiopathic thrombocytopenic purpura
A bleeding disorder caused by a shortage of platelets (clotting cells) in the blood. Symptoms include tiny blood spots or bruises in the skin and, occasionally, extensive spontaneous bleeding into the tissues. The underlying cause is an immune response, usually to a virus, drug, or toxin, in which the body's immune system attacks the blood platelets.

K

Kawasaki disease
A childhood disease of unknown cause characterized by fever, dryness and cracking of the lips, swollen lymph nodes, reddened eyes, red palms and soles, a measleslike rash, and swelling of the hands and feet. In most children, the symptoms go away in 2 weeks, but up to 2 percent die from a blood clot blocking a coronary artery supplying the heart.

L

Lymphoma
Any of a number of cancers affecting lymph tissue, such

as the lymph nodes or spleen. Doctors categorize lymphomas as Hodgkin's and non-Hodgkin's types, depending on whether a particular type of cell is present.

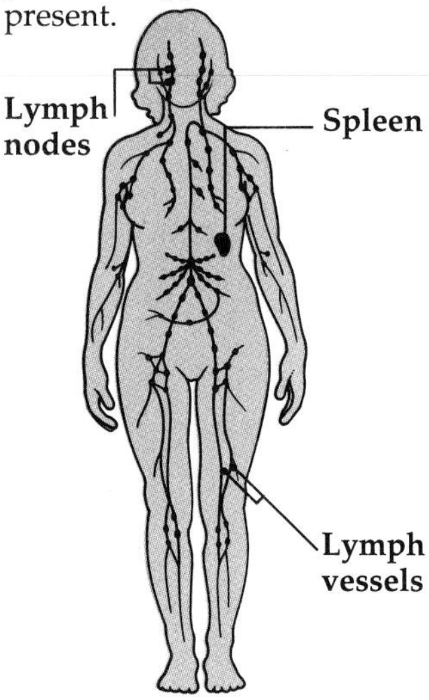

Lymphatic system
The lymphatic system plays a major role in the body's immune system. Lymph nodes trap and neutralize invading bacteria and viruses. The lymph vessels drain excess fluid (lymph) from body tissues and return it to the bloodstream.

M

Mesenteric lymphadenitis
A childhood abdominal disorder of sudden onset that is commonly mistaken for appendicitis. It causes inflammation of the lymph nodes in the mesentery, the membrane from which the intestines are suspended. It usually goes away without treatment.

Muscular dystrophy
An inherited progressively worsening muscle disorder that is classified according to its age at onset and rate of progress. All types feature gradual degeneration of muscle fibers and lead to increasing muscle weakness. The long-term outlook for children with muscular dystrophy varies according to the type they have.

N

Neuroblastoma
A tumor of the adrenal glands or that part of the nervous system that controls involuntary bodily functions. Neuroblastomas are the most common type of solid tumor of childhood that occurs outside the skull. Neuroblastomas range in severity from relatively harmless to highly malignant (cancerous).

O

Osgood-Schlatter disease
Inflammation of the bony protuberance of the shin just below the knee from overactivity of the muscles at the front of the thigh. The condition mainly affects active adolescent boys and responds well to rest or immobilization in a cast.

Osteosarcoma
The most common type of bone cancer in children, also known as an osteogenic sarcoma.

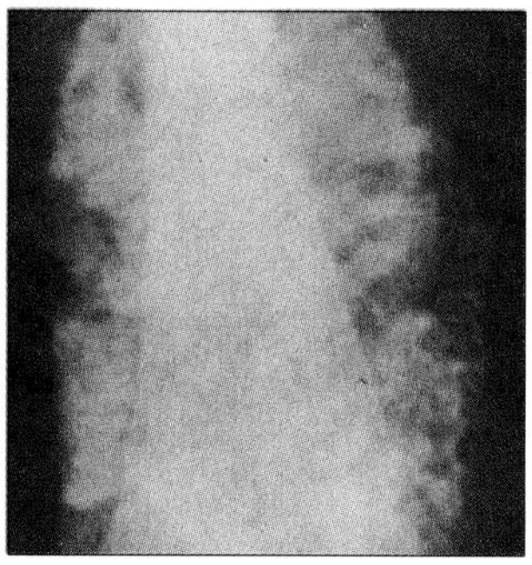

Bone cancer
Doctors use X-rays to detect the presence of bone cancer. Bone cancer shows up on an X-ray as a fuzzy area around the solid white bone.

P

Pigeon breast
A protrusion deformity of the breastbone caused by obstruction of breathing in infants or by rickets, a nutritional disease that causes bone deformity.

Pulmonary stenosis
Abnormal narrowing of the heart valve through which blood passes from the right ventricle on its way to the lungs. Sometimes the artery beyond the valve (the pulmonary artery) is also narrowed or dilated. If the narrowing is severe, the child may experience breathlessness on effort, blueness of the skin, and even heart failure.

R

Retinoblastoma
A malignant (cancerous) tumor of the retina at the back of the eye that affects infants and young children and is sometimes hereditary. The tumor may make the pupil appear white and may cause a squint. One or both eyes may be affected and blindness may occur. Unless treated early, the condition is usually fatal.

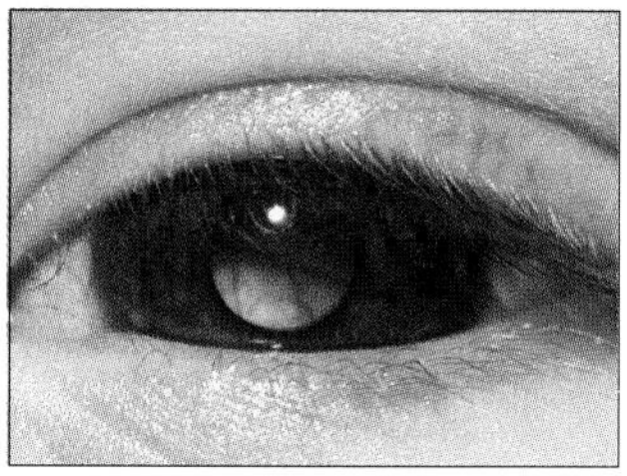

Tumor of the retina
In the above picture, a retinoblastoma appears as a flesh-colored area in the lower part of the pupil. Small tumors can be treated successfully with surgery and radiation therapy.

Rheumatic fever
A disease that may follow an untreated streptococcal throat infection and causes joint inflammation. It sometimes affects the heart, causing irregular rate or rhythm, valve damage, or heart failure. In rare cases, the disease affects the brain, causing a central nervous system disorder called Sydenham's chorea, which is characterized by involuntary jerking movements.

S

Schönlein-Henoch purpura
An allergic disorder that arises mainly in children and affects small blood vessels, causing spontaneous bruising of the buttocks, lower abdomen, and legs and joint swelling in ankles and knees. The condition usually heals in a few weeks without causing long-term damage.

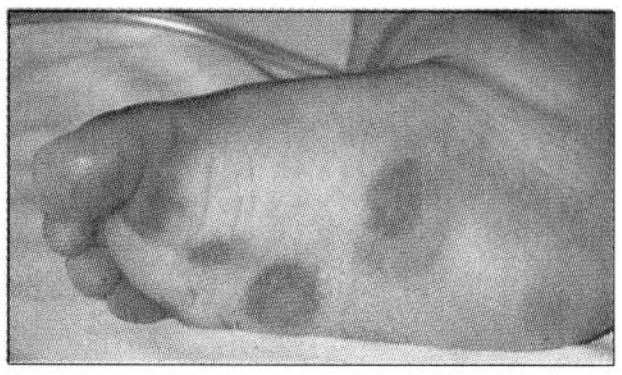

Purpura
Purpura is a purplish brown rash on the skin. This type of discoloration is usually produced by localized bleeding.

Scoliosis
An abnormal sideways curvature of the spine from muscular, nerve, or bone abnormalities. If detected early, doctors can correct the curvature with casts, exercises, a brace, or surgery.

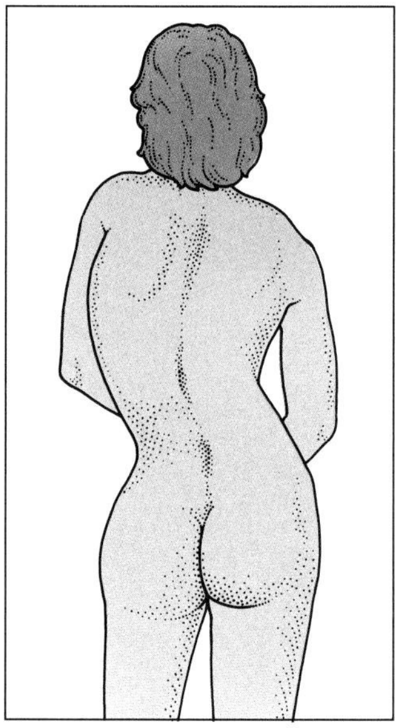

Abnormal spine curvature
If left untreated, the abnormal spine curvature of scoliosis can worsen during the growth spurt of puberty, producing a grossly hunched back.

Sickle cell anemia
A serious hereditary disorder, mainly affecting black children, characterized by abnormal hemoglobin (the oxygen-carrying pigment of red blood cells) that causes distortion and fragility of the red blood cells. The disorder can cause a severe, acute illness called a sickle cell crisis, in which many red blood cells break down and form masses that can obstruct small blood vessels. Anemia, extensive tissue damage, joint pain, and fever arise. Susceptibility to bacterial infection is common in sickle cell anemia and can be life-threatening.

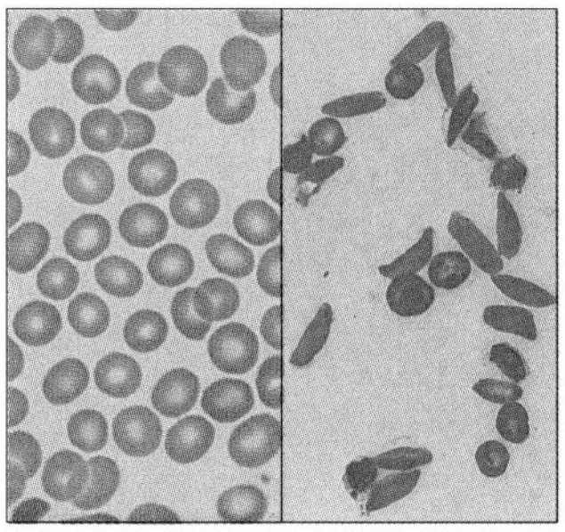

Spina bifida
A defect, present at birth, in the development of the bones of the spine and, in severe cases, of the spinal cord. The absence of part of the spinal column allows the spinal cord and its membranes to protrude through the skin. When this happens, the effects on nervous system functioning may be severe.

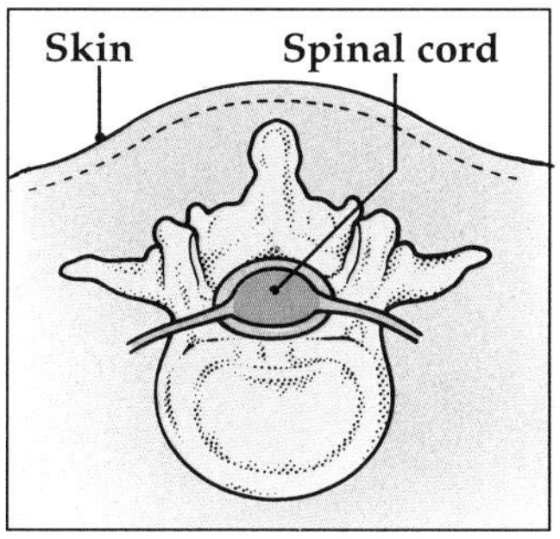

Normal spine
In a normal spine, the spinal cord is completely enclosed and protected by the back bone.

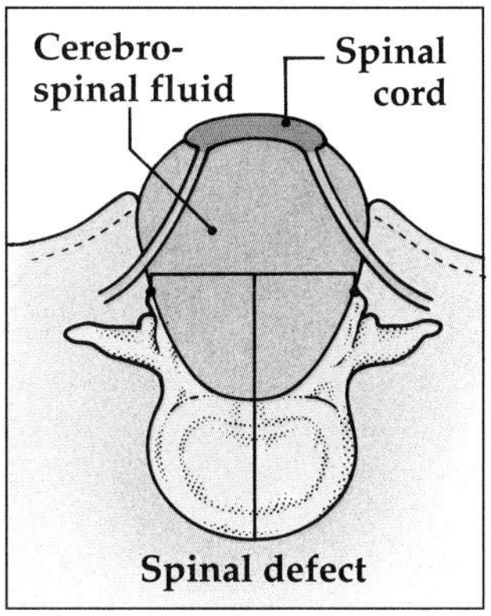

Defective spine
The spine defect spina bifida most commonly appears in the lower back. In severe spina bifida, there may be a swelling over the spine. The swelling contains a malformed spinal cord and excess cerebrospinal fluid. A child born with such a defect is likely to be severely handicapped.

Spinal muscular atrophy
A genetic disorder, also called Werdnig-Hoffman disease, that causes progressive weakness from gradual destruction of the nerves that carry signals to the muscles to initiate movement. The infantile form is usually fatal by the age of 2 years, but when the condition starts in later years, the disease progresses very slowly and usually does not shorten life.

T

Tetralogy of Fallot
The name for a collection of four heart defects present at birth. They include a hole in the wall between the ventricles of the heart, a narrowed valve in the artery from the right ventricle of the heart leading to the lungs, thickening of the wall of the lower chamber on the right side of the heart, and a displacement of the aorta (the main artery of the body) allowing blood to enter the artery from both lower heart chambers. Surgery must be performed to repair the defects.

Four heart defects
The four heart defects of the tetralogy of Fallot produce turbulence in the heart, causing murmurs that can be detected when a doctor uses a stethoscope. Affected children become increasingly breathless and may show poor physical development.

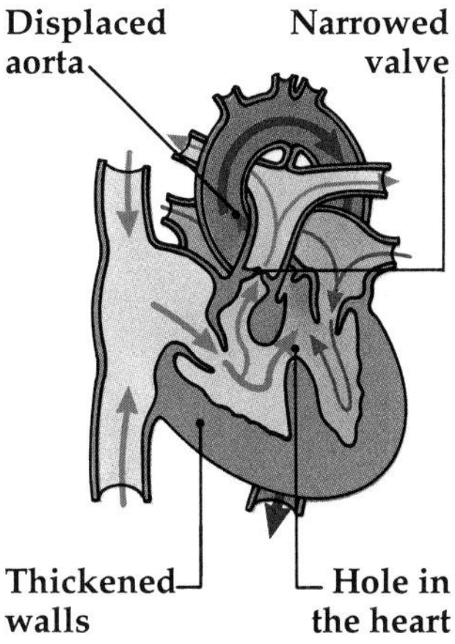

Thalassemia
A group of inherited blood disorders caused by the production of abnormal hemoglobin (the oxygen-carrying pigment in red blood cells). Blood cells may be fragile and easily broken down, causing anemia. Thalassemia major is a serious disease with many complications. Thalassemia minor causes only mild anemia.

Tics
Sudden, involuntary, repetitive, purposeless twitching movements of small groups of muscles, especially of the face or shoulders. Tics, or mimic spasms, are usually a sign of a psychological disturbance and do not suggest a muscular disorder. They are very common in childhood. Most eventually disappear without treatment.

Trichotillomania
A habit of pulling out of one's own hair that may signal psychological disturbance in children or an expression of anxiety or frustration.

V

von Willebrand's disease
An inherited disorder, similar to hemophilia, caused by a deficiency in the blood of a substance required for blood clotting. Both boys and girls may be affected by the disorder. Symptoms include spontaneous bleeding from the nose and gums and prolonged bleeding after injury. The menstrual periods of affected girls are very heavy.

W

Wilms' tumor
A malignant (cancerous) kidney tumor affecting children, usually before the age of 5. The tumor often enlarges and causes elevated blood pressure, blood in the urine, and a mass that can readily be felt through the wall of the abdomen. Prompt surgical removal of the affected kidney may cure the disorder. Affected children may need chemotherapy and radiation therapy.

Wryneck (torticollis)
An abnormal twisting of the neck caused by the contraction or shortening of the muscles on one side, causing the head to be pulled over to one side. Wryneck may be present from birth or may be caused by an injury or by sleeping in an awkward position.

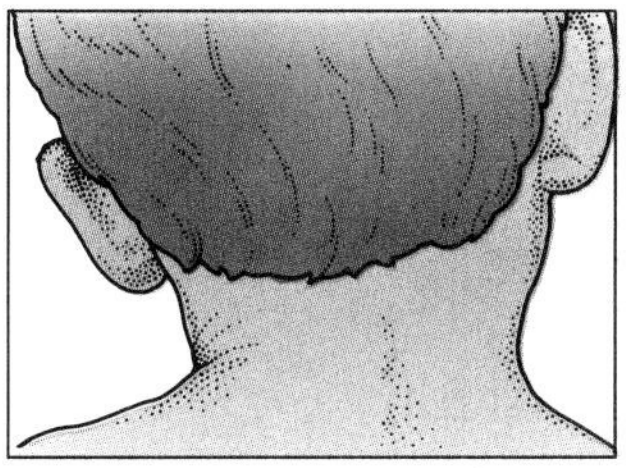

Child with torticollis
Torticollis can be treated surgically, with an orthopedic collar and physical therapy, or by injection of a drug.

INDEX

Page numbers in *italics* refer to illustrations and captions.

Photograph sources:
Audio Visual Department, St. Mary's Hospital **36**
Barts Medical Picture Library **38** (bottom center); **75** (bottom left); **100** (top left); **101**
Biophoto Associates **88** (center); **103** (center); **141**
Dr Tony Costello **25** (bottom)
Dr David Denhim, London School of Hygiene and Tropical Medicine **90** (bottom center)
The Hutchison Library **25** (top right)
The Image Bank **10**; **15** (top left); **24** (bottom); **48** (top left); **124** (top right); **130** (bottom left); **133** (top); **134** (top)
Institute of Child Health **103** (bottom left); **129** (center right); **138** (right)
Institute of Dermatology **104** (top right)
Moorefields Eye Hospital **80** (center)
National Blood Transfusion Services **113**; **135** (center)
National Medical Slide Bank **62** (top center); **62** (center right); **75** (top left); **76** (bottom center); **88** (top left); **88** (bottom left); **95** (right); **99**; **100** (bottom); **104** (center); **140** (center); **140** (top right)
OSF/Daniel J. Cox **74** (top right)
Pictor International Ltd **117** (center)
Reflections Photo Library **21**
Science Photo Library **37** (top center); **37** (top left); **103** (top); **133** (bottom); **138** (bottom left); **139**; **140** (bottom left)
Tony Stone Worldwide **17**; **61** (top left); **121**; **126** (bottom left)
Telegraph Colour Library **7**; **9**; **64**; **73**
Dr Ian Williams **37** (center); **62** (bottom); **74** (bottom right); **75** (top right); **75** (center); **76** (top right); **76** (center); **77**; **103** (bottom right)
Zefa **14**; **57** (top center); **65**; **75** (bottom right); **107** (top left); **110** (top right); **128**

Front cover photograph:
Jo Browne/Mick Smee/
Tony Stone Worldwide

Commissioned photography:
Steve Bartholomew
Jim Forrest
Susannah Price
Paul Venning

Airbrushing:
Paul Desmond
Roy Flooks

Illustrators:
Joanna Cameron
David Fathers
Tony Graham
Andrew Green
Kevin Marks
Philip Wilson

Index:
Sue Bosanko